DISMANTLING THE NHS?

Evaluating the impact
of health reforms

Edited by
Mark Exworthy, Russell Mannion, Martin Powell

First published in Great Britain in 2016 by

Policy Press
University of Bristol
1-9 Old Park Hill
Bristol
BS2 8BB
UK
t: +44 (0)117 954 5940
pp-info@bristol.ac.uk
www.policypress.co.uk

North America office:
Policy Press
c/o The University of Chicago Press
1427 East 60th Street
Chicago, IL 60637, USA
t: +1 773 702 7700
f: +1 773-702-9756
sales@press.uchicago.edu
www.press.uchicago.edu

© Policy Press 2016

British Library Cataloguing in Publication Data
A catalogue record for this book is available from the British Library

Library of Congress Cataloging-in-Publication Data
A catalog record for this book has been requested

ISBN 978 1 44733 023 3 paperback
ISBN 978 1 44733 022 6 hardcover
ISBN 978 1 44733 025 7 ePub
ISBN 978 1 44733 026 4 Mobi

The right of Mark Exworthy, Russell Mannion and Martin Powell to be identified as editors
of this work has been asserted by them in accordance with the Copyright, Designs and
Patents Act 1988.

Cover design by Andrew Corbett
Front cover image: iStock
Printed and bound in Great Britain by CMP, Poole
Policy Press uses environmentally responsible print partners

This book is dedicated to
Sarah, Dominic and Finnian
Judith, Lizzie and Catherine
Annette

Contents

List of tables, figures and boxes

Figures

Boxes

Glossary

A and E	Accident and Emergency
AQP	Any Qualified Provider
BCF	Better Care Fund
bn	Billion
CCG	Clinical Commissioning Group
CHS	Community health services
CMO	Chief Medical Officer
CQC	Care Quality Commission
CSR	Comprehensive Spending Review
DDRB	Review Body on Doctors' and Dentists' Remuneration
DH	Department of Health
DHA	District Health Authority
DPH	Director of Public Health/DsPH Directors of Public Health
FT	Foundation Trust
GP	General (medical) Practitioner
GPFH	GP fund-holding/fund-holder
GMS	General Medical Services
HCHS	Hospital and Community Health Services
HEE	Health Education England
HR(M)	Human Resources (Management)
HSCA	Health and Social Care Act (2012)
HSDR	Health Service and Delivery Research
HSCIC	Health and Social Care Information Centre
HWB	Health and Wellbeing Board
ISTC	Independent sector treatment centre
JSNA	Joint Strategic Needs Assessment
LA	Local Authority
NAO	National Audit Office
NHS	National Health Service
NHSE	NHS England
NICE	National Institute for Health and Care Excellence
NIHR	National Institute of Health Research
NPM	New Public Management
OECD	Organization for Economic Cooperation and Development
OOH	Out of hours
PbR	Payment by Results
PCG	Primary Care Group

PCT	Primary Care Trust
PFI	Private Finance Initiative
PHE	Public Health England
PMS	Personal Medical Services
QIPP	Quality, Innovation, Productivity and Prevention
QOF	Quality and Outcomes Framework
SHA	Strategic Health Authority
TDA	Trust Development Authority
WCC	World Class Commissioning

Notes on contributors

Pauline Allen is Reader in Health Services Organisation at the London School of Hygiene and Tropical Medicine and Head of the Department of Health Services Research and Policy. Her research interests include sociolegal theory, institutional economics, organisational theory and the structure and governance of the National Health Service in the UK. Current and recent research projects include studies of organisations delivering health services, competition between them and contracting for healthcare. She has published widely on these issues in peer reviewed journals and books.

Chris Bojke (PhD) is a Senior Research Fellow at the Centre for Health Economics at the University of York. His research has focussed on national and regional measures of NHS productivity, variation in patient outcomes and costs across hospitals, measuring the costs of specialised care and health labour force economic issues including the cost effectiveness of medical revalidation of consultants. Prior to rejoining CHE in 2009, Chris was a senior research consultant and director of Pharmerit Ltd

Adriana Castelli (PhD) is a Research Fellow at the Centre for Health Economics at the University of York, which she joined in 2004. She has an MSc and PhD in Economics, both awarded by the University of York. Her research interests include health policy reforms, performance measurement with a particular focus on the development of productivity measures of healthcare goods and services, and analysis of geographical/spatial variation in quality of life and health.

Anita Charlesworth joined the Health Foundation in May 2014. Previously, she was Chief Economist at the Nuffield Trust for four years where she led the Trust's work on health care financing and market mechanisms. Anita was Chief Analyst and Chief Scientific Advisor at the Department of Culture, Media and Sport from 2007 to 2010 and, prior to this, she was Director of Public Spending at the Treasury from 1998–2007, where she led the team working with Sir Derek Wanless on his reform of NHS funding in 2002. Anita has a MSc in Health Economics from the University of York and has worked as an Economic Advisor in the Department of Health and for SmithKline Beecham pharmaceuticals in the UK and USA. Anita is

Vice Chair of the Whittington Hospital NHS Trust and a Trustee of Tommy's, the baby charity.

Kath Checkland is Professor of Health Policy and Primary Care at the University of Manchester. Originally trained as a GP (and still working one day each week in a rural practice), her research focuses upon the interaction between health policy and organisations within the health service, with a focus on primary care. The research takes a qualitative approach. She is a co-lead for the Primary Care theme of the Greater Manchester CLAHRC.

Dr Anna Coleman is a Research Fellow in the Health Policy, Politics and Organisations Group at Manchester University, with extensive experience researching health policy, partnership working and commissioning.

Dr Surindar Dhesi is a Lecturer at the University of Birmingham, a Chartered Environmental Health Practitioner, and her PhD focussed on developing Health and Wellbeing Boards.

Mark Exworthy is Professor of Health Policy and Management at the Health Services Management Centre, University of Birmingham. His research interests focus on professional–managerial relations, governance, and decentralisation.

Robin Gauld is Professor and Head of the Department of Preventive and Social Medicine, University of Otago, New Zealand, where he is also Director of the Centre for Health Systems. Since mid-2013, he has been Independent Chair of Alliance South, an alliance between the Southern District Health Board and Primary Health Organisation. He was a Commonwealth Fund Harkness Fellow in 2008/09, and NZ–UK Link Foundation Visiting Professor at University of London in 2014.

Jon Glasby is Professor of Health and Social Care, and Head of the School of Social Policy at the University of Birmingham. A qualified social worker by background, he leads a national programme of research, teaching, consultancy and policy advice around joint working in health and social care.

Katja Grašič works as a Research Fellow at the Centre for Health Economics at the University of York. Her research has a specific focus on economic issues relating to the productivity of the healthcare sector, incentives related to financing of health care services (specialised services) and measurement of quality of care. Before joining CHE she was based in Ljubljana where she worked on projects dealing with performance of the Slovenian health care sector.

Ian Greener is Professor of Applied Social Sciences and Executive Director of the Wolfson Research Institute for Health and Wellbeing at Durham University. He has written for a range of international journals on health policy and politics, as well as authoring several books on those subjects, and is particularly interested in why governments continue to believe they can reorganise healthcare to make things better when almost every attempt to do so fails.

Scott L Greer (PhD) is Associate Professor of Health Management and Policy at the University of Michigan School of Public Health, and Senior Expert Advisor on Health Governance for the European Observatory on Health Systems and Policies. As a political scientist, he researches the politics of health policies, with a special focus on the politics and policies of the European Union and the impact of federalism on health care.

Daniel Howdon (PhD) is a Research Fellow in the Health Policy Team at the University of York's Centre for Health Economics. His research has covered topics including NHS productivity, equity in health outcomes, relationships between smoking and ill health, and healthcare costs in old age.

David Hughes is Professor of Health Policy at Swansea University, and has researched the divergent NHS policies of the UK home countries in areas such as patient choice, PPI and commissioning. He has studied Thailand's universal coverage reforms, and assisted in the government's 10-year assessment of that scheme. Hughes has also published extensively in the field of medical sociology and co-edits the Wiley journal *Sociology of Health and Illness*.

David J Hunter is Professor of Health Policy and Management and Director of the Centre for Public Policy and Health (CPPH), Durham University, and Deputy Director of Fuse, the Centre for Translational Research in Public Health. He is a non-executive director of the National Institute for Health and Care Excellence (NICE) and advises WHO Regional Office for Europe. CPPH is a WHO Collaborating

Centre on Complex Health Systems Research, Knowledge and Action. David has published extensively on public health policy and health system reform. The second edition of his 2008 book, *The Health Debate*, was published by Policy Press in early 2016.

Paula Hyde is Professor of Organisations and Society, and Director of the Health Services Research Centre at Manchester Business School, University of Manchester. Her critical-ethnographic research focuses on health service organisation and delivery, especially in organising care, sociology of work and critical and psychodynamic explorations of how care is organised.

Holly Jarman is Assistant Professor of Health Management and Policy at the University of Michigan's School of Public Health. Recent publications include *The Politics of Trade and* Tobacco Control (2015) and the co-authored *Everything you always wanted to know about European Union Health Policy but were afraid to ask* (2015).

Sarah Lafond joined the Health Foundation in August 2014 as an Economics Analyst. Sarah joined The Health Foundation from the Nuffield Trust where she conducted financial analysis of NHS funding. Previously, Sarah worked at the Health Analytical Services of the Scottish Government where she worked on a number of health and social care projects and publications such as the integration of health and social care project and the new social care survey. Sarah has an MSc in ecological economics from University of Edinburgh. Her dissertation was on the government cost of occupational cancer in Great Britain where she conducted a cost and benefits analysis of implementing a health policy to prevent occupational cancer. She graduated from McGill University in Canada with a degree in international development.

Russell Mannion is Professor of Health Systems at the University of Birmingham where he is currently Director of Research at the Health Services Management Centre. He also holds long-standing visiting professorial positions at the University of Oslo and the Australian Institute for Health Innovation based in Sydney.

Imelda McDermott is a Research Fellow at the University of Manchester, part of the Policy Research Unit in Commissioning and the Healthcare System (PRUComm). She has been researching the development of Clinical Commissioning Groups (CCGs) since its inception. Her research focus is on healthcare policy in commissioning. Her area of interest is the organisation of health services. She has an expertise in discourse analysis and has developed an interest in the use of realist evaluation

Robin Miller is a Senior Fellow and Director of Consultancy at HSMC and a Fellow of the School for Social Care Research. His research interests build on his practical experiences in the field, and centre on commissioning and development of integrated primary and community care services and the role of the voluntary and community sector. He leads on a variety of applied projects with health and social care organisations, with a particular focus on evaluating and learning from change initiatives. Robin is co-editor of the Journal of Integrated Care and an advisory group member of the European Primary Care Network.

Elias Mossialos is the Brian Abel-Smith Professor of Health Policy, and Director of LSE Health at the London School of Economics and Political Science. His particular research focus is European and comparative health policy, addressing questions related to financing health care, pharmaceutical policies, private health insurance and the impact of EU law on health care systems. In 1998, he co-founded the European Observatory on Health Systems and Policies, a major health policy research and knowledge transfer programme.

Dr Karen Newbigging is Senior Lecturer in Health Policy at the Health Services Management Centre, University of Birmingham. As a Clinical Psychologist and Fellow of the Royal Society for Public Health, Karen has thirty years' experience in the NHS. Her particular interests include service user agency and PPI. She provides advice to government bodies, development support to the health and care sector and is a Trustee of a service user organisation.

Professor Stephen Peckham is the Director of the Policy Research Programme Unit on Commissioning and the Healthcare System, Professor of Health Policy and Director of the Centre for Health Services Studies at the University of Kent, and Professor of Health Policy at the London School of Hygiene and Tropical Medicine.

Martin Powell is Professor of Health and Social Policy at the Health Services Management Centre, University of Birmingham. He has researched social and health policy for 30 years. He is the author of

Evaluating the NHS (Open University Press, 1997), the editor of a trilogy of texts examining the Labour governments of 1997–2010, and the author of over 80 journal articles.

Adam Roberts joined the Health Foundation in July 2014 as Senior Economics Fellow, exploring past, present and future trends for healthcare funding in the UK. Before joining the Health Foundation, Adam was a Senior Research Analyst at the Nuffield Trust where he worked on projects including the project funding gap facing the NHS in England and Wales, allocation of national resources to GP practices, lifetime cost for social care, travel distances for emergency care, and trends community prescribing. Prior to his time at the Nuffield Trust, Adam was responsible for the production of risk estimates of NHS organisations for the Care Quality Commission (and the former Healthcare Commission) to support the programme of targeted inspections. These estimates were generated by applying cutting edge methods to all relevant and available data sources, both quantitative and qualitative, to identify areas of possible concern for the commission to follow up. Adam graduated from Keele University in 2004 where he achieved a first class dual honours degree in Statistics and Economics.

David Rowland is a founding Director of the Centre for Health and the Public Interest thinktank. He has worked for the last 10 years as a Senior Policy Advisor within the field of Health and Social Care Regulation and previously as a Research Fellow at the School of Public Policy University College London.

Rod Sheaff is Professor of Health Services Research at Plymouth University, UK and founding member of the South West Collaboration for Leadership and Health Research in Care. His main research interest is in the relationship between organisational structures and the implementation of health policy, which he has studied in a number of countries. He trained, and has worked, as a NHS manager.

Andrew Street is Professor of Health Economics, Director of the Health Policy team at the Centre for Health Economics at the University of York and Director of the Economics of Social and Health Care Research Unit, a joint collaboration between the Universities of York and Kent and the London School of Economics. His current research interests include measurement of NHS productivity, hospital funding, integrated care and patient reported outcome measures (PROMs).

Martin Wenzl is a Research Officer at LSE Health at the London School of Economics and Political Science. His main research interests are in care for high-need/high-cost patients, financing of healthcare and equity of access as well as policy on non-pharmaceutical medical technology, in particular implantable devices. Prior to joining LSE Health in 2014, Martin received an MSc in Health Policy Planning and Financing (with distinction) from LSE and the London School of Hygiene and Tropical Medicine.

Foreword

In the history of the National Health Service, the period from 2010 to 2015 is remarkable for the transformation in the policy landscape that took place under the Coalition Government. By the time the Coalition Government left office, the preoccupations that had dominated its early years were overshadowed, indeed displaced, by a single issue: the £30 billion question. How was the NHS to cope with the twin pressures of unprecedented fiscal constraints and unprecedented demands?

In 2010 Andrew Lansley's White Paper, *Equity and Excellence*, was widely seen – and bitterly resisted – as an attack on the very essence of the NHS, threatening to bring about a period where privatisation and competition would end in disintegration. It was (at best) an exaggerated perception. Conceptually Lansley's proposals represented continuity – taking the logic of predecessor governments one step further – even while throwing the NHS into organisational turmoil. Nevertheless the perception shaped much of the debate leading up to the passage of the Health and Social Care Act in 2012, leaving a miasma of mistrust and apprehension.

Yet in 2015 when the Coalition Government left office, the scene had changed radically. In many respects the Lansley package had become something of a historical curiosity, reflecting the preoccupations of a bygone age. Concern about strategies for survival displaced ideology as a new policy agenda took shape. For not only were the Coalition years a period of unprecedented fiscal austerity for the NHS, with more of the same in prospect. On top of the demands generated by an ageing population and a creaking social care system, however, Coalition ministers added to the pressures on the NHS. In response to scandal more staff had to be hired by trusts already fending off fiscal deficits while ever more information advertising NHS shortcomings was published.

So we come to the £30 billion question: the gap between what the NHS expected to need by 2020 and was likely to get. It was in answering this question that NHS England set out the new, emergent agenda in the *Five Year Forward View*, the manifesto of the NHS's national leadership. The £30 billion gap by 'transforming' the NHS, as well as pursuing policies designed to reduce demands by improving population health.

Transforming meant not more competition or more privatisation but integrating services. So, on the one hand, acute trusts might move into providing primary care while, on the other hand, primary care providers might move into providing acute care in the community. No one model was prescribed. Furthermore, few thought that the £30 billion gap could be closed. The direction of travel was clear, though: the focus was to be on how local health communities served their communities, not on competing local health care providers.

This, of course, is a schematic, over simplified and contestable view of the evolution of policy under the Coalition Government. Policy rhetoric has clearly changed but institutional behaviour may be less adaptable. The chapters that follow therefore explore and set out a more complex reality which will allow the readers to judge for themselves. Read on.

Rudolf Klein

Section A:
Health reforms in context

ONE

Evaluating the impact of NHS reforms – policy, process and power

Mark Exworthy and Russell Mannion

Evaluating the state of the NHS in its seventh decade is the subject of this book. It specifically addresses the programme of reforms undertaken by the Coalition government (2010–2015) in England. Our particular focus is from a policy perspective. This book adds to the growing body of knowledge about the design and implementation of major health service reforms in the UK (for example, Greener et al, 2014). Although it takes as its specific focus the five year period of the Coalition government (between the Conservatives and the Liberal Democrats; 2010–2015), it sets these reforms within a wider social, political, financial and organisational context of reforms to the NHS over the previous 25 years.

When a major reform of the National Health Service is announced, it is often claimed to be the most significant, the most far-reaching, the most consequential re-organisation that has taken place since its inception in 1948 (for example, Margaret Thatcher's foreword to *Working for Patients*, Secretaries of State, 1989). Indeed this may be so. Yet the reforms of the Coalition government, whose apogee was the 2012 Health and Social Care Act, can truly meet this oft-quoted claim. In a speech in November 2010, David Nicholson, the then NHS Chief Executive, referred to these reforms as 'such a big change management, you could probably see it from space' (quoted in Greer et al, 2014, 3). Moreover, not only were they major health policy reforms in their own right, but they built on a series of successive pro-market reforms which date back to the mid-1980s.

Yet the scale of re-organisation was not mentioned in the Conservative party's manifesto (for the 2010 general election); instead, its emphasis was on decentralisation of power to clinical staff (including GPs) and enhancing autonomy for NHS providers. For example: 'We will decentralise power, so that patients have a real choice. We will make doctors and nurses accountable to patients, not to endless layers of bureaucracy and management' (Conservative Party, 2010, 45).

Nor did the Coalition partner, the Liberal Democrats mention large-scale NHS reform in their 2010 election manifesto. For example: 'We all know that too much precious NHS money is wasted on bureaucracy, and doctors and nurses spend too much time trying to meet government targets' (Liberal Democrats, 2010, 40).

Indeed, major reforms were also largely hidden in the Coalition Agreement, published in May 2010: 'We will stop the top-down reorganisations of the NHS that have got in the way of patient care. We are committed to reducing duplication and the resources spent on administration, and diverting these resources back to front-line care' (HM Government, 2010, 24).

Therefore, the absence of prior discussion of reorganisation, the scale of reforms and often evidence, presents a paradox of policy which, Timmins (2012) argues, reveals a 'subtle difference' in the meaning and interpretation of the term 're-organisation'.

Evaluating NHS reforms

Given the salience of the NHS to public life in the UK and the frequency of NHS reforms in recent years, it is surprising that major programmes of independent evaluation and research have not always been commissioned by the government, research funding bodies (such as the Economic and Social Research Council) or other research funders. In our period of inquiry (the last 25 years or so), the first book to compile extant evidence of NHS reforms was by Robinson and Le Grand (1994). In it, Robinson (1994) noted that there was an 'official lack of interest in monitoring the reforms' (1994, 1). Indeed, this went further than a 'lack of interest' as Kenneth Clarke, the then Secretary of State for Health 'denied the need for formal monitoring and evaluation and expressed the view that calling on the advice of academics in this way was a sign of weakness' (1994, 1), since he famously added that 'you buggers [the medical profession] will sabotage it' (that is, the reform) (quoted in Boyne et al, 2003, 78). Instead, the King's Fund, the independent health policy charity, sponsored an evaluation which formed the basis of the 1994 book.

The second book of this kind was by Le Grand et al (1998). Although it offered a 'systematic review of evidence', it again was undertaken by the King's Fund with some funding by the Department of Health (Acknowledgements; no page number). This book also reflected a series of evaluations undertaken in the 1990s such as Total Purchasing Pilots (Mays et al, 2001).

The third book, by Mays et al (2011), comprised the findings from studies undertaken by the Health Reform Evaluation Programme, funded by the Department of Health (2011, xii). Its focus was on the market-based reforms of the Labour government, so most attention was paid to the diversity of providers, commissioning, choice, pricing and reimbursement, and regulation and competition (as in Chapter 10).

Common to all three books are (perhaps understandably) the dominant discourses running throughout these major NHS reforms; namely, public choice theory and new public management (NPM) (Boyne et al, 2003; Ferlie et al, 2005). As such, there is a predominant focus on markets, competition, incentives, commissioning, and associated cultural changes. Less apparent are issues of equity, staffing (including managerialism and hybrid clinician managers), or public/ patient perspectives. Moreover, more critical perspectives of these reforms are largely absent.

This current book stemmed from a recognition of the scale of Coalition government reforms and the lack of a comprehensive programme of evaluation funded by central government (though some of the research reported here has been funded by the Department of Health or National Institute of Health Research). A smaller version of the Health Reform Evaluation Programme was commissioned by the Department in 2014/2015, comprising three projects). A number of other evaluations have been published which offer key insights into the performance and evaluation of the reforms which were designed and implemented during in an unusual period of coalition government and fiscal austerity (for example, Appleby et al, 2015; Gregory et al, 2012). The remit of this book, however, is broader.

Across this collection, chapter authors undertake three types of evaluation (Coulter, 1995). First, authors draw on a range of extant evidence relating to the monitoring of reforms. Second, they report on a series of different and distinct empirical evaluations usually relating to specific aspects of the reforms (such as commissioning or regulation of quality). These are largely process evaluations since it is too soon to provide a summative assessment. Third, they seek to apply, elaborate or test different conceptual perspectives, through theory-drive evaluation (Boyne et al, 2003). This third aspect is crucial since it allows a richer understanding and explanation of the broader trajectory of health policy, separate from the specific empirical case during the Coalition government. This trajectory can also be temporal in the sense that longer-term developments are put into an appropriate historical context.

Taken together, therefore, the chapters offer a synthesis and integration of knowledge and learning on different aspects of the reforms, from different (disciplinary) perspectives. The primary perspective taken in this collection is drawn from health policy. As necessarily an inter-disciplinary subject (Exworthy and Powell, 2011), it borrows much from related disciplines such as social and public policy, sociology, politics, economics, organisation studies and health services research (inter alia). As the sub-title of this chapter indicates, we are interested in issues of policy, process and power (Walt, 1994). It follows, therefore, that we are primarily concerned in conceptual topics such as agenda setting, implementation, stakeholders, organisational change, and policy impacts (including unintended and dysfunctional consequences).

Health reforms of the Coalition government

We offer a brief summary here of the salient features of the Coalition government NHS reforms (relating to England, see Table 1.1). Inevitably, we lose depth in search of covering the breadth of these reforms in this brief account.

Writing at the start of the Coalition government, Taylor-Gooby and Stoker (2011) noted that public sector reforms (and not just the NHS) seemed to comprise a 'coherent programme' beyond simply a deficit reduction exercise, prompted by austerity. The key features, they argued, consisted of: 'an emphasis on local decision making and budgeting, a shift in responsibility for outcomes from state to citizens, and the consistent promotion of the expansion of private and, in some areas, third sector provision' (2011, 9).

The five years of the Coalition government were marked by two distinct periods. Although fiscal austerity was common to both, the first period (2010–2012) comprised the preparations for and deliberations relating to the Health and Social Care Act (2012) (Timmins, 2012). The Act comprised 550 pages and 280 clauses; it was 'one of the longest and most controversial pieces of health legislation in the history of the NHS, which passed into law in March 2012' (Powell and Miller, 2014). The incumbent Secretary of State for Health was Andrew Lansley. The second period (since 2012) concerned the management of fiscal austerity and the consequences of reform implementation. It also entailed managing the consequences of the publications of the Francis Inquiry into Mid-Staffordshire NHS Trust. The incumbent Secretary of State was Jeremy Hunt. Charles Webster summarised these two periods thus:

Table 1.1: Health policy timeline (2010–2015)

2010	May	General election
		Coalition government: *Our programme for government*
	June	Full public inquiry into Mid-Staffs commissioned
		QIPP (reaffirmed in NHS Operating Framework for England, 2010–11)
	July	*Equity and excellence: liberating the NHS* white paper (cmd 7881)
	October	Comprehensive spending review (cmd 7942)
	November	*Healthy lives, health people* public health white paper (cmd 7985)
2011	March	Public Health Responsibility Deal launched
	November	Hart-Clywd report into NHS complaints
2012	March	Health and Social Care Act (royal assent)
	September	Lansley replaced by Hunt as Secretary of State for Health
	December	General Medical Council revalidation starts
2013	February	Final Mid-Staffs report published
	April	Public Health England formed; public health functions moved to local government and creation of Health and Wellbeing Boards; creation of CCGs
	July	Cavendish report into health-care assistant and support workers
	August	Berwick report into patient safety
2014	February	NHS 111 launched
	April	Simon Stevens starts as NHS Chief Executive
	May	Care Act (royal assent)
	September	Scottish independence referendum
	October	NHS England *Five year forward view* published
	Winter**	A and E crisis
2015	March	Manchester devolution of health and social care (memo of understanding)
	May	General election
		PM Cameron pledge on seven day working in the NHS (Cameron, 2015)
	November	Comprehensive spending review

** (last row 2014)

'If in the sixth decade the NHS seemed dominated by the turmoil of Labour's multiple reorganisations, the seventh was worse. The five years of the coalition government fell into two halves. The first was devoted to the debate on and passage of the Health and Social Care Bill, designed to increase competition and devolve decision making. The second was a damage limitation exercise following Andrew Lansley's disastrous reforms, with attempts to handle increasing financial problems, a process continuing under the Conservatives after election.' (Rivett, undated).

Explaining NHS reform: from 'not again' to 'never again'

A familiar refrain from NHS staff, the public and media is that the NHS has been subject to frequent reforms and re-organisations (Smith et al, 2001); 'not again' summed up the weariness of constant reform. Yet it has not always been thus. The first major reform of the NHS was in 1974, twenty-six years after its inception, the second after a further 8 years and then a further 9 years. During the Labour government (1997–2010), there were 26 Green and White Papers and 14 Acts of Parliament relating to the NHS (Thorlby and Maybin, 2010, 8). More recently, therefore, 'reform fatigue' has become an endemic feature of health policy. Yet, a continual process of reform was envisaged by Stevens (2004) (as one of the architects of recent reforms) who referred to this as a self-improving system. However, this does not account for dramatic periods of health policy-making such as that which took place during the period of the Coalition government. It was the first phase of this period which saw what was 'widely regarded as a 'car crash' of both politics and policy making' (Timmins, 2012, 6). Given the 'political damage' and 'complex mess' that resulted from this 'car crash', ministers (and indeed, many in the NHS) felt that reforms would 'never again' be designed or implemented in such a rushed and haphazard way.

Since the introduction of the NHS quasi-market in April 1991, we can identify a series of pro-market reforms, some of which have reinforced the original goals of the *Working for Patients* white paper (1989) but equally, others which have not. These waves of reforms revolve around key tensions which have faced the NHS since its inception. These tensions are the axes of interest, institutions and ideas; they include: the central–local axis, the public–private axis, and the state–profession axis (Exworthy and Freeman, 2009). These axes overlap and inter-lock with each other but they are useful heuristic devices to help understand and explain the health policy, process and power.

Our account of the Coalition health reforms presents four themes for explaining their significance.

Theme 1: Re-organisation within fiscal constraints

Undoubtedly, the fiscal constraints emanating from the 2008 financial crisis set the over-arching tone for the Coalition government and their reform of public services. Whilst political impulses encourage action, the combination of the (arguably) largest reform of the NHS and the fiscal constraints made a toxic mix.

Some existing organisations were abolished and new ones were created. The 152 English Primary Care Trusts (PCTs), as commissioners, were abolished and replaced by 211 Clinical Commissioning Groups (CCGs). Commissioning organisations have regularly been transformed since 1991, exacerbating the imbalance of power between commissioners and providers. With the demise of PCTs, public health functions were moved to local authorities, redolent of the pre-1974 reforms. Moreover, Strategic Health Authorities (SHAs), the regionally-based agencies, were also abolished. Whilst the newly formed NHS England put in place Local Area Teams, regions lost their traditional oversight and brokering role in the governance of local health systems.

Regards staffing, 45% cuts in management costs were initially planned, later recast as a one third cut. This accelerated management turnover, although some managers later re-joined the NHS. It also hastened longer-term trends in the loss of organisational memory across the service (Pollitt, 2009). The Coalition's emphasis on moving decisions to the 'front-line' of the NHS put GPs in leadership positions in CCGs; this added to their potential conflicts of interests in commissioning and providing services.

The most recent reform is NHS England's *Five year forward view*, a strategy designed and led by its Chief Executive, Simon Stevens. Working with the grain of existing service developments, this represents 're-organisation without reform.' Such change avoids the need for legislation or overt (top-down) political involvement, and captures developments, such as integration between health and social care, and new forms of primary care organisation, some of which had already been taking place.

Theme 2: Centralisation and localism

The tension between the centre and the locality has been a perennial issue in the NHS. Funded (mainly) by central taxation, the structure of decision-making has traditionally allowed a significant amount of local discretion and autonomy (Exworthy et al, 1999). This inevitably leads to questions of geographical rationing (postcode lottery), equity and accountability. In the period of the Coalition government, such issues were once again to the fore. Localism was espoused at a central tenet of the Coalition government, with an emphasis on (initially) the Big Society (including social enterprises) and (later) on devolution of power and resources to city regions.

Prompted by the demands of fiscal austerity and a rejection of NHS management (as the apparent cause of NHS ills), there was a strong emphasis on 'returning' decision-making to the so-called front-line. While the precise composition of the front-line was never fully clarified, the rhetoric was clear. In commissioning, this approach built on the experience of involving GPs in commissioning decisions, from fund-holding in the 1990s onwards.

Notwithstanding recent trends of decentralisation, the British state (including the NHS) has long been centralised (Greener et al, 2009). The re-assertion of powers at the centre has taken the form a fragmented centre, with many more actors involved. Symbolic of a network form of governance (Alvarez-Rosete and Mays, 2008), such diversity at the centre has become readily apparent in the NHS. Recent reforms have created or re-defined key agencies such as the National Institute for Health and Care Excellence, the Care Quality Commission, Monitor, Trust Development Authority, and NHS England (as an oversight body and commissioner of specialised services). In 2015, plans were announced to integrate the functions of Monitor and the TDA. Despite the 'bonfire of the quangos' promised by the Coalition (Dommett et al, 2014), many of their powers have been transferred to other arms-length bodies. The 'quango state [has thus been] reconfigured rather than abolished' (Dommett et al, 2014). This issue becomes crucial in understanding the ways in which system 'failures' are managed, especially as financial difficulties have become common (even among high performing NHS Trusts) and as the price (tariff) paid for procedures has fallen (under Payment by Results). For example, 88% of acute Trusts are forecasting a financial deficit in 2015–16 (Appleby et al, 2015). Local cases of 'failure' have included South London (NHS), Hinchingbrooke (Circle), Cornwall (SERCO), and Cambridge and Peterborough CCG (NHS), among others.

Theme 3: Marketisation

The NHS quasi-market has undergone various incarnations since it was introduced in 1991. The essence of the purchaser–provider split largely remains but much has changed. Whilst much of the 1990s was marked by 'steady state' approach (Le Grand, 2009), there has, in more recent years, been a heavy emphasis on stimulating diversity and pluralism in market provision. This stimulation has included Any Qualified Provider (Reynolds and McKee, 2012), Independent Sector Treatment Centre (Gabbay et al, 2011), and the private 'takeover' of public hospitals (for example, Hinchingbrooke hospital).

On the commissioning side, there has been much less emphasis on diversity. Whilst the distinction between health authority and GP fund-holding was seen, by some at least, as a form of purchaser competition, this was never allowed to develop fully. Beside, as many as 80% of patients did not know if their GP had fund-holding status or not (Kind et al, 1993). Moreover, the geographical basis of commissioners effectively reduced patients' ability to 'choose' their commissioner of services.

Whilst the marketisation creates an appearance of a self-sustaining system, forms of heavy steering have also been introduced through performance management, with some dysfunctional consequences (Hoque et al, 2004). Such was the scale of this during the 2000s that the period was termed 'targets and terror' (Bevan and Hood, 2006). Although the impacts of (provider) competition in the NHS are disputed (see Cooper et al, 2011; Pollock et al, 2012), it has damaged trusting relations between local actors (Hughes et al, 2011). It fostered, for example, a further fragmentation of relations in local health systems (Exworthy et al, 2009). The recent revival of interest in integration (especially between health and social care) is arguably a response to such previous fragmentation wrought by neo-liberal public choice policies. This might augur the demise of commissioning. After 25 years of commissioning, there is a case to be made that it is a failed experiment which has cost much but has delivered little in terms of enhancing quality and improving patient outcomes. The re-emergence of integration is arguably becoming the new organising narrative.

Theme 4: Health care quality and patient safety

Alongside funding, the quality and safety of NHS care is probably the biggest NHS issue that preoccupied the Coalition government most over their period of office. Whereas concerns over poor quality care date back at least as far as the mistreatment of long-stay patients at Ely hospital (Higgins, 2011; Secretary of State, 1969) and more recently at the tragic events at Bristol Royal Infirmary (Kennedy, 2001), the Stafford hospital scandal, which had first come to light under the previous Labour government, led to a number of high profile inquiries and reviews culminating in a raft of reforms designed to improve quality and safety across the NHS. In response to the Francis reports, the government appointed a new Chief Inspector of Hospitals and introduced a statutory duty of candour making it a criminal offence for providers to provide false information about quality of care. Other measures included a requirement on trusts to publish data on ward staffing levels a new, rigorous CQC inspection regime for hospitals, GPs and adult social care, new policies to protect whistleblowers from discriminationand a new special measures regime for failing trusts. Whereas the Coalition government had come to power promising a reduction in external systems of checking verification and audit, by the end of their term of office it had become clear that the corset of external control over providers and professionals had been tightened rather than loosened. Again, political rhetoric had not become reality for those working on the ground.

Although at this stage (about one year after the end of the Coalition government), evaluation of the Coalition government reforms might only offer a formative assessment of process, we can, however, place these reforms in a wider context of over 30 years of NHS general management, 25 years of markets and commissioning and 12 years of autonomous FTs and Patient Choice. These reforms, sedimented upon each other, build a complex picture of inter-relating policies. Here, we also consider issues which did not appear prominently in the reform programmes; this include patient and public involvement, for example. Each chapter in this collection offers a way to disentangle these multiple reforms, setting the Coalition reforms within a wider context of its antecedents.

The organisation of the book

This collection is organised into four sections. First, following this opening chapter, Powell offers an overview of the Coalition reforms in terms of Hall's 'orders of change' thesis. The second section examines the macro-level context of national health policy and politics. Often this perspective is overlooked in evaluation of reforms. The third section considers more meso- and micro-level factors associated with commissioning and service provision. This includes commissioning, provider diversity, public health and the equity implications of recent reforms. The third section considers the governance issue of reforms. This includes organisational systems and process as well as staffing and public involvement. A perspective of reform from abroad is also offered in this section. The final section draws out the conclusions from the preceding chapters and interprets them in conceptual terms using the multiple streams approach.

References

Alvarez-Rosete, A, Mays, N, 2008, Reconciling two conflicting tales of the English health policy process since 1997, *British Politics*, 3, 183–203

Appleby, J, Thompson, J, Jabbal, J (2015) 'How is the NHS performing'. *Quarterly monitoring report 17*. October 2015. London: King's Fund. http://qmr.kingsfund.org.uk/2015/17/

Bevan, G, Hood, C, 2006, What's measured is what matters: targets and gaming in the English public health system, *Public Administration*, 84, 3, 517–538

Boyne, G, Farrell, C, Law, J, Powell, M, Walker, RM, 2003, *Evaluating public management reforms*, Buckingham; Open University Press

Cameron, D. (2015) PM on plans for a seven-day NHS. Speech: 18 May 2015. https://www.gov.uk/government/speeches/pm-on-plans-for-a-seven-day-nhs

Conservative Party (2010) *Invitation to join the government of Britain: the Conservative manifesto*, The Conservative Party. https://www.conservatives.com/~/media/Files/Manifesto2010

Cooper, Z, Gibbons, S, Jones, S, McGuire, A, 2011, Does hospital competition save lives? Evidence from the English NHS patient choice reforms, *Economic Journal*, 121, F228–F260

Coulter, A, 1995, Evaluating general practice fundholding in the United Kingdom, *European Journal of Public Health*, 5, 233–239

Dommett, K, Flinders, M, Skelcher, C, Tonkiss, K, 2014, Did they 'read before burning'? The Coalition and quangos, *Political Quarterly*, 85, 2, 133–142

Exworthy, M, Powell, M, Mohan, J, 1999, The NHS: quasi-market, quasi-hierarchy and quasi-network? *Public Money and Management*, 19, 4, 15–22

Exworthy, M, Freeman, R, 2009, The United Kingdom: health policy learning in the NHS, in TR Marmor, R Freeman, KGH Okma (eds) *Comparative studies and the politics of modern medical care*. New Haven, CT: Yale University Press

Exworthy, M, Frosini, F, Jones, L, Peckham, S, Powell, M, Greener, I, Anand, P, Holloway, JA, 2009, *Decentralisation and performance: autonomy and incentives in local health economies*. Final report to the NHS NCC-SDO research and development programme

Exworthy, M, Powell, M, 2011, Case-studies in health policy: an introduction, in M Exworthy, S Peckham, M Powell, A Hann (eds) *Shaping health policy: case-study methods and analysis*. Bristol: Policy Press

Ferlie, E, Lynn, LE, Pollitt, C, eds, 2005, *Oxford handbook of public management*, Oxford: Oxford University Press

Gabbay, J, LeMay, A, Pope, C, Robert, G, Bate, P, Elston, M-A, 2011, *Organisational innovation in health services: lessons from the NHS Treatment Centres*, Bristol: Policy Press

Greener, I, Exworthy, M. Peckham, S, Powell, M, 2009, Has Labour decentralised the NHS? Terminological obfuscation and analytical confusion, *Policy Studies*, 30, 4, 439–454

Greener, I, Harrington, BE, Hunter, DJ, Mannion, R, Powell, M, 2014, *Reforming healthcare: what's the evidence?* Bristol: Policy Press

Greer, S, Jarman, H, Azorsky, A, 2014, *A reorganisation you can see from space: The architecture of power in the new NHS*. Centre for Health and Public Interest. http://chpi.org.uk/

Higgins, J, 2011, Hospitals in trouble, in M Exworthy, S Peckham, M Powell, A Hann (eds) *Shaping health policy: case-study methods and analysis*, Bristol: Policy Press

HM Government (2010) *The coalition: a programme for government*, London: Cabinet Office

Hoque, K, Davis, S, Humphreys, M, 2004, Freedom to do what you are told: senior management team autonomy in an NHS Acute Trust, *Public Administration*, 82, 2, 355–75

Hughes, D, Petsoulas, C, Allen, P, Doheny, S, Vincent-Jones, P, 2011, Contracts in the English NHS: market levers and social embeddedness, *Health Sociology Review, 20, 3, 321–337*

Kennedy, I, 2001, *Learning from Bristol: Public Inquiry into Children's Heart Surgery at the Bristol Royal Infirmary 1984–1995*, London: The Stationery Office

Kind, P, Leese, B, Hardman, G, 1993, *Evaluating the fundholding initiative: the views of patients*, York: Centre of Health Economics, University of York

Le Grand, J, Mays, N, Mulligan, J-A, eds, 1998, *Learning from the NHS internal market: a review of the evidence*, London: King's Fund

Le Grand, Julian, 2009, Choice and competition in publicly funded health care, *Health Economics, Policy and Law*, 4, 4, 479–488

Liberal Democrat, 2010, *Manifesto 2010*, Liberal Democrat Party. http://www.libdems.org.uk/manifesto

Mays, N, Wyke, S, Malbon, G, Goodwin, N, eds, 2001, *The purchasing of health care by primary care organizations: an evaluation and guide to future policy*, Buckingham: Open University Press

Mays, N, Dixon, A, Jones, L, eds, 2011, *Understanding New Labour's market reforms of the NHS*, London: King's Fund

Pollitt, C, 2009, Bureaucracies remember, post-bureaucratic organizations forget? *Public Administration*, 87, 2, 198–218

Pollock, A, Macfarlane, A, Greener, I, 2012, Bad science concerning NHS competition is being used to support the controversial Health and Social Care Bill, LSE blog: 5 March 2012. http://blogs.lse.ac.uk/politicsandpolicy/bad-science-nhs-competition/ (accessed 9.12.15)

Powell, M, Miller, R, 2014, Framing privatisation in the English National Health Service, *Journal of Social Policy*, 43, 3, 575–594

Reynolds, L, McKee, M, 2012, 'Any qualified provider' in NHS reforms: but who will qualify? *Lancet*, 379, 9821, 1083–1084

Rivett, G (undated) An uncertain path ahead: 2008-2017. Chapter 7. NHS History: http://www.nhshistory.net/chapter%207.htm

Robinson, R, 1994, Introduction, in R Robinson, J Le Grand, (eds) *Evaluating the NHS reforms*. London: King's Fund Institute

Robinson, R, Le Grand, J. (eds), 1994, *Evaluating the NHS reforms*, London: King's Fund Institute

Secretary of State, 1969, *Report of the Committee of Inquiry into Allegations of Ill- Treatment of Patients and other irregularities at the Ely Hospital, Cardiff*, Presented to Parliament by the Secretary of State of the Department of Health and Social Security by Command of Her Majesty, United Kingdom.

Secretaries of State, 1989, *Working for patients*, Cmd.855, London: HMSO.

Smith, J, Walshe, K, Hunter, DJ, 2001, The re-disorganisation of the NHS, *British Medical Journal*, 323, 7324, 1262–1263

Stevens, S, 2004, Reform strategies for the English NHS, *Health Affairs*, 23, 3, 37–44

Taylor-Gooby, P, Stoker, G, 2011, The Coalition programme: a new vision for Britain or politics as usual? *Political Quarterly*, 82, 1, 4–15

Thorlby, R, Maybin, J (eds), 2010, *A high performing NHS? A review of progress 1997–2010*, London: King's Fund

Timmins, N, 2012, *Never again? The story of the Health and Social Care Act 2012. A study in coalition government and policy-making*, London: King's Fund/Institute of Government

Walt, G, 1994, *Health policy: an introduction to process and power*, London: Zed Books

TWO

Orders of change in the ordered changes in the NHS

Martin Powell

Introduction

There does not appear to be a dominant approach to conceptualising or measuring change in health systems (Beland and Powell, 2016; Powell 2016), which makes it difficult to differentiate evolution from revolution. In other words, there is no clear dependent variable of change, but rather multiple and sometimes incommensurate criteria that defy attempts to come to neat conclusions.

There are many possible ways to examine these issues (Beland and Powell, 2016; Powell 2016), but this chapter draws on the influential account of Hall (1993) which differentiates between first, second and third order change. It views policymaking as a process that usually involves three central variables: the overarching goals that guide policy in a particular field, the techniques or policy instruments used to attain those goals, and the precise settings of those instruments. Hall regards change in settings as first order change; changes in instruments and settings as second order change; and changes in all three components – instrument settings, the instruments themselves and the goals – as third order or paradigm change. There are, however, a number of problems with this approach. First, it is not clear that first order change is always necessarily less important than second order change. For example, if the level of health spending was doubled or halved, this large first order change may be more important than a second order change in instruments. Second, it does not really capture outcomes, and so cannot explore the impact of 'change', which is complicated by issues of time lag and of causality and attribution.

This chapter tracks some of the main policy measures introduced by the Coalition's Health and Social Care Act (HSCA) of 2012 backwards to the Conservative government of 1979, which introduced market mechanisms into the NHS, using the framework of orders of change (Hall, 1993).

Orders of change: the challenge of evaluation in a complex service

This section explores some of the main changes since the Conservative government of 1979 (for details see, for example, Klein 2013a; Timmins, 2012; Powell, 2003, 2015a) in terms of first, second and third orders of change. Table 2.1 sums up the main points, which are developed in more detail below.

First order change

The main change in settings relates to expenditure. Spending in the United Kingdom (UK) on the National Health Service (NHS) has risen by an average of four per cent a year in real terms since it was formed

Table 2.1: Orders of change by government

	Conservative (1979–1997)	Labour (1997–2010)	Coalition (2010–2015)
First order change: Instrument settings			
Expenditure	Incremental	Significant	'Protected' but incremental
Second order change: Instruments	Purchaser/ provider split; internal market	Purchaser/provider split; external market	Purchaser/provider split; external market
	Largely internal competition	Internal and external competition	Internal and external competition
	Largely public provision	Growing private provision	Growing private provision
		Concordat	Any willing provider/Any qualified provider
	Largely 'collective' purchasing	Moves towards individual purchasing	Moves towards individual purchasing
	Price competition	Fixed price competition	Aim of moves towards price competition amended
		Competition law?	Competition law?
	Self-Governing Trusts	Foundation Trusts	Foundation Trusts

(continued)

Table 2.1: Orders of change by government (continued)

	Conservative (1979–1997)	Labour (1997–2010)	Coalition (2010–2015)
Second order change: Instruments (continued)	General Practitioner Fund Holding	Primary Care Groups/ Primary Care Trusts; Practice Based Commissioning; Total Purchasing	Clinical Commissioning Groups
		Private income limit of FT (capped at inception)	Private income limit of FT (capped at 49%)
	NHS Management Board		NHS England
		Regulation: Commission for Health Improvement/ Healthcare Commission/ Care Quality Commission; Monitor; Trust Development Authority	Regulation: Commission for Health Improvement/ Healthcare Commission/ Care Quality Commission; Monitor; Trust Development Authority
Third order change: goals	Stated that principles unchanged	Stated that principles unchanged	Stated that principles unchanged
	But critics state privatisation	But critics state privatisation	But critics state privatisation
	But critics state NHS will be abolished	But critics state NHS will be abolished	But critics state NHS will be abolished
			Duty of Secretary of State to promote rather than to provide?
Outcomes	Low in comparative terms	Low in comparative terms	Low in comparative terms

in 1948 (Roberts et al, 2012; Chapter 3). The 'Blair boost' following 'the most expensive breakfast in history' was followed by the 'Brown bust' associated with the financial crisis. Feast turned to famine with the 'Nicholson challenge' of delivering 'unprecedented levels of efficiency savings' of £20 billion by 2014/15 under the Quality, Innovation, Productivity and Prevention (QIPP) programme (see Chapter 4).

Although NHS spending was 'protected' by the Coalition government, it is generally considered that incremental increases will not keep pace with the requirements of demography, technology and expectations, and that a significant funding gap may occur (Roberts et al 2012; see Chapter 3). In comparative terms, spending on health is lower in the UK than the OECD average, with zero growth in health spending per person in real terms between 2009 and 2013. The UK also has a lower than average number of doctors and nurses, with 2.8 doctors per 1,000 population compared to the OECD average of 3.3, while the figures for nurses are 8.2 and 9.1 respectively.

Second order change

The Coalition maintained the purchaser/provider split, and the 'external market', with both internal and external competition (Powell, 2015a). Spencelayh (2015) points out that the HCSA did not introduce competition, marketisation or privatisation, although it may have increased all of them to some extent (see Chapter 11).

Labour's 'Concordat' between government and private providers arguably 'crossed the Rubicon' (Powell, 2003, 2015a), and provided the case of an irregular verb: we increased private sector capacity, but you are privatising the NHS (Powell and Miller 2013). The proportion of services delivered by private providers (including ISTC and social enterprises) slowly grew over time under Labour and Coalition governments. The data are disputed, but recent figures suggest anything from about 6 to 11 per cent (Spencelayh, 2015), which still falls short of the 15 per cent expectation by 2008 set out by Labour in the 'NHS Improvement Plan' (Department of Health, 2004).

The original Conservative internal market of 1991 allowed competition on both price and 'quality', but Labour introduced a fixed price tariff under the mis-named 'Payment by Results' (Bevan and Skellern, 2011; Spencelayh, 2015). The original Lansley Bill had included a degree of price competition, but this was amended (Timmins, 2012; Spencelayh, 2015). Timmins (2012, 80) points out that the NHS Operating Framework for 2011–12 allowed a limited amount of price competition over services covered by the NHS tariff, stating that the tariff would be a 'maximum' price in the coming year, which would be confirmed by the bill, but this had been trailed in the 2009 operating framework under Labour for 2010–11. At the time, however, 'no-one had picked that up in a way that made it a political issue.

This is hardly surprising, given the very subtle 'velvet glove' phrasing. The Labour Operating Frameworks states that 'After 2010/11, we shall move to a position where national tariffs represent the maximum price payable by a commissioner, as opposed to the mandated price for particular activity. (Department of Health, 2009, 35). According to the Coalition Operating Framework, 'The flexibilities set out in the 2010/11 NHS Operating Framework will remain largely in place for 2011/12. One new flexibility being introduced in 2011/12 is the opportunity for providers to offer services to commissioners at less than the published mandatory tariff price, where both commissioner and provider agree. Commissioners will want to be sure that there is no detrimental impact on quality, choice or competition as a result of any such agreement' (Department of Health, 2010b, 54).

In 2009, Labour Health Secretary, Andy Burnham announced an NHS 'preferred provider' approach, which was further explained in a letter from Sir David Nicholson, Chief Executive of the NHS (Spencelayh, 2015). There are some doubts, however, as to whether this was compatible with EU competition law (Timmins, 2012).

According to Timmins (2012, 78), competition law was one of the most furiously fought, if most misunderstood, elements of opposition to the changes. For example, Sarah Wollaston, the Conservative MP and then member and later Chair of the Health Select Committee, warned that the changes opened up the NHS to the stringencies of EU competition law. In the view of many lawyers, however, actions Labour had taken perhaps as far back as about 2006 meant that competition law already applied. A long war was to be fought to seek a way of 'protecting' the NHS from the application of a piece of legislation to which it was already subject (Timmins, 2012, 78–80). Davies (2013, 581) points to the 'juridification of the market', but writes that its impact is open to debate. On one level, it can be argued that the impact is small as competition law already applies to the NHS to some extent, but on another level, it can be argued that the reforms are more profound as they remove much of the doubt surrounding the applicability of competition law that may have served to shield NHS bodies from complaints and litigation in the past (2013, 584).

Many critics pointed to mandatory competition. For example, according to Toynbee and Walker (2015, 216), the key to the Bill was section 75 which 'ordained that every element of the NHS had to be competitively tendered.' Spencelayh (2015) considers that NHS commissioners are not required to put all clinical services out for competitive tender, however. She argues that the 2013 'Procurement, Patient Choice and Competition' Regulations have their roots in previous guidance documents issued by Labour in 2007, when the Department of Health (DH) published the Principles and Rules for Co-operation and Competition (PRCC). As Earl Howe put it in the

House of Lords, 'one area of the law that we have not changed one iota is the law relating to competitive tendering… these regulations usher in nothing new at all…' (in Spencelayh, 2015). While the CCG horses had been taken to water, it was unclear if they were forced to drink.

Moreover, the NHS was no stranger to compulsion. Under Labour, Independent Sector Treatment Centres (ISTC) and 'Darzi Centres' (or 'polyclinics') had been enforced on unwilling local areas, the 'Choose and Book' programme had to include at least one private provider Similarly, the Private Finance Initiative (PFI), which made a slow start under the Conservatives, expanded rapidly under Labour to become de facto 'the only game in town'. Labour Health Secretary Andy Burnham left his Coalition successor a shortlist of three private providers to take over Hinchingbrooke hospital, and then, with almost unbelievable hypocrisy, criticised him when he chose the private provider, Circle.

There has been a long history around greater autonomy for NHS providers. The Conservatives set up 'Self Governing Trusts', while Foundation Trusts (FT) represent one of the most protracted academic and political debates in health care under Labour. Timmins (2012, 105) explains that when Labour introduced FT, their private patient income was limited to the percentage they received at the time that the legislation was passed. This was a last-minute concession by the Blair government to Labour backbenchers who were concerned that the more independent nature of FT might let them concentrate on private care at the expense of public patients. While 'there were not many more than half a dozen hospitals where the cap was posing a problem', the Coalition government proposed to abolish the cap altogether, but in response to opposition, tabled an amendment that effectively placed the cap at 49% of a trust's income. Spencelayh (2015) argues that the HSCA increased the autonomy of FT by allowing trusts to increase their private income to 49%, but where a FT proposed to increase their private income by 5% or more in any financial year, the trust would require more than 50% of the council of governors to approve the proposal, and the FT would also be required in its annual report to explain the impact of private provision on its core NHS activity.

Commission has similarly been under discussion for a long while. The Conservatives' 1989 White Paper (Department of Health, 1989) provided the first attempt to insulate the NHS from day to day political meddling by giving responsibility for operational matters to an NHS Management Board, accountable for meeting the objectives set by the Secretary of State's Policy Board. The Coalition's independent board (NHS England) is the last in a long line of versions of 'take politicians out of the day-to-day management of the NHS' (such as the BBC Trust model) advanced by thinkthanks, the BMA and Labour under Brown (Timmins, 2012, 26).

Similarly, the Conservatives' aim (Department of Health, 1989) to move as much power and responsibility to the local level would be echoed in a succession of White Papers over the next decades, culminating in Lansley's promise that 'power will be given to the frontline clinicians and patients' (Department of Health, 2010a). The Conservatives' major and minor key commissioners of Health Authorities and GPFH were transposed under Labour to become Primary Care Groups and later Primary Care Trusts. Timmins (2012, 29) points out that GPFH had been voluntary, and had been rolled out in waves. Changes after 1997 that saw what remained of GP commissioning evolve into primary care trusts had been precisely that – a staged evolution, with Practice-based commissioning, in which GPs were intended progressively to take control of NHS budgets, had been launched in 2005 (Timmins, 2012, 26). Former Conservative Health Secretary and Chair of the House of Commons Health Committee, Stephen Dorrell, noted there were marked similarities between what Lansley was proposing and both the total purchasing pilots and Labour's first incarnation of GP commissioning, the primary care groups (in Timmins, 2012, 70). At one level, CCGs simply deliver the aim of Labour Health Secretary Frank Dobson's 1997 White Paper that 'Local doctors and nurses who are in the best position to know what patients need will be in the driving seat in shaping services' (Department of Health, 1997). The Coalition reforms may have settled a question, unanswered for 20 years, over who should be the key purchaser – GPs or health authorities – by the creation of something that is an amalgam of the two (Timmins, 2012, 124).

Finally, there have been a series of independent regulators on quality (CHI; HCC; CQC) and finance (Monitor, TDA). (Jarman and Greer, 2015; see also Chapter 5). It can, however, can be argued that Lansley wished to change the role of Monitor to be an economic regulator along the lines of utilities such as electricity and gas. Spencelayh (2015) argues that one of the main changes of the HCSA was to turn Monitor's role from regulator of NHS foundation trusts into a broader 'sector' regulator, but as it was passed, the Act had a different emphasis to the original bill, with a weaker focus on economic regulation than was originally envisioned. In 2014 it was announced that 2014 CQC and Monitor would be working together with a Memorandum of Understanding, while in 2015 Monitor and TDA would be renamed NHS Improvement.

Third order change

There has been a great deal of debate over the multiple and unclear goals of the NHS. In particular, critics argue that stated goals are untruthful, and that 'real' goals are much more malevolent.

All of the main reform documents under different governments (Department of Health 1989, 1997, 2000, 2010a) have asserted that the 'principles' of the NHS, such as being available to all, funded by taxation, fair, and free at the point of use) remain unchanged. There have always been debates about their precise meanings and about the extent to which they have been maintained, however (see Powell 1996, 1997). For example, the DH and BMA has consistently repeated their support for the founding principle of the NHS of 'free at point of use' and their opposition to charges, conveniently forgetting that the 'charging horse' bolted over 60 years ago when dental, optical and prescription charges were introduced.

Critics have argued that these reassuring statements camouflage the 'real aims' of reform – privatising, ending or Americanising the NHS (see, for example, Leys and Player, 2011, 2, 143, 145). While many commentators have regarded the Coalition reforms as a continuation or acceleration of trends by New Labour on the basis of criteria such as marketisation, provider pluralism, choice and competition (see, for example, Ham et al, 2015; Timmins, 2012), some commentators claim that the NHS is being privatised (see, for example, Davis et al, 2015; Hunter, 2013a, b). According to Davies (2013, 585–7), despite substantial continuity between the 2012 reforms and pre-existing government policy, the HSCA does contain various elements that may encourage greater private-sector involvement, but there are some important limitations on private-sector involvement in NHS provision. She concludes that the HSCA does create highly favourable conditions for greater private participation, and it is 'indeed possible that there may be gradual privatisation in the NHS without proper public debate'. Klein (2013b) states, however, that the NHS in England is being neither privatised nor destroyed. According to Ham et al (2015), the reforms have certainly resulted in greater marketisation in the NHS, but claims of mass privatisation were and are exaggerated. Powell and Miller (2013) argue that the term privatisation is multidimensional, and definitions and operationalisations of the term are often implicit, unclear, and conflicting (see also Spencelayh, 2015; Vizard and Obolenskaya, 2015), resulting in conflicting accounts of the occurrence, chronology, and degree of privatisation in the NHS.

There appears to be no clear 'tipping point' of privatisation. Moreover, private firms may be drawing back from secondary care due to the difficulty of making money out of the NHS. This can be illustrated by the failure of the 'iconic case of privatisation', where Hinchingbrooke hospital was handed over to a firm called Circle in February 2012, but handed back in January 2015 after a negative CQC report which resulted in the trust being put into special measures (Jarman and Greer, 2015). While further management franchises by private sector providers now seem unlikely (Ham et al, 2015; Klein, 2013b; Jarman and Greer, 2015), any future cherries left to pick are likely to be individual services or pathways within acute services, and in community services (Davis et al, 2015; Spencelayh, 2015).

It has been claimed that the 'legal basis for the abolition of the NHS' can be found in the change of wording of the duty of the Secretary of State to 'promote rather than provide' services (see, for example, Davis and Tallis, 2013). As Timmins (2012, 102–3) explains, it was argued that this 'hands off' or 'autonomy' clause effectively allowed the health secretary to 'wash his hands' of responsibility for provision of the NHS, handing that duty over to the board and the commissioning groups. He continues that to some critics, this was a core issue, but to other commentators it appeared a sideshow. The brute political reality, they argued, was that whatever the law said, in a tax-funded NHS the health secretary would remain ultimately accountable for the provision of services, even if this is 'accountability by telephone' (Jarman and Greer 2015.) As Stephen Dorrell had repeatedly put it – and as the former Conservative health minister Tony Newton was to argue in the Lords, seeking changes to the bill – if services got into trouble, it would be impossible for the health secretary of the day to say it was 'nothing to do with me, guv'. Spencelayh (2015) states that the HSCA, like previous legislation before it, requires the Secretary of State to promote a comprehensive health service and states that services provided as part of the health service in England must be free of charge (bar a few exceptions, such as prescription charges), and that the NHS constitution specifies that access to NHS services is based on clinical need and not an individual's ability to pay. While the Secretary of State remains formally accountable for the NHS, the HSCA has the potential to undermine this accountability in significant ways. There remains considerable central government control over the NHS, albeit in more complex and cumbersome form (Davies, 2013).

Outputs and Outcomes

Hall's (1993) framework tends to focus attention at political and legal interpretations of legislation, and largely ignores issues of implementation and impact. In other words, it takes a 'Webbsian' view that discursive analysis ends with the Parliamentary Act, with little interest in its implementation.

There are a number of possible evaluation templates of the NHS under the Coalition: temporal (is the NHS getting better over time?); intrinsic (is it delivering its aims, or being consistent with its principles?) and extrinsic/comparative (how does it compare to other health systems?) (see Powell, 1997, 2016b).

This gives a wide range of approaches, dimensions and indicators. For example, Gregory et al (2012) focus on nine dimensions of care that makes an effective health care system, while Gardner (2015) examines nearly 300 indicators which can be used to monitor changes over time in the quality of services provided.

There are many bodies that provide an 'official' view on NHS performance with a large variety of different perspectives (see, for example, CQC 2015; Monitor 2015; NHS England 2015a). In NHS England Annual Report (2015a), NHS Chief Executive Simon Stevens writes that 2014–15 was a year in which the Health Service responded – largely successfully – to wide-ranging operational pressures. The document claims that 'unprecedented numbers of patients were treated by the NHS last year' for both urgent and planned care. Although NHS hospitals missed their A&E target during the winter, overall NHS A&E Services delivered the best performance measured by a major industrial country. The document claims that most of the 25 objectives of the Government's Mandate for 2014–15 'were met or were close to being met'. It is difficult to judge this claim from the material given, however (see Appendix 1 of the Mandate, p 12). For example, Objective 1 (Improvement against the NHS Outcomes Framework) provides 48 metrics with data available from 2013 onwards. Of these, it is claimed that notable progress has been made in 40 per cent of metrics, a further 40 per cent have remained fairly static and deterioration has been shown in 20 per cent.

Department of Health (2015) provides an annual assessment of NHS England's performance during 2014–15, based on evidence from NHS England's own annual report and accounts for 2014–15, available data, feedback from stakeholders and the discussions that the Secretary of State and his departmental team have held with NHS England's team throughout the year. It agrees with the assessment of the annual report for 2014–15 (NHS England 2015) that NHS England has made good progress against the mandate. In a challenging year, NHS England has made progress on the majority of the mandate objectives, with the majority of the 68 indicators of the NHS outcomes framework showing improvements in outcomes over the past year.

The Care Quality Commission (2015) reported the results of its 'new tougher approach' of inspection. It focused on higher risk acute trusts first: of the 38 acute trusts, nine were rated as 'good', improvement was required in 24, and five were rated as 'inadequate'. Safety was the biggest concern: four out of every five safety ratings were 'inadequate' or 'requires improvement'. It stated that this variation in the quality and safety of care in England is too wide and unacceptable.

According to Monitor (2015), the financial performance of FTs 'revealed an exceptionally challenging year'. For the first time, they reported an overall deficit of deficit of £345 million, which was £479 million worse than 2013/14, with over 50 per cent of foundation trusts in deficit at the end of the year. Many FTs did not meet key operational performance standards, and by the end of March 2015, 29 FTs (or 19 per cent of the total) were in breach of their licence and subject to regulatory action by Monitor.

There are a number of 'unofficial' assessments. Ham et al (2015) consider that 'Historians will not be kind in their assessment of the coalition government's record on NHS reform.' According to the Kings Fund 'mid-term' assessment, it appears that the performance of the NHS is holding up despite financial pressures and the disruption of reforms, but cracks are now emerging (Gregory et al, 2012, 56). The overall verdict of the final assessment (Appleby et al, 2015) is that NHS performance held up well for the first three years of the parliament but has now slipped, with waiting times at their highest levels for many years and an unprecedented number of hospitals reporting deficits. Despite this, patient experience of the NHS generally remains positive and public confidence is close to an all-time high. Vizard and Obolenskaya (2015, 108) point to some adverse movements against a number of key indicators which raise the prospect of retrogression and moving backwards.

QualityWatch (2015) presents three main conclusions in an 'an independent view of how patterns of quality have changed over time'. First, care services are improving in many markers of quality. Second, there are nonetheless clear signals that performance in many areas is declining, and it seems that the NHS has been unable to reverse the trends of deteriorating access to hospital, mental health and social care services that were identified in the 2014 report. Third, given the relationship between engaged staff and good quality care, there is a substantial risk that the current staffing situation in both health and social care may be reducing the quality of care received by patients and service users, with worrying indications of stress, high vacancy rates and increases in instances of bullying.

Gardner (2015) writes that there are two sides to every story and measures that could be viewed as an overall proxy for how well the NHS is performing are incomplete and potentially misleading. He concludes that the NHS has done extraordinarily well to maintain and improve quality across a range of areas in the face of growing pressure from increased demand and financial constraints. Progress on improving quality has stalled in some areas, though, and may even be starting to unravel, while information gaps in a range of other areas mean we simply do not know whether quality is getting better or worse.

Finally, the NHS can be compared to other health systems. First, the English NHS can be compared with other systems within the UK (see Chapter 7). Bevan et al (2014) state that there is little sign that one country is consistently moving ahead of the others. Second, the English NHS can be compared to health systems outside the UK (see Chapter 17). There are many different studies (see Kossarova et al, 2015), but international comparisons are problematic, with different studies at different times stressing different measures, which have produced rather different results. The NHS has tended to do well in the annual Commonwealth Fund study, with the latest study (Davis et al, 2014) placing the UK best of 11 countries on overall rank and for 9 of the 11 criteria. Niemietz (2014) claims, however, that this study is mostly based on inputs and procedures as opposed to outcomes, and on doctors' and patients' survey responses as opposed to clinical data. Only one category is concerned with outcomes, and in that category, the UK comes out second to last. He cites the Guardian's (presumably non-ironic) verdict that 'The only serious black mark against the NHS was its poor record on keeping people alive.' Moreover, the data relates to 2011–3, and it is possible that a future ranking may show a sharp decline. The Economist Intelligence Unit (2014) produced a report measuring population outcomes and spending across 166 countries. The UK came 23rd, which was a fairly mediocre performance for a wealthy country. This was followed by a study of 30 countries with a wider range of measures based on data from around 2012 (Economist Intelligence Unit, 2015). The UK was ranked 3rd on equity and access; 14th on disease outcomes 16th on expenditure; 17th on healthcare costs; 19th on population health outcomes; and 28th on healthcare resources. Kossarova et al (2015) use Organisation for Economic Co-operation and Development (OECD) data to explore care in four sectors – primary care, hospital care, cancer care and mental health – across 15 countries over the period 2000–2013. The UK does not consistently over-perform or underperform when compared with the pool of the other 14 countries. Absolute and relative trends – that is, whether the UK is improving or deteriorating and how it is performing in relation to other countries – are also mixed. While it is encouraging that the UK is stable or improving on 25 out of 27 indicators, it is worrying that the UK performs worse than most countries on 14 out of 27 indicators and performance is deteriorating on two indicators. Finally, OECD (2015) compares the quality of healthcare across 34 countries. It notes low level of expenditure and staffing (see above), and claims that quality of care in the NHS is 'poor to mediocre' compared to other developed nations. The UK lags behind on a number of measures, coming 22nd out of 25 countries on cervical cancer survival, 21st out of 25 countries on breast cancer survival, 20th out of 23 countries on bowel cancer survival, and 19th out of 31 countries on stroke survival.

Evolution or revolution?

The debate of continuity versus change or evolution versus revolution remains unclear (Vizard, and Obolenskaya, 2015). As early as June 2010, Sir David Nicholson privately stated that Lansley's plans were 'really, really revolutionary' (in Timmins, 2012, 12), and later related a phrase told to him: 'It is the only change management system you can actually see it from space – it is that large' (in Timmins, 2012, 74). Similarly, according to Nigel Edwards, then acting chief executive of the NHS Confederation, 'I do not think most people have grasped the scale of this change. By 2014, the NHS will no longer be a system which still contains the characteristics of an organisation. Instead it will be a regulated industry in which that management chain no longer exists' (in Timmins, 2012, 78). According to D'Ancona (2014, 105) 'the revolutionary principle at the heart of the reform was the transfer of commissioning powers to family doctors'.

Timmins (2012, 124) suggests that the combination of five factors in the HSCA turned evolution into something that can be seen as revolution. There were three new elements: the insistence that all GPs had to be in GP consortia (CCG); the extent to which Lansley wanted to turn the NHS into a version of a regulated industry, creating a form of self-improving machine that required minimal ministerial oversight;

and his determination to legislate for all this in such a way that it would take further legislation to change the key building blocks in the new dispensation. Added to that was speed and the complete dismantling of the PCTs and SHAs – a by- product of coalition politics.

Other commentators, however, suggest a broad continuity or evolution thesis. Some stress continuity with Labour. For example, according to Jarman and Greer (2015), the core ideas contained in the White Paper (Department of Health 2010a) maintain continuity with the previous government's reform agenda. The reforms represent evolution, 'finishing Labour's dirty work' (Davis and Tallis, 2013, 12–13). Leys and Player (2011, 142) write that the HSCA does not represent a major break with the policy of the Blair and Brown governments. Cameron and Lansley advanced 'evolutionary' or 'going with the grain' arguments (Timmins, 2012, 28). Similarly, former Labour advisers have argued that Coalition reforms essentially complete Labour business. For example, commentators such as Julian Le Grand argued that the reforms were 'a logical, sensible, extension of [changes] put in place by Tony Blair' (Le Grand quoted in Timmins, 2012, 84), while Simon Stevens stated that 'What makes the Coalition's proposals so radical is not that they tear up that earlier [Blair] plan. It is that they move decisively towards fulfilling it' (Stevens quoted in Timmins, 2012, 67). Timmins points out that sections in the original draft had emphasised that continuity, pointing out that Labour had been doing the right things but had failed to implement its reforms properly or see them through. That evolutionary perspective got stripped out in favour of a revolutionary one (Timmins, 2012, 64), however. Similarly, Seldon and Snowdon (2015, 186) see Coalition reforms as essentially a continuation of the Blair reforms, but presented by Cameron and Lansley as a paradigm shift.

The reforms can be seen, instead, as having longer term continuity with the Conservatives governments of 1979–1997. Stephen Dorrell stated that

> health policy hasn't changed. Frank Dobson would like to have changed it and wasn't able to. But apart from him, no health secretary has wanted to change policy since 1991, which is the day when it really did change. We used to have a provider-led system; we now have a commissioner-led system. That is different, but it's the last time anybody fundamentally changed health policy. (Timmins and Davies, 2015, 164)

According to Timmins (2012, 9) the HSCA is by far the most contentious change to the way the service functions since the introduction of the purchaser/provider split in to the NHS in 1991 – a change arguably far more revolutionary than Lansley's reforms, given where the NHS then was. He continues that there is marked continuity between what it provides and the direction in which Blairite health policy was heading. It can easily be seen as an extension, a logical outcome even, not just of what Blairite health ministers had been up to but of what was intended – or at least implied – way back in 1989 when Working for Patients first introduced a quasi- market into the National Health Service. In the great long sweep of history, it can certainly be viewed that way (Timmins, 2012, 123).

There has not been a neat or linear pattern of evolution, however. Timmins (2012, 34) argues that since 1991 these market-like reforms to the NHS had gone through a repeated process of two steps forward and one step back, depending on the ministers in charge. Although the steps back included Dobson (abolition of GPFH and the NHS was told to use the private sector 'as a last resort') and Burnham (proposed NHS as 'preferred provider'), the broad direction of travel is towards a market. Former Conservative Health Secretary, Ken Clarke advances the 'Nixon goes to China' argument that

> Labour secretaries of state have got away with introducing private sector providers into the NHS on a scale which would have led the Labour Party onto the streets in demonstration if a Conservative government had ever tried it. In the late 1980s I would have said it is politically impossible to do what we are now doing. (Ken Clarke, in Timmins, 2012, 6)

Conclusion

It is difficult to evaluate 'reform so complex it made the Schleswig-Holstein question seem simple' (D'Ancona, 2014, 110) using a complex template of multiple and sometimes incommensurate criteria and evidence that has been interpreted in different ways (see Vizard and Obolenskaya, 2015) The orders of change framework, however, suggests that health reform over the last 25 years of so in the UK appears to be characterised more by evolution rather than revolution. The 1991 reforms seem to be closer to third order or paradigm change than the 2010 reforms (Timmins, 2012).

Former Labour Health spokesperson, Robin Cook regarded the 1991 Conservative reforms as a series of 'Granny's footsteps' or increments (in Powell, 1996). These footsteps, in varying size but broadly in the direction of market-based reform, seem to have continued over the past 25 years.

Part of the reason for the 'revolution' of the HCSA was the sheer size of the legislation in terms of the size of the Bill, the number of clauses, the days of debate, or the number of amendments. Leys and Player (2011, 107) note that, with the exception of FT, none of the main steps towards the transformation of the NHS into a healthcare market down to 2010 have required legislation.

Andrew Lansley once remarked that 'I could have done most of this without the legislation' (in Timmins, 2012, 120). Ken Clarke stated that the enormous bill was 'just hubris. I argued to him that he didn't need a bill. That all of it, certainly almost all of it, could have been done within his existing powers' (in Timmins and Davies, 2015, 63). Timmins (2012, 136–8) suggests that the 'no legislation' or 'minimal legislation' routes legislating for the board and the regulator in one bill, or two spread over time would not have been without large-scale controversy, and would clearly have been an evolution rather than the revolution that it came to be seen. In the words of Dorrell, it essentially gave all the different interests permission to go back into their trenches, and to refight all the battles that had been fought over the previous 20 years since Working for Patients (in Timmins, 2012, 82). Put another way, it provided another chance to fire 20 years of ammunition for Klein's (2013, 2015) 'indignant' or 'NHS fundamentalists'.

As suggested above, however, the Hall (1993) framework tends to ignore issues of outputs, outcomes and impact. It is unclear if and how outcomes are causally related to reform. This can be highlighted by some apparent paradoxes in the evidence advanced by some critics. For example, it has been claimed in terms of outcomes that the NHS closed the gap with other health care systems [during a period of market-based reform] and that the NHS was rated as the best health care system by the Commonwealth Fund *after* the 2010 reforms (see, for example, Leys and Player 2011, 10; 148–9; Davis et al 2015, 37–41; Toynbee and Walker, 2015, 213–4). There are a number of possible explanations for this apparent paradox. First, market-based reform is associated with improved outcomes. Second, there is no clear relationship between reform and outcomes. Third, outcomes have improved despite market-based reform. This may be possible due to the resilience of the NHS, where staff, not patients, have absorbed the pain of change (Klein, 2015). Put another way, NHS staff act as institutional shock absorbers, who may attenuate negative (and possibly also positive) elements of reforms. It is unclear how long this 'finger in the dam' approach can hold back any approaching torrent, though. If staff act as the canary in the coal mine, there are some worrying signs in terms of staff stress, high vacancy rates and increases in instances of bullying (QualityWatch, 2015). Finally, time lags make it difficult to link interventions with outcomes. For example, the data in the Commonwealth Fund study (Davis et al, 2014) data relates to 2011–2013, before any impact associated with the 2012 HSCA. There may be a lagged effect, and it is possible that any recent improvements may be due to Labour reforms, such as increased expenditure. If this is the case, the effect of this inheritance may soon end, and it follows that – due to the time lag effect– the full impact of the Coalition reforms is yet to be felt.

References

Appleby, J, Baird, B, Thompson, J, Jabbal, J, 2015, *The NHS under the coalition government. Part two: NHS performance*, London: King's Fund

Baggott, R, 2016, 'Health policy and the coalition government' in H. Bochel and M. Powell, eds, *The coalition government and social policy*, Bristol: Policy Press, pp 99–126

Beland, D, Powell, M, 2016, Continuity and change in social policy, *Social Policy and Administration*, 50, 2, 129-147

Bevan, G, Skellern, M, 2011, Does competition between hospitals improve clinical quality? A review of evidence from two eras of competition in the English NHS. *British Medical Journal*, 343, d6470

Bevan, G, Karanikolos, M, Exley, J, Nolte, E, Connolly, S, and Mays, N, 2014, *The four health systems of the United Kingdom: how do they compare?* London: Health Foundation/Nuffield Trust

Carrier, J, Kendall, I, 2015, *Health and the National Health Service*, 2nd edn, London: Routledge

CQC (Care Quality Commission), 2015, *The State of Health Care and Adult Social Care in England 2013/14*, London: CQC

D'Ancona, M, 2014, *In it together: the inside story of the Coalition Government*, London: Penguin

Davies, A, 2013, This time, it's for real: the Health and Social Care Act 2012, *Modern Law Review*, 76, 3, 564–588

Davis, J. and Tallis, R, eds, 2013, *NHS SOS*, London: OneWorld

Davis, J, Lister, J, Wrigley, D, 2015, *NHS for Sale*, London: Merlin Press

Davis, K, Stremikis, K, Squires, D, Schoen, C, 2014, *Mirror, Mirror on the Wall, How the Performance of the U.S. Health Care System Compares Internationally* [internet]. New York: Commonwealth Fund, 2014, www.commonwealthfund.org/ publications/fund-reports/2014/ jun/mirror-mirror

Department of Health, 1989, *Working for patients*, London: The Stationery Office

Department of Health, 1997, *The New NHS*, London: The Stationery Office

Department of Health, 2000, *The NHS plan*, London: The Stationery Office

Department of Health, 2002, *Implementing the NHS plan*, London: The Stationery Office

Department of Health, 2004, *The NHS improvement plan*, London: The Stationery Office

Department of Health, 2009, *The operating framework for 2010/11 for the NHS in England*, London: DH

Department of Health, 2010a, *Equity and excellence: Liberating the NHS*, London: The Stationery Office

Department of Health, 2010b, *The operating framework for the NHS in England 2011/12*, London: DH

Economist Intelligence Unit, 2014, *Health outcomes and cost: A 166-country comparison*, London: EIU

Economist Intelligence Unit, 2015, *The NHS: How does it compare?* London: EIU

Gardner T, 2015, *Swimming against the tide? The quality of NHS services during the current parliament*. London: The Health Foundation, 2015

Gregory, S, Dixon, A, Ham, C, eds, 2012, *Health policy under the coalition government. A mid-term assessment*, London: King's Fund

Hall, P, 1993, Policy paradigms, social learning and the state, *Comparative Politics*, 25, 3, 275–96

Ham, C, Baird, B, Gregory, S, Jabbal, J, and Alderwick, H, 2015, *The NHS under the Coalition Government, part one: NHS reform*, London: King's Fund

Jarman, H, Greer, S, 2015, The big bang: health and social care reform under the Coalition, in M Beech and S Lee, eds, *The Conservative–Liberal Coalition*, Basingstoke: Palgrave

Klein, R, 2013a, *The new politics of the NHS*, 7th edn, Abingdon: Radcliffe Medical

Klein, R, 2013b, The twenty-year war over England's National Health Service: a report from the battlefield, *Journal of Health Politics, Policy and Law* 38, 4, 849–69

Klein, R, 2015, England's National Health Service: Broke but not broken, *The Milbank Quarterly*, 93, 3, 455–458

Kossarova, L, Blunt, I, Bardsley, M, 2015, *Focus on: International comparisons of healthcare quality: what can the UK learn?* Health Foundation/Nuffield Trust

Leys, C, Player, D, 2011, *The plot against the NHS*, Pontypool: Merlin

Monitor, 2015, *Annual report and accounts 1 April 2014 to 31 March 2015*, HC 237, London: The Stationery Office

National Health Service (NHS) England, 2014, *Five Year Forward View*, London: NHS

National Health Service (NHS) England, 2015, Annual Report and Accounts 2014–15, HC 109, London: The Stationery Office

Niemietz, K, 2014, *Health check: IEA discussion paper No. 54*, London: Institute of Economic Affairs

OECD, 2015, *Health at a Glance*, Paris: OECD

Powell, M. 1996, Granny's footsteps, fractures and the principles of the NHS, *Critical Social Policy*, 16(1): 27-44

Powell M, 1997, *Evaluating the National Health Service*, Buckingham: Open University Press

Powell, M, 2003, Quasi-markets in British health policy, *Social Policy and Administration*, 37, 7, 725–41

Powell, M, 2015a, Making markets in the English National Health Service, *Social Policy and Administration*, 49, 1, 109–27

Powell M, 2015b, Who killed the English National Health Service? *International Journal of Health Policy and Management*, 4, 5: 267–269

Powell, M, Miller, R, 2013, Privatizing the English National Health Service: an irregular verb? *Journal of Health Politics, Policy and Law*, 28, 5, 1051–9

Powell, M, 2016, Reforming a health care system in a big way? The case of change in the British NHS, *Social Policy and Administration* 50, 2: 183-200

Powell, M, Miller, R, 2013, Privatizing the English National Health Service: an irregular verb? *Journal of Health Politics, Policy and Law*, 28, 5, 1051–9

QualityWatch, 2015, *Closer to critical?* London: Health Foundation/ Nuffield Trust

Roberts, A, Marshall, L, and Charlesworth, A, 2012, *A decade of austerity?* London: Nuffield Trust

Seldon, A, Snowdon, P, 2015, *Cameron at 10*, London: William Collins

Spencelayh, E, 2015, *Evolution, revolution or confusion? Competition and privatisation in the NHS*, London: Health Foundation

Timmins, N, 2012, *Never again? The story of the Health and Social Care Act 2012*, London: The King's Fund and the Institute for Government

Toynbee, P, Walker, D, 2015, *Cameron's coup*, London: Guardian Faber

Vizard, P, Obolenskaya , P, 2015, *The Coalition's record on health: Policy, Spending and Outcomes 2010–2015*, Social Policy in a Cold Climate, Working Paper 16, Centre for Analysis of Social Exclusion, LSE: London

Section B:
National health policy

THREE

NHS finances under the Coalition

Anita Charlesworth, Adam Roberts and Sarah Lafond

The English NHS faced a number of challenges over the five years of Coalition Government. Some were new and unique to the period, such as the major system reforms introduced with the Health and Social Care Act (HSCA) 2012 (The Stationery Office, 2012). Others were a continuation of underlying challenges such as the growing and ageing of the population, along with the rising burden of chronic disease. All were affected by a substantial shift in the financial pressure facing the NHS, however, as it had to adapt from a decade of real-terms budget increases of 7% each year on average, to five years of receiving budget increases of less than 1%. With demand for services rising, the NHS in England faced the daunting task of making efficiency savings of £20bn in five years.

The NHS was not alone in facing austerity – many other European health care systems faced similar challenges in the aftermath of the 2008 recession (OECD, 2015). The policies implemented in the English NHS mirror those used elsewhere. There was national action to reduce input costs through mandated reductions in administrative budgets, a national public sector pay policy which reduced real wage increases and measures to constrain drug prices. Alongside this, the NHS was asked to deliver improved technical efficiency through a reduction in the prices paid to hospitals under the national tariff system and attempts were made to improve system efficiency with policies to better integrate health and social care (NAO, 2011; Department of Health and Department for Communities and Local Government, 2014).

The Nicholson challenge

The global economic crisis in 2008 would have a substantial impact on public finances, and therefore the budget for the NHS. In 2009 Sir David Nicholson, the head of the English NHS, anticipated the forthcoming period of austerity, suggesting that the NHS would need to make around £15–20 billion of efficiency savings over the coming

5 years (Nicholson, 2009). This was then turned into a more specific objective of £20 billion of efficiency savings over the 4 years from 2011/12 to 2014/15 (Gregory et al, 2012), which came to be known as 'The Nicholson Challenge'. The NHS established a programme, Quality, Innovation, Productivity and Prevention (QIPP), to deliver these efficiency savings (NAO 2011).

The Coalition Government committed to increase NHS funding in England throughout the parliament (Cameron and Clegg 2010) and so NHS funding was protected from the overall reduction in public spending. Funding nonetheless rose at a lower rate than the cost of rising demand and inputs. This resulted in the need to bridge the potential funding gap. In the Coalition Government's first spending review in autumn 2010, the government set out spending plans for the financial years 2010/11 to 2014/15. Table 3.1 shows the total budget plans for the NHS through this period. After allowing for inflation this was a planned average increase of 0.4% a year over the spending review period. Within this budget the NHS was required to allocate part of this funding to local government to support social care services. The required transfer began in 2011/12 with £0.8 billion ring-fenced within the NHS Resource Departmental Expenditure Limit (RDEL) for social care, followed by £0.9 billion in 2012/13, £1.1 billion in 2013/14 and £1 billion in 2014–15 (HM Treasury, 2010).

Although funding for the English NHS rose in real terms, this settlement required the NHS to make substantial efficiency savings if access to, and quality of care was not to suffer. The reason for this is that pressures on health spending were projected to increase at a much faster rate than the funding growth committed to in the 2010 spending review (Roberts et al, 2012). Equally, the rate of increase was much lower than the NHS had received in previous years (Lloyd 2015). In the decades preceding the recession of 2008, public spending

Table 3.1: Health spending plans in Spending Review 2010 (£bn)

	2010/11	2011/12	2012/13	2013/14	2014/15
Resource DEL	98.7	101.5	104	106.9	109.8
Capital DEL	5.1	4.4	4.4	4.4	4.6
Total DEL	103.8	105.9	108.4	111.4	114.4
Total DEL, (2015/16 price[1])	112.8	113.3	113.9	114.7	116.0
Resource DEL excludes depreciation					

Note: [1] Real terms figures adjusted for inflation using HM treasury GDP deflator published on 08/01/2016 www.gov.uk/government/statistics/gdp-deflators-at-market-prices-and-money-gdp-december-2015-quarterly-national-accounts

Source: HM Treasury Spending Review 2010 Cm 7942 October 2010

on health care increased faster than whole economy inflation and GDP growth in all OECD countries (OECD, 2015). The pressures on health spending arise from a mix of changes to the demand for health care including an ageing population and increasing income per capita. Changes affecting the supply of health care also influence health care spending. Principal among these are new technologies and treatments, increasing relative prices and the rate of productivity improvement (Chernew and Newhouse, 2011).

In the first decade of the 21st century, publicly-funded health spending in England increased by an average of 8.3% a year. This reflected the additional investment under the previous Labour Government following the review of health funding pressures undertaken by Sir Derek Wanless (Wanless, 2002). The Wanless review estimated the funding pressures facing the NHS over two decades ending in 2022–23. It developed three scenarios which varied according to the assumption made over different domains: health seeking behaviour, the prevalence of risk factors for chronic disease and productivity. The 'fully engaged' scenario assumed productivity growth between 2012–13 and 2022–23 of 3% a year compared, to productivity growth of 1.75% a year in the 'slow uptake' scenario. These different assumptions about productivity, combined with different demand-side assumptions, produce significant differences in the pressures on health funding. Table 3.2 compares the funding pressures projections for the three scenarios from the Wanless Review. The low productivity, high demand scenario (slow uptake) results in pressure on health funding which are two percentage points of GDP higher in 2022–23 than the high productivity, low demand scenario (fully engaged).

As the table shows, the Wanless Review scenarios projected that NHS funding would need to increase by between 4.4% and 5.6% a year at the mid-point of the Coalition Government (2012–13). In practice, funding increased by less than a quarter of this rate.

In 2010, McKinsey estimated that the English NHS would face a potential funding gap of between £10–15bn by 2013/14 (in cash terms), based on their projections for demand pressures and possible allocation to Department of Health (DH). This analysis formed the basis of Sir David Nicholson's estimate of the efficiency challenge facing the NHS. McKinsey estimated that the English NHS could capture efficiency savings of between £13–20bn over 3–5 years, through a combination of technical efficiency, allocative efficiency through decommissioning interventions with lower value added, and shifting management of care from towards out-of-hospital alternatives (McKinsey and Company, 2012; Monitor, 2013).

Table 3.2: The 2002 Wanless Review projections of English NHS funding pressures

	2002–03[1]	Projections			
		2007–08	2012–13	2017–18	2022–23
Total health spending (per cent of money GDP)[2]					
Solid progress	7.7	9.4	10.5	10.9	11.1
Slow uptake	7.7	9.5	11.0	11.9	12.5
Fully engaged	7.7	9.4	10.3	10.6	10.6
Total NHS spending (£ billion, 2002–03 prices)					
Solid progress	68	96	121	141	161
Slow uptake	68	97	127	155	184
Fully engaged	68	96	119	137	154
Average annual real growth in NHS spending (per cent)[3]					
Solid progress	6.8	7.1	4.7	3.1	2.7
Slow uptake	6.8	7.3	5.6	4.0	3.5
Fully engaged	6.8	7.1	4.4	2.8	2.4

Notes:
[1] Estimates.
[2] All figures include 1.2 per cent for private sector health spending.
[3] Growth figures are annual averages for the five years up to date shown (four years for the period to 2002–03).
Source: Wanless, 2002, p 75

Subsequent work found that health spending pressures in England were projected to be rising at around 4% a year above inflation over the Coalition Government's term in office, leading to a potential funding gap of £16bn for the NHS in England by 2014/15 (2010/11 prices) (Roberts et al, 2012). This projected increase in spending pressures is very similar to the long-term increase in health funding – indeed, since the NHS was founded in 1948, health spending across the UK grew by an average of 3.7% a year in real terms (Lloyd, 2015). The rate of increase in funding has fluctuated in the past with periods of relatively low growth corresponding to previous periods of relative economic hardship. The budget allocations set out in the Spending Review of 2010, however, represented the lowest rate of real terms funding increase since at least 1955 (Lloyd, 2015).

The QIPP programme was introduced to help bridge the projected gap between rising funding pressures and the much slower rate of growth in the NHS budget. It consisted of a mix of:

• National initiatives to reduce cost growth – most notably the government's public sector pay restraint policy and reduced administrative costs through a centrally imposed ring-fenced budget for administration which imposed a real terms reduction of a third on administrative costs. As part of the changes introduced with the HSCA 2012, a tier of system management (Strategic Health Authorities; SHAs) was abolished.

- Improved provider productivity – the Government reduced the prices paid by the commissioners of healthcare (Primary Care Trusts until April 2013, when Clinical Commissioning Groups began operating) to hospitals under the 'payment by results' tariff based on its estimates of the efficiency and productivity improvements required to balance the NHS budget.
- Improvement system efficiency – the Government set up a series of workstreams – initially supported by a national programme (although this ceased in 2013 with the implementation of the Health and Social Care Act) to improve system wide performance. These included new ways of managing and paying for services for people with long-term conditions and redesigning access to urgent care.

Overall it was anticipated that central initiatives on input costs and provider productivity savings would make up the bulk of the QIPP savings in the early years as the NHS began to implement the more transformative changes required to deliver improvements in system efficiency (see Chapter 4). System efficiency savings were therefore expected to form a larger part of the QIPP savings over time. In 2010 Sir David Nicholson told the Health Select Committee that:

> If you look at those savings, about 40% of them will come from essentially a mixture of things which are much more under our central control. So, for example, the pay savings, the management costs savings, the administrative cost savings, the savings on central budgets of the Department – all of those things – come to about 40% of the total savings. The second group of savings – about 20% – come from service change... the movement from secondary to primary care and that sort of thing. The third lot is about 40%, which is the savings you get through the tariff in the acute sector, so driving efficiency in hospitals.' (Health Committee, 2010)

Although the Coalition Government planned to increase funding for the NHS by 0.4% a year on average over the parliament, the actual real-terms funding increase was higher. Table 3.3 shows the outturn

Table 3.3: Health expenditure (TDEL excluding depreciation) in England from 2011/12 to 2014/15

	2009–10	2010–11	2011–12	2012–13	2013–14	2014–15
Health expenditure, cash terms (£m)	98,419	100,418	102,844	105,222	109,777	113,300
Annual change, cash terms (%)		2.0	2.4	2.3	4.3	3.2
Health expenditure, 2015/16 prices (£m)	110,164	109,125	110,054	110,572	112,998	114,886
Annual change, real terms (%)		–0.9	0.9	0.5	2.2	1.7

for the years covered by the 2010 spending review – this was an annual average of 1.4% in real terms. Over the parliament as a whole the NHS budget grew by an average of 0.9% a year in real terms, from £110.2bn in 2009/10 to £116.6bn in 2015/16 (Table 3.3). This was the lowest rate of increase in funding since 1955 (Lloyd, 2015).

Administrative costs

The cost of NHS administration fell sharply through the Coalition Government. The 2010 spending review introduced ring-fenced administrative budgets across the government. As part of this system of administrative cost control health was required to reduce administration costs by one third against 2010/11 baseline in real terms (Department of Health, 2014).[1] The ring-fenced administration budget fell from £5.9 billion in 2010/11 to £2.9 billion in 2014/15 (in 2015/16 prices) – an annual average reduction of 16.2 (PESA 2015). The greatest reduction in spending was between 2010/11 and 2011/12 where spending fell by 36%.

Better Care Fund

There is a strong recognition of the interdependence between the NHS and the provision of adult social care (see Chapter 9). Public spending on adult social care is provided by local government according to an individual's ability to pay. While the budget for NHS was protected, however, funding for local government was not, and spending on adult social care fell by an average of 2% a year in real terms between 2009/10 and 2013/14 (The Health Foundation, 2015).

The Better Care Fund (BCF) was announced in June 2013, to help limit the impact of the reduced budgets on social care provision, and improve the level of service integration. The BCF required NHS clinical commissioning groups and local authorities to create local pooled budgets to encourage staff to work more closely together to provide more person focused health and care services. The BCF originally included a requirement for the pooled budgets to be worth at least £3.8bn in 2015/16, but local agreements meant that the true figure rose to £5.3bn (NAO, 2014).

Managing Pay

Pay is the largest single cost for the NHS. It accounted for 63% of provider expenditure in 2013/14 (Lafond et al, 2015). Therefore decisions made nationally about public sector (and therefore NHS) pay has major implications for NHS funding pressures. Historically NHS staff pay has risen by an average of 2% a year in real terms (authors' calculations, based on Department of Health, 2011), broadly in line with the trend in whole economy earnings. With the need to make substantial savings to meet the Nicholson challenge, limiting increases in pay was seen as a key method to restrict the growth in costs. Therefore, instead of rising in line with the historic rate, average earnings fell by an average of 0.3% a year in real terms between June 2010 and June 2014.

The extent of the pay restraint varied by staff type (Figure 3.1, and also see Chapter 13). Earnings for doctors fell by an average of 1.3% a year, while nurses qualified nursing, midwifery and health visiting staff fell by an average of 0.6% a year, and ambulance staff by an average of 1.5% a year.

The impacts to costs of the national pay award are complex, as they depend on factors such as the change in skill mix and the extent of promotions. Accounting for this using the electronic staff record shows that average spending on permanent staff fell by around 1.1% in real terms between 2010/11 and 2014/15 (data supplied to authors by NHS England).

Although the pay offer was comparatively lower than NHS staff had received previously, it did compare favourably to the private sector (Figure 3.2). So, although despite the relatively low pay increase for NHS staff, there was a low pull from other sectors on staff.

Partly due to this, staff numbers continued to rise over the period, despite the restricted pay. The number of full time equivalent nurses rose by 1.7%, from 310,400 in 2010/11 to 316,600 in 2014/15, and the number of clinical staff rose by 2.8%. The number of ambulance staff, however, fell by 0.2% over the same period. The rising number

Figure 3.1: Average annual change in earnings per person, 2010–2014

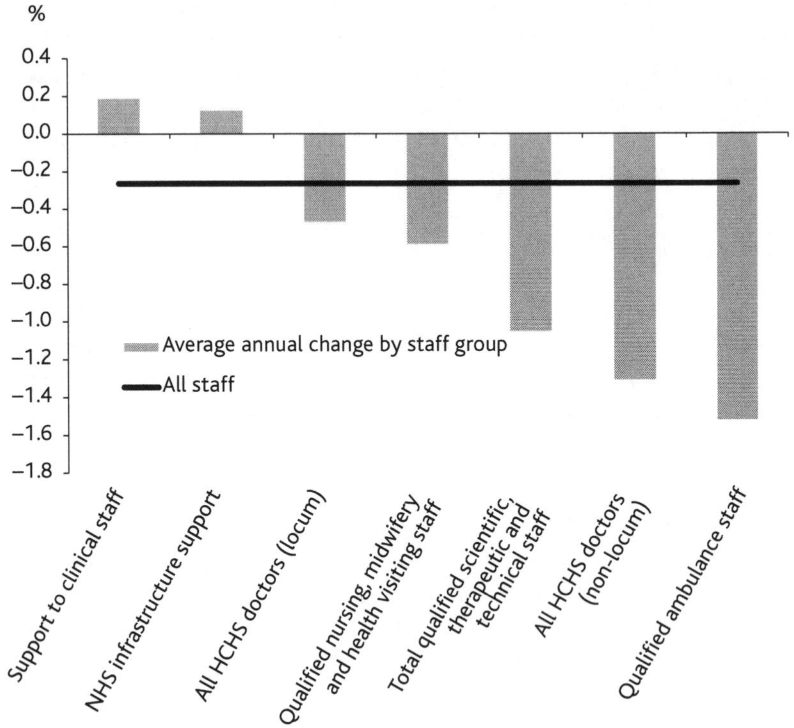

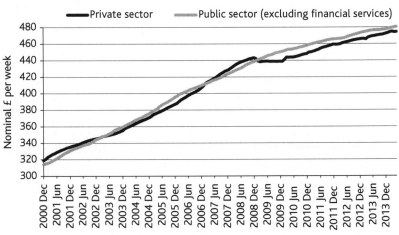

Figure 3.2: Average weekly earnings in the public and private sectors 2000–2014 (rolling 12-month averages)

Note: Measured as a 12-month rolling average of monthly (not seasonally adjusted) average weekly earnings. Includes bonuses.

Source: IFS: http://www.ifs.org.uk/uploads/publications/comms/r97.pdf

of staff (0.8%) is in stark contrast to the reaction to austerity in some other countries. For example in Ireland, the number of nurses fell by 4.2% between 2009 and 2010 (Thomas et al, 2012). So while the pay restraint will have impacted on employed staff, it is possible that a higher rate of pay increase would have had an adverse effect on the number of staff that NHS organisations could employ.

Agency Staff

Alongside the national pay restraint for permanent staff, this period saw an increase in the number and cost of temporary and agency staff, particularly towards the end of the period. In 2013/14 spending on temporary and agency staff rose by 20% in real terms from £3.1bn to £3.8bn (Department of Health, 2015; see Chapter 13).

In part, this was due to some staff opting to work as agency staff (rather than permanent staff) due to improved pay, and the opportunity to work more sociable hours (Gainsbury, 2015). There was also a substantial increase in the demand for nursing staff following the inquiry into Mid Staffordshire NHS Foundation Trust by Robert Francis QC (Francis, 2013; see Chapter 16). One of the key findings was that key staff, especially nurses, were overworked due to understaffing of some wards. As a result of this, there was a sudden increase in the demand for nurses, without a corresponding increase in the supply. Equally, the national pay structure made it difficult for NHS organisations to increase pay to encourage new staff, or people who used to be nurses to re-join. Therefore, trusts had to increasingly use agency staff to ensure that wards were appropriately staffed.

Cost of existing and new medications

The period covered by the Coalition Government coincided with two major factors that helped reduced total NHS spending on pharmaceuticals. First, a large number of proprietary medicines came to the end of the period covered by their patent. This meant that generic alternatives were introduced to the market, and at a much reduced cost. As a result, while the numbers of prescriptions dispensed during the period, the total cost fell in real terms (Figure 3.3).

Non-NHS Providers

Under the Coalition Government the proportion of NHS funding used to purchase care from non NHS providers (independent and

Figure 3.3: Cost and number of prescriptions dispensed in the UK, 2002–2014

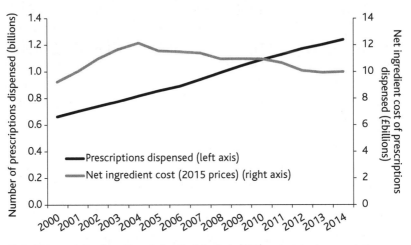

Note: Data are taken from Prescription Cost Analysis (PCA) and relates to prescriptions dispensed in the community only. Data excludes dressings and appliances.

Sources: England, Health and Social Care Information Centre (HSCIC); Wales, NHS Wales Informatics Service (NWIS); Scotland, Information Services Division of NHS National Services Scotland (ISD); Northern Ireland, Health and Social Care Business Services Organisation (HSCBSO). Data from abpi: http://www.abpi.org.uk/industry-info/knowledge-hub/medicines/Pages/community-prescribing.aspx

voluntary sector) continued to increase (see Chapter 11). In 2010/11 the NHS spent £9.4bn billion on NHS funded care provided by non-NHS providers. By 2014/15 this had increased to £10.5 billion, an increase of 12% in real terms (Department of Health 2015 and Lafond et al 2014). As a result non NHS providers accounted for an increasing share of spending on NHS care, rising from 9.3% in 2010/11 to 10.6% in 2014/15. In part this reflected the impact of policy decisions introduced under the previous Labour government – most notably from 2008 the role of the independent and voluntary sector was expanded with the development of the Any Qualified Provider (AQP) policy (Arora et al, 2013). This extended patient choice for elective care to all providers registered with what was then known as the Care Quality Commission, with a PCT or national contract, willing to provide services at the NHS tariff. The second change was the decision to require all PCTs to divest themselves of the direct provision of community services by 2010/11 under the Transforming Community Services Programme (Nicholson, 2010).

Following the introduction of AQP, there was a rapid increase in spending with independent sector providers of acute hospital care as more patients chose alternative providers common elective procedures such as hip replacement (Arora et al, 2013). A portion of this appears to be substitution from care that was previously funded privately. Following the recession in 2008, private medical insurance coverage fell from 12.4% of the population covered by either company or individual policies to 10.9% in 2012 (LaingBuisson, 2007–12). This was part of a wider fall in private spending on health care following the recession. This change meant that independent sector providers had capacity and were more willing to take NHS funded patients at the NHS national tariff payment rate. For patients, the recession coincided with historically low NHS waiting times and an opening up of treatment options through the AQP system.

Since 2012, however, the role of the independent sector in providing acute care has been relatively stable. Although it has increase as a share, over 90% of NHS spending is received by NHS owned and run organisations.

Through the Coalition Government the bigger changes have been in the growing role of the independent sector in the provision of community health services and the substantial expansion of local authorities' role in public health. Spending on independent sector provider for the provision of community health care rose by 70.5% in real terms from £1.1bn in 2010/11 to 1.8bn om 2012/13 accounting for 18% of all NHS funded care (Lafond, 2015). Local authorities now play a greater in the provision of health care services. Services provided by local authorities account for 28% of the total spend on non-NHS providers (an average increase of 18.4% a year in real terms). After the 2012 HSCA, parts of the public health budget were transferred over to local authorities for them to provide more services.

Performance against the efficiency targets

The Coalition Government established a system of reporting from local NHS bodies against the overall QIPP target. As Table 3.4 below

Table 3.4: QIPP savings, 2011–12 to 2014–15

Year	Outturn/forecast	Saving (£ billion), cash terms	Saving (£ billion), 2013/14 prices
2011–12	Outturn	5.8	5.9
2012–13	Outturn	5.0	5.1
2013–14	Outturn	4.3	4.3
2014–15	Forecast	4.8	4.7
Total		19.9	20.0

Source: correspondence with NHS England, 2014

shows, the Department of Health reports the NHS as having met the aggregate target through the period of the Coalition Government.

There are substantial problems with the approach to measuring savings under the QIPP programme, however (Appleby et al, 2014). The savings are the estimate of the gross value of the impact of specific schemes identified by NHS organisations to deliver savings. Therefore any counter-veiling costs or new pressures beyond the scheme boundaries are not considered. They do not represent a measure of the overall organisation or system efficiency. Various studies have attempted to measure efficiency and/or productivity performance through the Coalition Government. The table below shows the findings of some of the key studies through the period.

Studies vary in the extent to which they allow for differences in the quality in addition to the volume of health care delivered, in the range of health services (hospitals or sectors), whether they measure efficiency or productivity and whether England or UK wide. What all studies have in common, however, is that they show levels of efficiency performance which are substantially below the 4% a year implied by the QIPP programme.

A number of studies find that hospital productivity varied substantially from one hospital to another, and that this variation has persisted through the Coalition Government (Castelli et al 2014, Lafond et al 2015, Aragon et al 2015) (see Chapter 4). Following the HSCA in 2012, Monitor was tasked with responsibility for setting prices under the NHS tariff system. They commissioned Deloitte Economic Consulting to undertake research into the efficiency of NHS providers in order to provide a more robust, evidence base

Table 3.5: A comparison of estimates of NHS efficiency and productivity improvement

	Scope	Annual average change (%)
University of York, 2014	England, NHS-wide Total Factor Productivity (TFP) with quality adjusted output, 2004/05–2011/12	1.5
ONS, 2015	UK NHS-wide TFP with quality adjusted output, 1995–2012	0.8
Deloitte, 2014	English NHS acute hospitals efficiency frontier shift, 2008/09–2012/13	1.2
The Health Foundation, 2015	Acute care in English NHS hospitals, 2009/10–2013/14	0.4

Source: Roberts et al, 2015

for setting the efficiency factor in the tariff. Deloitte employed a range of econometric techniques to identify efficiency performance between 2008/09 and 2012/13. They found efficiency for the hospital sector had increased by an average of 1.2% a year (Deloitte, 2014); however, they also found substantial variation and estimated the scale of potential for 'catch-up' efficiency gains. Deloitte estimated that if all NHS hospitals were able to match the productivity performance of the best-performing hospitals, there was an efficiency opportunity of 5–5.5%. The scope to realise these 'catch–up' efficiency savings was a key part of the rationale for a much higher efficiency factor than had been achieved historically.

The relative productivity performance of most hospitals changed little through the period, and past productivity performance was most predictive of subsequent performance (Lafond 2015, Aragon et al 2015) (Chapter 4). Some elements of hospital characteristics may influence productivity – for example, there is some evidence that larger hospitals are less productive, while Foundation Trusts, which have greater freedom from central government in their spending decisions, are usually associated with either lower productivity or in other studies found to have no impact. Aragon et al (2015) found that Foundation Trusts status was associated with a statistically significantly lower total factor productivity between 2010/11 and 2012/13, but this result is not replicated for labour productivity.[2] Their hypothesis was that this may be because these hospitals are able to invest more heavily in capital resources that are costly but may improve productivity in future. Studies find relatively few factors which are associated with positive productivity differences but there is some limited evidence that a richer skill mix (more medical staff as a proportion of the workforce) may be associated with higher productivity (Jones and Charlesworth, 2013).

All studies find that the constant productivity differences over time cannot be fully explained by the characteristics of the hospital or types of patients they treat. While none of the studies were able to control for all the possible factors which might be associated with variations in productivity, the existence of persistent and large differences between NHS providers has been taken to imply that there is scope to improve the performance of hospitals with low productivity is present.

Narrowing the variations in productivity between providers was a key plank of the Coalition Government's plan to bridge the gap between funding pressures and available resources. Benchmarking tools were developed – most notably the Better Care, Better Value indicators (NHS Improving Quality, 2015) aimed to help providers understand the potential areas for improvement. NHS providers were then required to develop Cost Improvement Plans (CIPs) which detailed their organisational specific proposals to improvement productivity and realise savings. These plans were reported to Monitor (the national regulator for Foundation Trusts) and the NHS Trust Development Authority for providers who had not attained Foundation Trust status. Organisation's CIPs were then subject to performance management and then NHS reported the scale of CIP targets and delivery against those targets in its financial management systems locally and nationally.

The emphasis of policy, however, remained focused on a reliance on the previous government's model of autonomous providers incentivised to improve efficiency and performance by a combination of financial incentives. The evidence would suggest that this policy had limited success. NHS financial performance deteriorated sharply over the period of the Coalition Government from a net surplus of £8.1bn in 2009/10 to £0.1bn in 2014/15. The deficit is concentrated among providers where the net surplus fell from £0.7bn to −£0.8bn. As a result NHS spending increased by more than initially planned.

Figure 3.4: Annual change in financial performance of providers and commissioners from 2009/10 to 2014/15 (2015/16 prices)

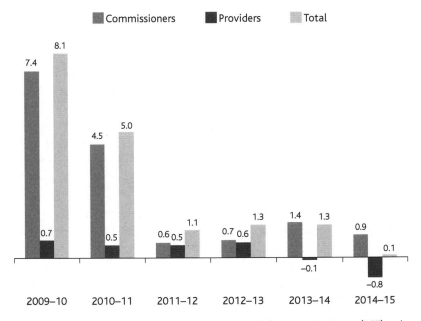

Note: Commissioners from 2009/10 to 2012/1 consisted of Primary Care Trusts (PCT) and NHS England from 2013/14; therefore the data is not fully comparable between the two periods.

While this may reflect fundamental weaknesses at the heart of the model for delivering improved productivity performance, part of the explanation for the financial pressures is changing policy priorities during the Coalition Government. From 2012/13 onwards, following concerns about staffing and quality of care in acute hospitals arising from the Francis Report into the Mid Staffordshire NHS Foundation Trust, staffing numbers were significantly increased with the effect that the labour input into an episode of care was increased. This was designed to improve safety and address concerns about compassion and dignity (see Chapter 16). These aspects of quality of care are often poorly measured in analyses of productivity and efficiency and the impact of staffing levels on observed quality may take time to feed through. There is also limited evidence on the precise nature of the relationship between staffing and quality of healthcare (Griffiths et al, 2014). Analysis of crude productivity and efficiency measures shows that acute hospital productivity and efficiency fell from 2013 onwards and financial performance deteriorated. From 2009/10 to 2014/15, hospital productivity measured at an input output ratio rose at average of 0.19% per year. Figure 3.5 shows that since 2012/13 input cost rose faster than activity leading to a declining productivity index.

Reducing Prices through the Payment by Results (PbR) tariff

Over the last decade, the way NHS Commissioners pay for care provided by NHS hospitals has evolved. Prior to 2003/04 hospitals

Figure 3.5: Change in hospital productivity from 2009/10 to 2014/15

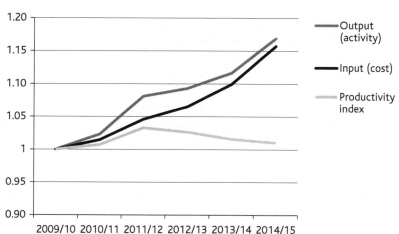

were predominately funded by block contracts. In 2003/04 the then Labour Government introduced the Payment by Results system – a prospective, nationally fixed, case-mix adjusted payment for each episode of care (Marshall et al, 2014). This is also known as the tariff system. This payment system is similar to those used in other countries (Busse et al 2011). The tariff links the income of a hospital to the volume and case mix of the hospital's activity, with the result that money follows the patient through the NHS. By fixing the payment level for each episode of care nationally it is designed to incentivise providers to compete on quality and not cost and encourages providers bring their costs into line with the national prices. Prospective, fixed price, case-mix adjusted payment systems have also been associated with changes in the volume of care. The impact depends on the system of payment in place prior to case-mix adjusted payment systems. In those countries which historically relied on fee for service payments, the volume of care tends to fall. In those which had previously used block budgets (such as the NHS) volumes tended to increase (Busse et al 2011). The national prices are based on benchmarks of providers' costs across England these are then adjusted to reflect known cost pressures in the system from pay and prices, nationally mandated quality improvements and an efficiency factor.

Reducing the tariff paid to providers of NHS care was a key plank of the Coalition Government's plan to deliver the £20 billion of QIPP savings. Around 40% of the total savings were expected to come from provider efficiencies and the tariff was the principle policy lever used to incentivise this improvement in productivity and efficiency. £32bn of commissioner budget is covered by this national tariff, worth around 40% of all commissioned spend (figures supplied to authors by Monitor, 2015).

Evidence suggests that prospective, fixed price, case-mix adjusted episodic payment systems do provide greater incentives for efficiency than many of the alternative payment systems (Busse et al 2011). The evaluation of the introduction of PbR into the NHS from 2003 onwards found that – at least in the early years – the tariff system was associated with reductions in length of stay in hospitals and increases in the proportion of patients treated as day cases across most groups of patients, providers and HRGs (Farrar et al, 2010). The overall resource saving attributable to the introduction of PbR is estimated to be between 1% and 3% over a five-year period. It was also accompanied by an increase in activity and increased administrative costs associated with administering the scheme (Marini and Street, 2007). These findings are consistent with international evidence which does find that case-mix adjustment payment systems may improve the productivity and efficiency of providers of care (Street et al 2011).

It should be borne in mind, however, that these results were comparing PbR with alternative payment systems. There is no robust evidence on the potential of tariff based systems to drive forward year-in, year-out efficiency gains and certainly not those on the level required for QIPP. Table 3.6 shows the components of the annual change in Payment by Result prices for the 4 years covered by the QIPP programme.

Moreover, the theoretical literature on health care payment systems suggestions that if prices are set below cost quality will be impacted (Street et al 2011). Over the period of the Coalition Government, the efficiency requirement for NHS providers was set at 4% a year. This is substantially above the evidence of past rates of efficiency or productivity improvements. It is also almost double the Office of Budget Responsibilities' estimates of the trend rate of productivity improvement for the economy as a whole (OBR, 2015).

Impact on different sectors

The total commissioner's budget, held by Primary Care Trusts (PCTs), fell in real terms each year between 2009/10 and 2012/13, at an average rate of 0.9% per year. The impact that this had differed by type of service, spending in primary care fell by an average of 2.9% a year, and spending on mental health care fell by an average of 1.0% per year in real terms. Spending on hospital services fell in both 2010/11 (0.8%) and 2011/12 (0.4%) but then rose by 1.7% in 2012/13.

Since April 2013, NHS England became responsible to commission healthcare services through allocations to Clinical Commissioning Groups (CCGs) and direct commissioning. Figure 6 shows that between 2013/14 and 2014/15, commissioner budget rose by £0.6bn

Table 3.6: The components of the annual change in payment by results prices

	2011/12 (%)	2012/13 (%)	2013/14 (%)	2014/15 (%)
Pay and prices	2.4	2	2.5	1.9
Revenue cost of capital	0.2	0.2	0.2	0.2
Service Development	0.0	0.0	0.1	0.4
Clinical Negligence Scheme for Trusts (CNST)				0.4
Efficiency factor	−4.0	−4.0	−4.0	−4.0
Net price adjustment	−1.5	−1.8	−1.3	−1.2

Source: Monitor and NHS England 2013b; Department of Health 2010, 2012a, 2013b

(0.7%) in real terms. The greatest increase in spending in this year was in community services, which rose by 4.4% (£0.4bn). Spending on both mental health and hospital services were reduced by −1.5% (£0.1bn) and 1.1% (£0.5bn) respectively (see Figure 3.6).

NHS budget for devolved countries

While the UK Coalition Government opted to protect the budget for the NHS in England, the outcome for Scotland, Wales and Northern Ireland was determined by the devolved government in each country (see Chapter 7). Each country receives an allocation for devolved services determined by the change in spend on these services in England, calculated using the Barnett consequentials formula

Figure 3.6: Annual change in Commissioner spending from 2009/10 to 2014/15 (2015/16 prices)

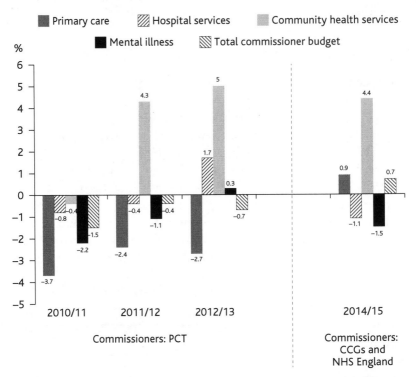

Note: Data between 2012/13 and 2013/14 are not comparable due to change the way services are commissioned. In 2013/14 and 2014/15 includes both CCGs spend and direct commissioning, hospital services include specialised care. Specialised services also include provision of some mental health care.

Source: PCT financial account and correspondence with NHS England

(HM Treasury, 2010). The respective countries then determine how best to allocate this funding across the devolved areas to best meet the requirements of their respective populations.

In contrast to England, the NHS budget in Scotland and Wales budget fell in real terms during this period. Both fell by a similar amount between 2009/10 and 2014/15, 2.0% in Scotland and 2.4% in Wales, but the timing of the change was different.

In Scotland, under the Scottish National Party led by Alex Salmond, the budget remained relatively flat in real terms, at £11.9bn until 2012/13. After 2012/13, the budget began to fall, reaching £11.6bn by 2014/15 (PESA, 2015).

The Labour Government in Wales under Carwyn Jones, however, opted to apply reductions to public services equally in the early years, including the NHS. This meant that in the early years the budget for the NHS fell by 5% in real terms, from £6.6bn in 2009/10 to £6.5bn in 2012/13 (2015/16 prices). Although this led to a substantial financial challenge in the Welsh NHS compared to the rest of the UK, it meant that other public services were relatively protected. Furthermore, while spending on public services fell in real terms, the extent of the reduction was lower. For example funding for local government in Wales fell by 4.5% in real terms between 2010/11 and 2013/14; compared with 7.6% in Scotland and 9.5% in England (Institute for Fiscal Studies, 2013). In 2014 the Welsh government announced an increase in the funding for the NHS following the publication of the 'A Decade of Austerity' report (Roberts et al, 2014), which showed a possible funding gap for 2014/15 and 2015/16 of around £200m in each year. This saw funding begin to rise again, reaching £6.5bn by 2014/15.

In Northern Ireland, as in England, the NHS budget increased in real terms during the period. The total increase was 2.8%, from £3.9bn in 2009/10 to £4.0bn in 2014/15, an average increase of 0.5% a year. A large part of this rise in spending was driven by a substantial increase in capital investment in 2012/13, rising by 59% from the investment in 2011/12 (see Figure 3.7).

International comparisons

The UK was not alone in seeing a sharp slowdown in the growth of healthcare spending in the first years of this decade. Across the OECD health care spending grew by around 4% a year for the period 2000–2008. Within that period, however, it fell by −0.4% in 2010, the increasing by just 0.3% in 2011 and 1% in 2012. As a result, two-

Figure 3.7: Real-terms change in NHS budget for the devolved countries as an index of the budget in 2009/10

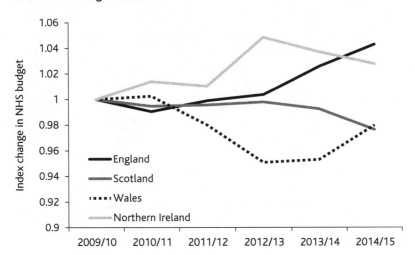

thirds of OECD countries have seen health spending increase at below the rate of economic growth since 2009 (OECD, 2015). A number of countries (Spain, Ireland Portugal and Greece), faced with significant economic challenges, cut more sharply (see Figure 3.8).

Countries across the OECD used a mix of supply-side and demand-side measures to constrain costs. Almost all countries have introduced policies to constrain the growth in pharmaceutical spend – some efficiency-orientated (increasing the use of generic medicines and renegotiating prices for branded products) others cost-shifting (raising the levels of co-payment). Constraining pay and staff numbers has also featured in the policies of those countries hardest hit by economic crisis, alongside reduced administrative costs, but also a reduction in spending on public health and disease prevention. While OECD countries have put in place some sensible strategies to achieve greater efficiency, for example in relation to pharmaceuticals, 'other policies are likely to have more detrimental impacts, such as cuts in prevention spending' (OECD, 2015). Moreover all countries have struggled to find savings on the scale and pace required for budgetary purposed. This highlights the challenge associated with realising the potential improvements that could flow from reducing variation in medical practice, improving coordination of care, reforming payment systems and focusing spending on care which represents best value.

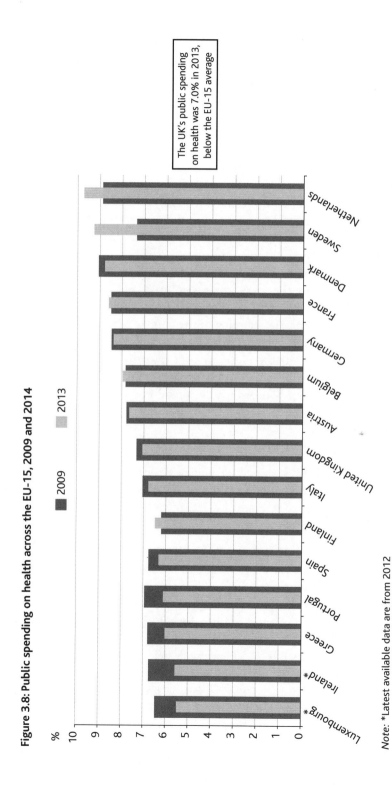

Figure 3.8: Public spending on health across the EU-15, 2009 and 2014

■ 2009   ▨ 2013

The UK's public spending on health was 7.0% in 2013, below the EU-15 average

Note: *Latest available data are from 2012

Conclusion

The Coalition Government's experience of managing the health budget through austerity is very similar to that of other countries. The UK has not seen any major redefining of the boundary between public and private spending and there has been no formal change to the scope of NHS care. Instead, the response to austerity has been dominated by short-term cost control measures, and efforts to improve technical and allocative efficiency have proved much harder. This is despite the NHS identifying the scale of the challenge it faced very early in the period. The QIPP programme was an attempt to ensure that the NHS focused on the underlying potential for efficiency savings. The aim was to use short-term cost control measures to create headroom for the more fundamental system efficiencies to be realised. While headline savings were reported, though, underlying efficiency improvements were not delivered at the scale or pace required, and by the end of the Coalition Government NHS finances were under severe pressure once again. In part this may reflect changing agendas with two significant events which diverted managerial and political focus from the existing financial challenge: first was the system reforms and restructuring associated with the HSCA and second the Francis Report into the quality failings at Mid Staffordshire Hospital Foundation Trust.

Note
[1] DH annual accounts 2014.

[2] Labour productivity is output per unit of labour (or output per person employed). Total factor productivity is output per unit of labour and capital.

References
Appleby, J, Galea, A, Murray, R, 2014, *The NHS productivity challenge: Experience from the front line*, London: The Kings Fund

Arora, S, Charlesworth A, 2013, *Public payment and private provision: The changing landscape of health care in the 2000s*, Nuffield: London, www.nuffieldtrust.org.uk/publications/public-payment-private-provision-2000s

Aragon, MJM, Castelli, A, Gaughan, JM, 2015, Hospital trusts productivity in the English NHS: Uncovering possible drivers of productivity variations, *Centre for Health Economics (CHE) Research Paper* 117, York: University of York

Busse, R, Geissler, A, Quentin, W, Wiley, M, 2011, Diagnostic-related groups in Europe: Moving towards transparency, efficiency and quality in hospitals, *European Observatory on Health Systems and Policies Series*, Geneva: WHO

Cameron, D, Clegg, N, 2010, The Coalition: Our programme for government, *The Cabinet Office*, 20 May, London: Cabinet Office

Castelli, A, Street, A, Verzulli, R, Ward, P, 2014, Examining variations in hospital productivity in the English NHS, *European Journal of Health Economics*, 16, 3.

Chernew, M, Newhouse, J, 2011, Health care spending growth, in M Pauly, T McGuire, P Barros (eds) *Handbook of health economics, Volume 2*, Oxford: Elsevier

Deloitte, 2014, Method for efficiency factor estimation, London: Deloitte, www.gov.uk/government/uploads/system/uploads/attachment_data/file/317572/Supporting_document_A_-_Deloitte_Efficiency_Factor_for_publication352b.pdf

Department of Health, 2011, *HCHS pay and prices*, Series 2010–11, www.info.doh.gov.uk/doh/finman.nsf/af3d43e36a4c8f8500256722005b77f8/276315c0677bf5478025796b00418a4d?OpenDocument

Department of Health, 2015, *Annual report and account 2014–15*, www.gov.uk/government/uploads/system/uploads/attachment_data/file/447002/DH_accounts_14-15_web.pdf

Department of Health and Department for Communities and Local Government, 2014, Better Care Fund, Policy Framework, www.gov.uk/government/uploads/system/uploads/attachment_data/file/381848/BCF.pdf

Farrar, S, Chalkley, M, Yi, D, Ma, A, 2010, Payment by results: Consequences for key outcomes measures and variations across HRGs, providers and patients, *Report to the Department of Health*, Aberdeen: Health Economics Research Unit

Francis, R, 2013, *Report of the Mid Staffordshire NHS Foundation Trust public inquiry*, London: The Stationery Office

Gainsbury, S., 2015, The use of temporary clinical staff in the NHS, *HSJ Workforce Investigation*, London: HSJ

Gerdtham U, Jonsson, B, 2000, International comparisons of health expenditure: Theory, data and econometric analysis, in A Culyer, J Newhouse (eds) *Handbook of health economics*, Vol 1, London: Elsevier

Gregory, S, Dixon, A, Ham, C, 2012, *Health policy under the Coalition Government: A mid-term assessment*, London: The Kings Fund

Griffiths, P, Ball, J, Drennan, J, Jones, J, Reccio-Saucedo, A, Simon, M, 2014, *The association between patient safety outcomes and nurse/healthcare assistant skill mix and staffing levels and factors that may influence staffing requirements*, Southampton: University of Southampton

Health Committee, 2010, Second Report of the Session 2010–11, *Public expenditure*, HC 512

Health Committee, 2013, Eleventh Report of Session 2012–13, *Public expenditure on health and care services*, HC 651

Health Committee, 2014, Seventh Report of Session 2013–14, *Public expenditure on health and care services*, HC 793

HM Treasury Public Expenditure Statistical Analysis (PESA), 2015, www.gov.uk/government/uploads/system/uploads/attachment_data/file/446716/50600_PESA_2015_PRINT.pdf

HM Treasury, 2010, Funding the Scottish Parliament, *National Assembly for Wales and Northern Ireland Assembly*, London: The Stationery Office

Jones, N, Charlesworth, A, 2013, *The anatomy of health spending 2011/12: A review of NHS expenditure and labour productivity*, London: Nuffield Trust

Institute for Fiscal Studies, 2013, *Hard choices ahead for government cutting public sector employment and pay*, London: IFS

Lafond, S, 2015, *Current NHS spending in England,* London: The Health Foundation

Lafond, S, Arora, S, Charlesworth, A, McKeon, A, 2014, *Into the red? The state of the NHS finances*, London: Nuffield Trust

Lafond, S, Charlesworth, A, Roberts, A, 2015, Hospital finances and productivity: In a critical condition? The Health Foundation

LaingBuisson, 2007, *Health cover UK market report: 2007.*

LaingBuisson, 2008, *Health cover UK market report: 2008.*

LaingBuisson, 2009, *Health cover UK market report: 2009.*

LaingBuisson, 2010, *Health cover UK market report: 2010.*

LaingBuisson, 2011a, *Healthcare market review 2010–2011.*

LaingBuisson, 2011b, *Health Cover UK Market Report: 2011.*

LaingBuisson, 2012a, *Laing's Healthcare Market Review 2011–2012.*

LaingBuisson, 2012b, *Health Cover UK Market Report: 2012.*

Lloyd, T, 2015, Historical trends in the UK, *The Health Foundation*, January 2015, London: The Health Foundation

Marini, G, Street, A, 2007, A transaction costs analysis of changing contractual relations in the English NHS, *Health Policy* 83, 1, 17–26

Marshall, L, Charlesworth, A, Hurst, J, 2014, *The NHS payment system: Evolving policy and emerging evidence*, London: Nuffield Trust

McKinsey and Company, 2010, *Achieving world class productivity in the NHS 2009/10 – 2013/14: Detailing the size of the opportunity*, London: Department of Health, www.nhshistory.net/mckinsey%20report.pdf

Monitor, 2013, *Closing the NHS funding gap: How to get better value health care patients*, London: Monitor, www.gov.uk/government/uploads/system/uploads/attachment_data/file/284044/ClosingTheGap091013.pdf

NAO (National Audit Office), 2011, *Delivering efficiency savings in the NHS*, London: National Audit Office National Audit Office, 2015, Planning for the Better Care Fund, London: National Audit Office, www.nao.org.uk/wp-content/uploads/2014/11/Planning-for-the-better-care-fund.pdf

National Institute for Health and Clinical Excellence, 2014, *Safe staffing for nursing in adult inpatient wards in acute hospitals*, London: National Institute for Health and Clinical Excellence www.nice.org.uk/guidance/sg1/chapter/2-evidence

NHS Improving Quality, 2015, *NHS better care, better value indicators*, www.productivity.nhs.uk/Content/Introduction

Nicholson D, 2009, *The year: NHS Chief Executive's annual report 2008/09*, London: Department of Health www.dh.gov.uk/en/Publicationsandstatistics/Publications/PublicationsPolicyAndGuidance/DH_099689

OECD, 2015, Fiscal sustainability of health systems: Bridging the health and finances perspectives, Paris: OECD

Roberts, A, Marshall, L, Charlesworth, A, 2012, *A decade of austerity? The funding pressures facing the NHS from 2011–12 to 2021–22*, London: Nuffield Trust

Roberts, A, Thompson, S, Charlesworth, A, Gershlick, B, Stirling, A, 2015, *Filling the gap: Tax and fiscal options for a sustainable UK health and social care system*, London: The Health Foundation, ,www.health.org.uk/publication/filling-gap

Street, A, O'Reilly, J, Ward, P, Mason A, 2011, DRG-based hospital payment and efficiency: theory, evidence and challenges, in R Busse, A Geissler, W Quentin, M Wiley (eds) *Diagnosis-related groups in Europe: Moving towards transparency, efficiency and quality in hospitals, European Observatory on Health Systems and Policies Series*, Geneva: WHO

The Health Foundation, 2015, *Health Foundation Representation to the 2015 Comprehensive Spending Review*, September, www.health.org.uk/sites/default/files/HealthFoundationRepresentationTo2015CSR.pdf

The Stationery Office, 2012, *Health and Social Care Act 2012*, Chapter 7, London: The Stationery Office, www.legislation.gov.uk/ukpga/2012/7/pdfs/ukpga_20120007_en.pdf

Thomas, S, Keegan, C, Barry, S, Layte, R, Jowett, M, Portela, C, Normand, C, 2012, Resilience of the Irish Health System: Surviving and utilising the economic contraction, *Year 1 Report of the Resilience Project*, Dublin: Centre for Health Policy and Management, Trinity College Dublin www.medicine.tcd.ie/resilience4health/assets/pdf/Resilience-Year-1-Report-2012.pdf

Wanless D, 2002, *Securing our future health: Taking a long-term view, Final report*, London: HM Treasury

FOUR

Did NHS productivity increase under the Coalition government?

*Chris Bojke, Adriana Castelli, Katja Grašič,
Daniel Howdon and Andrew Street*

Introduction

In the light of seemingly inexorable pressures to increase NHS expenditure year on year, it is not surprising that the productivity of the health system looms large in political debate. It has long been argued that the impacts of an aging population and the development of new technologies place ever greater demands on the health system. The question is whether these demands should translate directly into greater allocation of resources, or whether better use can be made of the resources already devoted to the NHS though improved productivity. Unsurprisingly, politicians presume that there is scope for the latter, and in the first section of this chapter we summarise some of the key political measures claimed to promote NHS productivity improvements over the past ten years.

Productivity is a conceptually simple construct, relating the amount of output produced to the amount of inputs used in the production process. NHS outputs include the amount and quality of care provided to patients. Inputs include the number of doctors, nurses and support staff providing care, the equipment and clinical supplies used, and the hospitals and other premises where care is provided. This ratio of outputs to inputs can be constructed at national level to assess the productivity of the entire NHS or of different parts of the system, or sub-nationally to look at the productivity of hospitals or other organisations engaged in producing health care. The productivity ratio simply divides outputs by inputs at any particular point of time. Productivity growth can also be calculated, by comparing the change in outputs produced to the change in inputs utilised from one period to the next. Political interest is focused primarily on productivity growth. Maximising productivity is a necessary but not sufficient condition for attaining overall efficiency: merely maximising output from available inputs does not necessarily imply an optimum mix of outputs. Assessing this broader concept of efficiency is, however, problematic in the context of a free-at-the-point-of-use health service such as the NHS, where willingness to pay for the output generated is not directly assessed by the conventional means of market prices. As individuals are not able to forgo NHS outputs – treatment – in order to purchase other goods in a market, we cannot directly assess in this conventional sense the overall economic efficiency of the health service.[1] Our approach is therefore a narrower, but valuable, assessment of the outputs produced from the health service's inputs.

Although conceptually straightforward, calculating productivity ratios and productivity growth for the NHS raises practical challenges. We provide a brief description of these challenges, and how they might be overcome, in the second section. Readers interested in more technical details are referred to our annual reports (Castelli et al, 2007b, Castelli et al, 2008, Castelli et al, 2011, Bojke et al, 2016).

Third, we describe the growth in outputs, inputs and productivity between 2004/05 and 2013/14. 2004/05 is taken as the starting point, because it marks the date at which the most comprehensive data were first available. We segment our description into the financial years that correspond most closely to three parliamentary terms: 2004/05 to 2007/08 when Tony Blair was in his final three years as Labour Prime Minister, 2007/08 to 2010/11 when Gordon Brown was Labour Prime Minister, and 2010/11 to 2013/14 when David Cameron was Prime Minister of a Conservative–Liberal Democrat Coalition government.

We conclude with a discussion of whether the key political measures highlighted in the first section appear to have had an influence on NHS productivity growth.

Productivity policy in the NHS over time

While our analysis centres on the performance of the NHS under the coalition government elected in 2010, providing context for this requires some attention to both past policies regarding the NHS. Much of the pre-history of the last six years of the Labour government (the last three years of Tony Blair's period in office, and Gordon Brown's three years in power) lies in the landslide election of the newly styled 'New Labour' in 1997, and the decisions taken by this government in their early years in power.

The coming to power of New Labour initially saw a reversal of many of the market-led NHS reforms introduced in 1991, following the publication, by the Conservative then–Health Secretary Ken Clarke, of the *Working for Patients* White Paper (Department of Health, 1989). Labour's first Health Secretary Frank Dobson scrapped many of the Conservatives' initiatives, and finessed other elements. GP fundholding was, for instance, abandoned but the purchaser–provider split was maintained. Purchasers were, however, renamed as 'commissioners', with an extended role of shaping rather than just purchasing services (Mays et al, 2011). By 2002, under new Health Secretary Alan Milburn, Labour had reintroduced and strengthened many elements of the internal market. Key elements included the introduction of Payment by Results (PbR), increased hospital financial autonomy, greater patient choice, and a small role for private sector provision of NHS-funded services.

In addition to the changing underlying policy rhetoric regarding the use of market mechanisms to drive efficiency, the Labour government also announced via the 1999 Budget 'an unprecedented increase in NHS UK funding of 6.1% average annual real terms growth over the four years to 2003–04 ... the longest period of sustained high growth in the history of the NHS' (HM Treasury, 2000). The April 2002 Budget saw this commitment increased to an average of 7.4% annual real terms growth for the years to 2007–08 – a rate of growth almost double the NHS's historical average of 3.8% (Emmerson and Frayne, 2002). While the 2004 Spending Review reaffirmed this commitment to sustained investment, the government, with John Reid as Health Secretary (2003–2005), combined this with top-down centrally-determined targets. Prominent among these targets were those to address long waiting times with the commitment to an 18-week 'referral-to-treatment' target for all conditions treated by a consultant, to be achieved by the end of 2008 and a commitment to halve hospital acquired infections (HAI) such as MRSA and *C. difficile* over the same period.

2004 also saw the introduction of a new contract for General Practitioners (GPs). In the face of decreasing job satisfaction and increased intentions to quit (Sibbald et al, 2003), GPs were offered a new contract with the NHS which enabled them to opt out of 24 hour care for patients for a 6% reduction in basic salary. GPs were able to top up salaries by hitting targets in a voluntary performance related bonus scheme – the Quality Outcomes Framework (QOF). The response in both the number of GPs adopting the scheme and their ability to meet targets vastly exceeded the government's predictions leading to estimates that the average GP's salary had increased by some 30%

despite shifting the burden of care during evenings and weekends to Primary Care Trusts (PCTs) (Oliver, 2009).

While the early 2000s had seen a period of large and sustained growth in NHS funding, policy changes had begun to take place in a context of plateauing expenditure as the end of the decade neared (Harker, 2012), both in line with planned cooling off of historically high rates of expenditure growth, and due to pressures brought about by the onset of the financial crisis of the late 2000s. Changes in Secretary of State for Health every two years (Rivett, undated) during the 2000s also coincided with a reduction in the intensity of NHS reform (Vizard and Obolenskaya, 2013). The establishment of the NHS Constitution in 2008 enshrined the rights of patients to choose care from any willing provider, both registered with the Care Quality Commission and contracting with the NHS to provide services at the national tariff. This had the effect of further extending private sector involvement within the NHS. (Cooperation and Competition Panel, 2011).

Further, the NHS Annual Report for 2008/09 heralded the Quality, Innovation, Productivity and Prevention (QIPP) programme, also known as 'The Nicholson Challenge' (House of Commons, 2010)(see Chapter 3). This was purportedly aimed at delivering efficiency savings of some £15–20 billion between 2011 and 2014, and was estimated to require 4% year-on-year productivity gains. This was acknowledged as being extremely challenging when seen in the context of traditionally flat, or even negative, productivity growth over a sustained historical period. Indeed, Nicholson himself commented in 2010 that 'It is huge. You don't need me to tell you that it has never been done before in the NHS context and we don't think, when you look at health systems across the world, that anyone has quite done it on this scale before' (House of Commons, 2010)(see Chapter 2).

The Nicholson Challenge was ultimately implemented under the Coalition government formed following the May 2010 general election. The implications of the Challenge were reflected in the 2010 Comprehensive Spending Review, one of the first major acts of the Coalition government (HM Treasury, 2010). Despite government policy of overall cuts to public sector spending, the NHS was shielded from real reductions, following an election campaign pledge by the Conservative Party (The Conservative Party, 2015). The spending review outlined plans of £3.8 billion real growth between 2010/11 and 2014/15 which – due to additional realignments of budgets, transfers and lower than expected inflation – materialised as a total real growth of £4 billion, a 3.95% overall increase from 2010/11

(Appleby et al, 2015). While positive, this annual input growth of less than 1% per annum was substantially below the aforementioned historical average of 3.8% (Emmerson and Frayne, 2002).

The other major NHS initiative undertaken by the Coalition government was the development and passing into legislation of the 2012 Health and Social Care Act. Initially proposed by new Health Secretary Andrew Lansley, the route from policy paper to legislation was long and torturous (Timmins, 2012)(see Chapter 6). The main elements of the Act were to restructure the NHS, extend choice of services to any public or private 'willing provider' and place GPs at the heart of commissioning services. Despite the knowledge that the NHS was simultaneously undergoing a period of growing demand and severely restrained input growth, there was surprisingly little direct mention in the Act of productivity per se. This may stem from the implicit proposition that competition and choice drive productivity gains – as had been previously claimed regarding the telecommunication and water utility privatisations in the 1980s, during Lansley's time as private secretary in the Department of Trade and Industry (Ham et al, 2015).

Direct references to productivity in the Act are limited to mention of the role of Monitor as an independent economic regulator in either improving quality or the efficiency of provision of services. Even then, the extent to which Monitor was required to promote competition has been argued to have been watered down during the lengthy consultation period which occurred during the passage of legislation through parliament (Ham et al, 2015). In this respect, the Act may be seen as a continuation of the promotion of choice and competition as purported drivers of productivity improvement, consistent with the Conservatives' 1991 NHS reforms (Chapter 2). This is despite there being little evidence that competition works as a driver of either greater quality or productivity (Street, 2013).

In addition to the incentives for efficiency provided by competition and choice, the government also applied pressure to amenable 'contractual levers' – principally by imposing a 4% real reduction in the national tariff payable for hospital activity and a two-year pay freeze for all public sector workers starting from April 2011 (National Audit Office, 2012). While the reduction in tariff prices does not automatically generate greater productivity, it was claimed that this would promote an environment in which there are stronger incentives for hospitals to seek productivity improvements (National Audit Office, 2012).

Measuring productivity

The key to understanding the impact of Coalition policy on productivity is to understand how the actions of the government have played out on the inputs and outputs of healthcare production across the NHS. In this next section we briefly describe the methods and intuition underpinning the measurement of NHS productivity.

While in principle being little different to the measurement in any other sector, in practice, measurement of NHS productivity is problematic. This is principally due to: the difficulty in defining, measuring and valuing the output that the health system produces; the lack of granular input data; and changes in data recording and activity definitions over time (Castelli et al, 2011).

Measuring output

It is commonly argued that the objective of the health care system is to produce improved health related quality of life (HRQoL) and, consequently, that this should be the defining form in which output is described. Indeed, this is the perspective adopted by the National Institute for Health and Clinical Excellence (NICE) (National Institute for Health and Clinical Excellence, 2013) in evaluating new technologies which are assessed on the basis of whether the extra HRQoL, as measured by Quality Adjusted Life Years (QALYs) produced by the new technology, is greater than the opportunity costs of the provision of such a new technology. In principle, this measure of output could be applied to a productivity measure: instead of focusing on a few new technologies, we could attempt to assess the QALYs produced across the whole NHS, and how such a measure changes over time. Unfortunately, very little is known about the QALY consequences of the vast majority of activity. Despite initial steps in the direction of such assessment, with the routine collection since 2009 of patient reported outcomes for a small number of conditions, a comprehensive account of the health gains produced by every type of NHS activity is unlikely to be available in the near future. Further potential complications arise if the aim of the health service is seen as not only improving population health, but also contributing to a broader construction of social welfare. Indeed, recent proposals regarding the use of value-based pricing in NICE decision-making have sought to move the NHS in the direction of taking into account 'other attributes of benefit' when making decisions regarding the cost-effectiveness of new health technologies (Claxton et al, 2015).

Even if it were possible to measure the QALYs and wider social welfare consequences for each activity, there may nonetheless be an argument for not using QALYs (or a similar measure or health benefit) as the principal measure of output. Triplett (Triplett, 2011) argues that, although the case for using a QALY measure seems appealing in principle, it ultimately mixes two distinct processes: the generation of health care services and the generation of health itself. Problems occur if there are determinants of health above and beyond that generated by NHS activity, such as environment, housing or education. It may be possible that the NHS could provide exactly the same quantity and quality of services at the same cost from one year to the next, but for this to still be associated with an apparently higher QALY output, if there are sufficient improvements in the other determinants of health. In such a scenario, it is possible that a QALY-based productivity growth measure could yield a positive measure of growth even though healthcare system productivity was unchanged. Triplett argues that, unless it is possible to disentangle these effects, it may better to focus on measuring and valuing health care service activity than to 'inter-mingle and confound separate conceptual systems'.

An alternative approach, and one adopted for national accounting purposes, is to use NHS activity as the measure of output. In practice, thanks to the comprehensive and routine collection of data regarding the volume of NHS activity, this is a more pragmatic alternative to measuring output in terms of QALYs. The Reference Costs (RC) database and Hospital Episode Statistics (HES) database, for instance, comprehensively cover both inpatient and outpatient secondary care activity in hospital trusts. The adoption of this an approach still poses some challenges, however, such as the lack of consistent and comprehensive detailed coverage of primary care activity. Researchers can attempt to overcome such problems by estimating activity from survey or sample data.

Health care activities are diverse, and some means of aggregation is required in order to produce an overall index of NHS output. If perfectly competitive free markets existed for these activities, then it could be argued that the price of each activity signals value. The vast majority of NHS care, however, is provided free of charge; the remainder is heavily subsided. In the absence of prices, it is standard national accounting practice to use costs as relative values. Annual costs for each health care activity are available from a number of sources, such as reported by hospitals and collated in the RC database or those published in the Unit Costs of Health and Social Care (PSSRU) (Curtis, 2014).

A measure of health service productivity growth aims to compare growth in the aggregate value (as proxied by costs) of outputs with growth in the aggregate value of inputs. This is, however, complicated by year-on-year changes in the value attributed to individual outputs. A common method of obviating this problem is to construct a Laspeyres index of output growth (Goodridge, 2007). In short, this uses the *previous* year's costs in valuing both current and the previous year's output, thus ensuring that changes in measured output reflect changes in the amount of activity and are not driven by changes in the costs of individual types of activity.

While, in the context of perfectly functioning free markets, prices may be claimed to reflect the value that people attach to traded goods and services, costs are less likely to reflect the values of NHS activities. For instance, over and above its cost, activities of higher quality are likely to be more highly valued than those of lower quality, even though their costs may be the same. In recognition of this, after weighting activity according to costs, our measure of NHS output also captures changes in the quality of health care activities. All other things being equal, for instance, reductions in waiting times and improvements in blood pressure control and in 30-day survival rates following hospital admission contribute to increased output over time.

Insofar as data allow, our NHS output index captures all activities provided to NHS patients by either NHS organisations or independent sector organisations. Data for both the amount of hospital activity and for the measures of the quality of elective, non-elective and mental health care delivered in hospitals are derived from the HES dataset. Activity performed in all NHS settings, other than hospitals and primary care, is captured in the Reference Cost returns. In particular, RC data cover activity conducted in outpatient and accident and emergency departments, mental health and community care settings, and diagnostic facilities. The RC dataset also contains information on reported costs for these activities, including activity performed in hospitals.

Comprehensive data on primary care consultations are unavailable. In their absence, nationally representative survey data have been used instead. Data about the quality of primary care activity are obtained from the Quality and Outcomes Framework (QOF), which reports disease prevalence and achievement in reducing blood pressure for patients with coronary heart disease, transient ischaemic attacks or stroke and hypertension. Community prescribing data are taken from the Prescription Cost Analysis (PCA), supplied by the Prescription Pricing Authority.

There have been substantial changes over time in some of the source datasets: in particular the roll-out of Reference Costs has allowed coverage to become progressively more comprehensive. The disbanding of Primary Care Trusts, though, appears to have led to a recent reduction in the capture of some data. There have been regular periodic changes in the way that activities are defined and categorised. Our output index is designed to accommodate these categorisation changes (Castelli et al, 2011b, Castelli et al, 2011).

Measuring inputs

Inputs into the health care system consist of labour, intermediate goods and capital. The distinction between capital and intermediate categories depends on the timescale over which they are utilised. For example, Magnetic Resonance Imaging (MRI) scanners – used over several years – would be classed as capital, whereas bandages and other items – put to single use – would be classed as intermediate inputs.

In principle, the input measure could be constructed in much the same manner to the output measure: by directly counting and valuing each element of input used in the production process. There are few data sources that capture the use of distinct types of inputs, however.

For the NHS, such data are available only for labour inputs, with the Electronic Staff Record (ESR) containing detailed information about full time equivalents by staff type and grade. The ESR data allow us to construct a Laspeyres direct measure of labour growth. To do this, the number of full time equivalent (FTE) staff in the current year are first multiplied by the previous year's labour costs and summed for all staff categories. This is then divided by the product of the previous year's FTEs and the previous year's costs, summed for all staff categories.

For other inputs, we are constrained to using expenditure data derived from organisational accounts. Expenditure data are subject to cost inflation, however, so a simple comparison of expenditure over time will conflate general cost increases with increases in the volume of resource use. To isolate the volume effect, it is necessary to convert nominal expenditure into constant expenditure using a deflator. Growth in the volume of input use for a specific category may then be calculated by comparing expenditure measured in constant terms from one period to the next.

Measuring productivity over time

The final major practical hurdle in measuring productivity over time is the lack of consistency in activity definition and data collection. Major revisions to how hospital activity is described and to the definitional codes used in the RC database cause significant difficulties in comparing activity on a like-for-like basis from one year to the next.

One way of tackling this problem is to adopt a basket of activities that remain consistently defined every year, to which a single set of weights can be applied. This basket may become very unrepresentative over time, however, and the single set of weights may not reflect recent values particularly well.

The alternative is to use a 'chain-linked' index whereby the series is constructed by linking individual pairwise comparisons of two consecutive individual years. In each link a specific year-to-year index is constructed with the earlier year acting as the base period. The whole time series index may be updated by adding this new link to the end of the existing chain. Over time the link that compares two years at the very beginning of the time series may contain very different types of activities to the link at the end of the chain. Nevertheless, this pragmatic approach allows a meaningful comparison over time. This approach is best able to accommodate fundamental changes to how either outputs or inputs are described from one period to the next.

Output growth over time

For each of the three parliamentary terms we present output growth for the NHS as a whole, and for each of the following settings: hospital admitted care (which contributes approximately 30% to overall output growth); outpatient care (11%); community mental health care (9%); community care (5%); primary care (14%) and prescribing (12%). The remaining 19% covers a wide range of diverse activities conducted in various settings. Average annual growth rates by parliamentary term are presented in Table 4.1 while growth by setting from a 2004/05 baseline is shown in Figure 4.1.

Output growth for the NHS as a whole was greatest during Blair's final three years in office, averaging 5.76% per annum (pa) between 2004/5 and 2007/8. Growth was particularly strong for hospital and community mental health care services, averaging more than 12% over the period, and almost 7% for prescribing.

Output growth fell to 4.80% pa under Gordon Brown's administration, with outpatients and prescribing being the settings with the highest growth rates of 6.6% and 6% respectively. We observe negative output growth in primary care, though, averaging –0.18% per annum over the three years between 2007/8 and 2010/11.

The annual growth in NHS output fell even further under the Coalition government between 2010/11 and 2013/14, averaging just

Table 4.1: Average annual output growth by setting (%)

	Overall	Hospital admitted care	Outpatient	Hospital and community mental health	Community care	Primary care	Prescribing
Blair's 3rd term	5.76	5.83	3.85	12.96	4.36	3.05	6.88
Brown's term	4.80	3.46	6.55	3.83	2.97	−0.18	6.01
Coalition term	2.71	2.25	3.24	0.92	−1.70	2.24	3.20

Figure 4.1: Output growth by setting

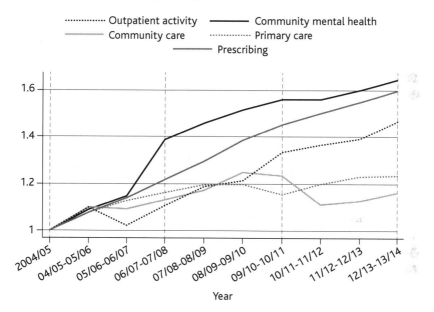

2.71% per annum. In no setting was the average annual growth rate in excess of 3.3%, and in community care this growth was negative, averaging −1.7% per annum. This is partly due to reorganisation, as PCTs that provided the majority of community care activity ceased to exist.

We can look in more detail at some of the elements that contributed to output growth in each of these settings. Growth in admitted hospital care is driven mainly by the number of patients admitted to hospital, but also by the quality of care these patients receive. Figure 4.2 shows growth in the number of patients admitted to hospital, according to whether they were elective or non-elective admissions. There has been an almost linear upward trend in the number of elective admissions,

Figure 4.2: Inpatient activity: elective and non-elective inpatient stays

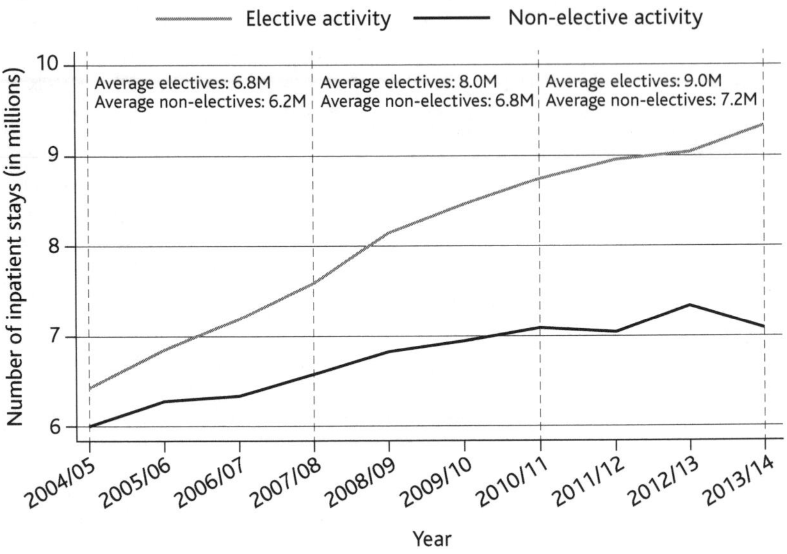

rising from 6.43 million in 2004/05 to 9.34 million in 2013/14. There has been a rise in non-elective activity, from 6.01 million admissions in 2004/05 to 7.11 million in 2013/14. The upward trend has not been completely smooth and, indeed, there was a 2.97% fall in non-elective activity between 2012/13 and 2013/14.

Changes in those measures of the quality of hospital activity that are incorporated in the output index are summarised in Table 4.2, again for elective and non-elective activity. For elective admissions, the average 30-day survival rate was 99.45% during Blair's 3rd term, rising to 99.74% under Brown, but falling back slightly to 99.54% under the Coalition, although this may be more a function of a move

Table 4.2: Average annual Inpatient quality adjustment components

	Elective			Non-elective		Outpatients	
	30-day survival rate (%)	Mean life expectancy	80th percentile waiting times	30-day survival rate (%)	Mean life expectancy	Average waiting times*	Average waiting times**
Blair's 3rd term	99.45	23.67	96.00	95.43	34.33	46	n/a
Brown's term	99.74	23.37	66.33	95.90	34.57	23	36
Coalition term	99.54	23.23	93.50	96.36	34.40	n/a	38

Sources: *DH; **HES

to a more complex patient case-mix rather than a decline in quality of care. Similarly, while life-expectancy has marginally fallen over time, this is a result of treating older patients rather than any direct reflection of Coalition policy. For non-elective activity, 30-day survival rates improved progressively under each parliamentary term, from 95.43% under Blair to 96.35% under the Coalition.

Changes in waiting times reflect very closely the policy emphasis placed on them over time under government, as expressed through the targets that hospitals were expected to meet. 80th percentile waiting times, rather than the mean or median statistic, are used to capture the disutility from having long waiting times (Castelli et al, 2007a). The pattern in terms of 80th percentile waiting times is one of year-on-year reductions until 2008/09, followed by subsequent increases, as shown in Figure 4.3. Elective waiting time, measured at the 80th percentile of the distribution, was 96 days for hospital admission under Blair, but only 66 days during Brown's term in office. Under the Coalition, average elective waiting times had increased to 94 days, peaking at 120 days in 2012/13.

The average waiting time for an outpatient appointment fell progressively from 52 days in 2004/5 to 24 days in 2008/9. A change was made in the form in which outpatient data were recorded during

Figure 4.3: Waiting time changes by setting; average values are reported on the annual basis

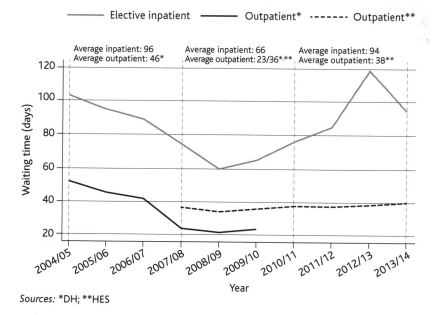

Sources: *DH; **HES

the Brown administration, with the new system showing a very slight upward trend in output waiting times between 2008/9 and 2013/14.

Input growth over time

As reported in Table 4.3, total input growth amounted to an average of 4.33% pa during Blair's final three years in office. The largest driver of this growth was in use of capital and intermediate inputs, where we observe an average growth of 13.12% pa. Labour growth was much smaller at 1.57% pa while there was a decrease in utilisation of agency staff of −3.60% pa.

High input growth continued in Brown's term of office, with average growth of 3.66% pa. We observe a big increase in labour inputs, with an average 3.35% pa growth in NHS staff and 18.10% pa for agency staff. While growth in the utilisation of capital and intermediate inputs was lower than had previously been the case, this still amounted to 4.62% pa.

Input growth was slowest during the Coalition's parliament. Average growth was 1.14% pa, most notably because of a negative growth of −0.60% pa in labour inputs. Growth in the use of other inputs remained positive, with a large growth of 7.55% pa in use of agency staff and 16.89% in the use of capital and intermediate inputs.

Growth in the use of labour inputs is presented from a baseline of 2004/05 in Figure 4 for NHS staff and in Figure 4.5 or agency staff. Figure 4.4 shows that growth in NHS staff increased gradually under Blair, substantially under Brown, and then turned negative under the Coalition.

Meanwhile, as shown in Figure 4.5, there have also been substantial year-on-year fluctuations in the use of agency staff. While there has been increased use of agency staff over the full series, there have been periods of retrenchment, notably between 2004/5 and 2006/7, coinciding with the period in which the hospital sector was struggling to reduce deficits. As might be expected, in times of austerity, savings were first made in agency staff before any reduction in regularly employed NHS staff.

Table 4.3: Average annual input growth by type (%)

	Overall	NHS staff	Agency staff	Capital and intermediates
Blair's 3rd term	4.33	1.57	−3.60	13.12
Brown's term	3.66	3.35	18.10	4.62
Coalition term	1.14	−0.60	7.55	16.89

Figure 4.4: Labour input growth

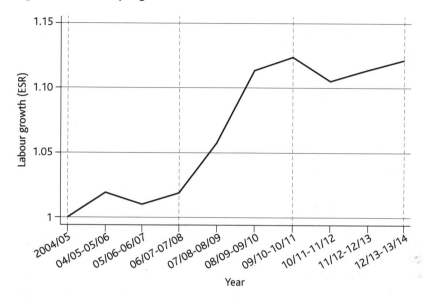

Figure 4.5: Growth in agency staff; average values are reported on the annual basis

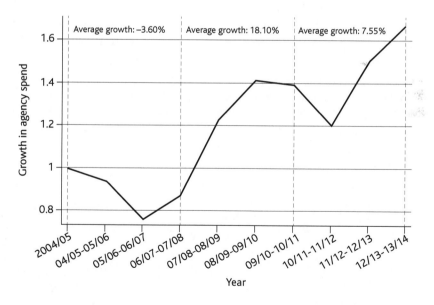

Productivity

Table 4.4 reports output, input and productivity growth averaged across each of the parliamentary terms. Under the last three years of

Table 4.4: Output, input and productivity growth by parliamentary term (%)

	Average output growth	Average input growth	Average productivity
Blair's 3rd term	5.76	4.33	1.41
Brown's term	4.80	3.66	1.13
Coalition term	2.71	1.14	1.56

the Blair government, average annual productivity growth amounted to 1.41%. Input growth was greatest during this period, averaging 4.33% per annum, but this was outstripped by output growth averaging 5.76% a year. Under the Brown administration, input growth slowed to 3.66% per annum, and output growth also slowed to 4.8% a year, with average productivity growth amounting to 1.13% a year. There was a greater slowdown in both input and output growth under the Coalition. The general economic climate of austerity had an impact on the NHS, with input growth averaging just 1.14% a year. Output growth also slowed, to 2.71% per year over this period. With input growth being slower than output growth, however, annual productivity growth averaged 1.56% under the Coalition, the highest rate achieved under the three parliamentary terms.

Figures 4.6 and 4.7 disaggregate these average figures, with Figure 4.6 illustrating year-on-year growth rates in output and inputs,

Figure 4.6: Output and input growth; hatch-shaded area (output line above input line) represents positive productivity growth; dark grey solid-shaded area represents negative productivity growth (input line above output line)

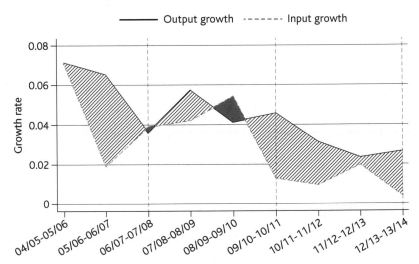

Figure 4.7: Output, input and productivity indices

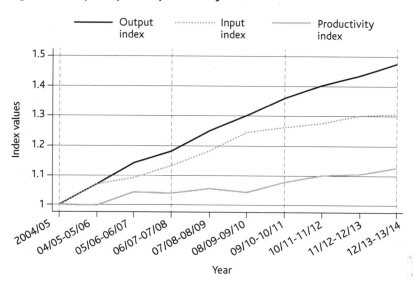

and Figure 4.7 illustrating growth in indices of inputs, outputs and productivity (2004/5 indexed at 100 in all cases). While the Blair years were characterised by the largest average output and input growth of the period under consideration, a fall in output growth was observed during his third term of office, from 7.11% in 2004/5–2005/6 to 3.66% in 2006/7–2007/8. A general fall in input growth is also evident in the data, with a slight increase in his final year of office enough to produce a small negative divergence between output and input growth in 2009/10. The Brown years saw a growth in productivity on average, but also featured the only occasion in this nine year period in which output growth lay appreciably below input growth: with a divergence of −1.32% observed between 2008/9–2009/10.[2] The austerity of the years of the coalition government saw generally falling output growth, but even lower input growth, producing an overall picture of year-on-year productivity increases, at least in this short period observed.

Discussion

Measuring NHS productivity over time is a challenge. The NHS produces a wide range of services and there are no unequivocal measures of value or quality. Furthermore, changes in data definitions and coverage are a major obstacle in any analysis covering an extended period of time. The main features of our measure are that all inputs and outputs are covered as comprehensively as possible, and a long-term chained index can be constructed by linking together year-by-year comparisons of like-for-like data. As usual there are a few caveats to our analysis that need to be considered. The major one is that the data on primary care over the entire period are especially limited and it is difficult to say with any degree of certainty just how primary care output has changed over time. That said, we do not believe that there are any reasons to believe our conclusions would change dramatically with better data. In addition to poor primary care data, the major re-organisation of the NHS prompted by the Health and Social Care Act 2012 has recently limited our ability to comprehensively measure all inputs and outputs – for example the outputs obtained from the increasing spend on non-hospital community and mental health services from non-NHS providers. The increasing proportion of spend on non-NHS organisations means a larger proportion of input and corresponding outputs are not included in our measure.

The time series shows a general declining but fluctuating input growth over time from historically high growth during the Blair years to consistently low growth during the Coalition government. Output growth has also followed a downward trend, though over time the trend has generally been smoother than for input growth. Visual inspection of the time series suggests that there may be a link between outputs and lagged inputs as the most pronounced falls in input growth appear to precede the more pronounced falls in output by one year. Similarly, increases in input growth appear to lead to a rebound in output growth in the following year.

Over the whole time series, the overall picture is that growth in inputs has been exceeded by growth in outputs. There has, however, been a systematic difference in productivity growth over the whole period. In the initial years of Brown's period in office there was relatively large input growth, and this explains the brief period of negative productivity growth observed from 2008/09 to 2009/10, after which productivity growth reverted to being positive.

Although there are quite large differences in average input and output growth across the three parliamentary terms, average productivity has remained relatively stable – a range of 0.43%, while the highest average productivity growth of 1.56% was observed under the Coalition government.

These recent productivity gains have been obtained largely through replacing PCTs with more numerous but less costly Clinical Commissioning Groups (CCGs) and strict input control via manipulation of the contractual levers such as setting tariff prices and freezing of public sector pay. These policies have not come without cost. The majority of trusts are now reporting deficits (National Audit Office, 2015), there has been a large scale rejection of the 2015/16 tariff proposals (National Health Executive, 2015) and there are issues with staff recruitment which lead to increased use of expensive agency staff (NHS England, 2015). As such it is difficult to see this approach as being sustainable in the long term, and while productivity growth has been positive, at an average of 1.56% pa it falls some way short of the estimated 4% pa required to meet the Nicholson Challenge.

In terms of what has previously worked, it is difficult to pin down precisely the changes in productivity to specific policies. Observed patterns do conform to the more predictable elements of the policies, though, and we observe different patterns across settings: for instance, the increase in hospital activity which might be expected as a result of Payment by Results and reductions in waiting time that match the targets hospitals were set. Similarly primary care quality has responded up to the point at which it has been rewarded by QOF, but no further. There is no corresponding face value evidence in the figures that the market-influenced policies of choice have had any marked effect.

Our overall conclusion is that the Coalition government has produced a sustained period of positive NHS productivity growth, primarily generated by keeping a tight rein on input growth. There are however two main points of note. First, it is not clear how long a policy of input restriction is likely to be sustainable. Indeed with 76% of hospital trusts reporting deficits in the first 6 months of 2015–16 (National Audit Office, 2015), there is prima facie evidence that the existing restrictions may already be untenable. Second, although there has been a consistent period of productivity growth, it has failed to meet the challenging targets set by the Nicholson Challenge. Consequently, future demands on the health service are unlikely to be met by a simple continuation of Coalition policies, and pressure to increase NHS funding is likely to remain or increase.

Acknowledgements

This chapter draws on an independent study commissioned and funded by the Department of Health in England as part of a programme of policy research at the Centre for Health Economics (070/0081 Productivity; 103/0001 ESHCRU). The views expressed are those of the authors and not necessarily those of the Department of Health. The Hospital Episode Statistics are copyright © 2004/05 – 2013/14, re-used with the permission of The Health & Social Care Information Centre. All rights reserved.

Notes

[1] While a full discussion of the overall merits of this approach is beyond the scope of our research, such discussions exist in, for example, Claxton et al (2007).

[2] Small negative differences between output growth and input growth were observed in 2004/5–2005/6 (–0.08%), and in 2006/7–2007/8 (–0.22%).

References

Appleby, J, Baird, B, Thompson, J, Jabbal, J, 2015, *The NHS under the coalition government. Part two: NHS performance*, London: The King's Fund

Bojke, C, Castelli, A, Grašič, K, Howdon, D, Street, A, 2016, Productivity growth in the English National Health Service from 1998/99 to 2013/14, *Health Economics,* DOI: 10.1002/hec.3338 http://onlinelibrary.wiley.com/doi/10.1002/hec.3338/full

Castelli, A, Dawson, D, Gravelle, H, Jacobs, R, Kind, P, Loveridge, P, Martin, S, O'Mahony, M, Stevens, P, Stokes, L, Street, A, Weale, M, 2007a, A new approach to measuring health system output and productivity, *National Institute Economic Review* 200, 1, 105–117

Castelli, A, Dawson, D, Gravelle, H, Street, A, 2007b, Improving the measurement of health system output growth, *Health Economics*, 16, 10, 1091–1107

Castelli, A, Laudicella, M, Street, A, 2008, Measuring NHS Output Growth, *Centre for Health Economics Research Paper 43*, York: University of York

Castelli, A, Laudicella, M, Street, A, Ward, P, 2011, Getting out what we put in: Productivity of the English National Health Service, *Health Economics, Policy and Law* 6, 313–335

Claxton, K, Sculpher, M, Culyer, AJ, 2007, Mark versus Luke? Appropriate methods for the evaluation of public health interventions, *CHE Research Paper 31*, York: University of York, www.york.ac.uk/media/che/documents/papers/researchpapers/rp31_evaluation_of_public_health_interventions.pdf

Claxton, K, Sculpher, M, Palmer, S, Culyer, AJ, 2015, Causes for concern: Is NICE failing to uphold its responsibilities to all NHS patients? *Health Economics* 24, 1, 1–7

Cooperation and Competition Panel, 2011, *Review of the operation of 'Any Willing Provider', for the provision of routine elective care*, London: Cooperation and Competition Panel

Curtis, LE, 2014, Unit Costs of Health and Social Care 2014, *Personal Social Services Research Unit*, Kent: PSSRU, www.pssru.ac.uk/project-pages/unit-costs/2014/

Department of Health, 1989, *Working for Patients*, London: Department of Health

Emmerson, C, Frayne, C, 2002, *Challenges for the July 2012 spending review*, London: Institute for Fiscal Studies

Goodridge, P, 2007, Methods explained: Index numbers, *Economic and Labour Market Review* 1, 3, 54–57

Ham, C, Baird, B, Gregory, S, Jabbal, J, Alderwick, H, 2015, *The NHS under the Coalition government*, London: The King's Fund

Harker, R, 2012, *NHS funding and expenditure*, London: House of Commons Library

HM Treasury, 2000, *Comprehensive spending review 2000*, London: HM Treasury, www.gov.uk/government/publications/comprehensive-spending-review-2000

HM Treasury, 2010, *Comprehensive spending review 2010*, London: HM Treasury, www.gov.uk/government/publications/ spending-review-2010

House of Commons, 2010, *The spending review settlement for healthcare*, London: Hansard, House of Commons, www.publications.parliament.uk/pa/cm201011/cmselect/cmhealth/512/51208.htm

Mays, N, Dixon, A, Jones, L, 2011, *Understanding New Labour's market reforms of the English NHS*, London: King's Fund

National Audit Office, 2012, *Progress in making NHS efficiency savings*, London: National Audit Office, www.nao.org.uk/report/progress-in-making-nhs-efficiency-savings/

National Audit Office, 2015, *Sustainability and financial performance of acute hospital trusts*, London: National Audit Office, www.nao.org.uk/report/sustainability-and-financial-performance-of-acute-hospital-trusts/

National Health Executive, 2015, *'Disarray' as providers resoundingly reject 2015–16 tariff proposals*, London, National Health Executive, www.nationalhealthexecutive.com/Health-Care-News/disarray-as-providers-resoundingly-reject-2015-16-tariff-proposals-

National Institute for Health and Clinical Excellence, 2013, *Guide to the methods of technology appraisal 2013*, London: National Institute for Health and Clinical Excellence, www.nice.org.uk/article/pmg9/chapter/foreword

NHS England, 2015, *Overcoming the challenges facing NHS providers*, London: NHS England, www.england.nhs.uk/2015/09/02/nhs-challenges/

Oliver, A, 2009, Update on the impact of the 2004 GP contract, *Health Policy Monitor, Survey 2009(14)*,www.hpm.org/en/Surveys/LSE_-_UK/14/Update_on_the_impact_of_the_2004_GP_contract.html

Rivett GC (undated) National Health Service History, retrieved 3 May 2016 from www.nhshistory.net

Sibbald, B, Bojke, C, Gravelle, H, 2003, National survey of job satisfaction and retirement intentions among general practitioners in Enland, *British Medical Journal* 326, 7379, 22–4

Street, A, 2013, An overview of competition in UK health care, in A Charlesworth and E Kelly (eds), *Competition in UK health care: Reflections on an expert workshop*, London: Institute for Fiscale Studies and Nuffield Trust research report

The Conservative Party, 2015, *The Conservative Manifesto 2015*, London: The Conservative Party, https://s3-eu-west-1.amazonaws.com/manifesto2015/ConservativeManifesto2015.pdf

Timmins, N, 2012, *Never again? The story of the Health and Social Care Act 2012*, London: The King's Fund and Institute for Government

Triplett, JE, 2011, Health system productivity, in PC Smith, SA Glied (eds), *The Oxford handbook of Health Economics*, Oxford: Oxford University Press

Vizard, P, Obolenskaya, P, 2013, *Labour's record on Health (1997–2010)*, London: Centre for Analysis of Social Exclusion, London School of Economics and Political Science

FIVE

The central management of the English NHS

Scott L Greer, David Rowland and Holly Jarman

The English NHS, serving over fifty million people, is one of the largest health care systems in the rich world (Greer 2006). It is no wonder that making it respond to its political direction has been a long-time preoccupation of its political directors. Since its creation in 1948, there have been constant attempts by Ministers to keep the NHS under central political control in ways which are commensurate with the political salience of the service, and the high levels of taxpayer funds which pay for it. NHS professionals, working in a service which is necessarily local, complex and made up of a diverse set of organisations, have tended to resist central control and political interference. The centralisation of the English NHS has thus been a decades-long project, with the Coalition government's 2012 reforms of the NHS forming a dramatic new chapter in this pull between central control and local autonomy. This chapter focuses on the central management of the NHS: the central organisations in Westminster charged with making and implementing NHS policy. It quickly reviews the central management of the NHS in 2010, then focuses on the architecture proposed for it by the Coalition reforms and its subsequent evolution. It concludes by arguing that the Coalition reforms might best be seen as part of a cycle in central management that has been happening for decades in the NHS and perhaps other public services.

State of the topic in 2010

The impact of the Coalition's policies on the central management of the NHS, and the role and shape of that centre, make sense in the context of this decades-long struggle and the organisational tools that previous governments have employed in their efforts to manage the NHS. The later Blair years, after a period of forceful central direction by Secretary of State Alan Milburn, had seen the introduction of more 'mimic market' (Klein, 1998) mechanisms. These included a centrally set tariff, increased openness to (and welcome for) private and social sector providers, and independence for the trusts, which could if they wanted to become more autonomous Foundation Trusts (FTs). In 2004, the government created a special central regulator for the FTs, Monitor, whose task was to be the gatekeeper to FT status and then monitor the financial stability of trusts that successfully became FTs. Labour also created a set of quality regulators which eventually became the Care Quality Commission (CQC) in 2008.

According to this logic, Monitor would be responsible for the finances of FTs and the quality regulators for the quality of FTs. Most hospital trusts would become FTs, and the system would no longer require exhausting performance management from the centre. Instead, local commissioners would drive quality improvements through their contracting arrangements with Trusts. The government therefore slowly stripped away tiers of territorial management and slimmed down the performance management.

NHS policy in 2010, when the coalition government came to power, was thus focused on making the NHS a complex and autonomous market. A significant number of providers had become Foundation Trusts with Monitor responsible for monitoring their finances. The DH was orchestrating much NHS policy and finances centrally and through Strategic Health Authorities, whose work was a blend of performance management and efforts to coordinate and direct local health economies.

The Coalition reforms

Andrew Lansley's Health and Social Care Act 2012 (HSCA) was a particularly radical attempt to resolve this conflict between central aspirations and NHS diversity. The HSCA introduced key reforms, completing the elimination of territorial units by wiping out regional Strategic Health Authorities and Blair's local Primary Care Trusts and replacing them with a purer version of a mimic market which would be managed by national regulators. In this model, there would be no more performance management based on targets. Instead, regulators would police the quality, financial, and anti-competitive aspects of a system underpinned by a series of contracts struck between CCGs and health care providers, many of whom would be private providers or those from the third sector. In what for many became a symbol of the radical nature of the reforms (Powell, 2015), the HSCA removed the Secretary of State's responsibility for providing a comprehensive healthcare service for the population and instead transferred significant responsibilities for day-to-day management to a quasi-autonomous national Commissioning Board (see Chapters 2 and 6).

The intention of the Lansley White Paper appeared to be to establish the same type of relationship between the Secretary and the Health Service which the Chancellor of the Exchequer has with the Independent Bank of England. In particular, the Act intended that a tripartite structure should be established with each of the following institutions central to how the NHS would be managed in the future.

Monitor gained a new role leading to substantial turnover in the senior management team. In addition to its existing role as the financial guardian of FTs, it would become an economic regulator responsible for ensuring competition in the newly opened NHS market and would jointly set prices within the market with the NHS Commissioning Board. Its role would also include preventing barriers to entry or anti-competitive behaviour. As the economic regulator, furthermore, it would also license providers to provide NHS services in the new NHS market, including providers from the private sector.

The Care Quality Commission (CQC) had started to operate in 2009. It was formed out of the Healthcare Commission (regulating healthcare providers), the Commission for Social Care Inspection and the Mental Health Act Commission. It was left largely unchanged under the HSCA. The continuity reflected agreement that in a more competitive, contestable market an independent care quality regulator would be necessary and that it was a virtue to combine regulation of different sectors as well as public and private in one organisation. The quality assurance role played by Monitor, however, and Monitor's role licensing non-NHS providers in the new NHS market, clearly had the potential for overlap between the two regulatory bodies.

The Commissioning Board, which quickly renamed itself NHS England (NHSE) became the central player in managing the new NHS envisioned in the HSCA. Under the new arrangements it would be given almost the entire NHS budget to commission services in accordance with the mandate set by the Secretary of State. It would pass on most of that budget CCGs but it would also have responsibility for commissioning complex services itself as well as General Practice provision, dentistry, ophthalmic services and pharmacy, which had previously been commissioned by Primary Care Trusts.

NHSE therefore combined a large-scale commissioning role of its own with a variety of system-preservation and coordination tasks that the DH and the SHAs had previously carried out. Unlike the regulators, its resources (commissioning power and staff) were not constrained by a formal role other than that set out in the mandate, and it absorbed many of the policy tools and responsibilities of the old DH structure and before that the Management Executive.

Evidence

The most effective way of evaluating the Lansley reforms is through assessing whether the central aim of liberating the NHS from political interference was successful. The structures put in place by the HSCA should also, if the theory behind them was correct, lead to greater clarity about where power and accountability lie. We can also assess the Lansley reforms in terms of whether the new organisational structure of the NHS evolved as intended, particularly once Lansley, as the architect of the new structure, was replaced by a different Secretary of State – Jeremy Hunt – in September 2012.

In carrying out this analysis, we proceed organisation by organisation, looking at both the functions and roles played by each part of the new system as well as the biographies of the key players – directors and board members – within each of them. In doing so we are acknowledging that the politics of the centre can be intensely personal rather than simply bureaucratic. Our account also relies on reports of activities in order to capture the general orientation of the different organisations. We have conducted a series of studies of the organisation charts and biographies of NHS leadership (Greer and Jarman, 2007, 2010; Greer et al, 2014; Jarman and Greer, 2010), building on earlier work (Day and Klein, 1997). Much of this account draws on these studies.

An initial look at the data shows that following the reforms the Department of Health, the traditional tool of Ministers to shape the NHS had become, as one Labour Secretary of State for Health had previously described it, a 'very thin rim' around the NHS, with just 7% of the total staffing for ensuring health and social care delivery falling directly under its control (Jarman and Greer, 2010). In terms of policy capacity – at least in numbers – Table 5.1 also shows that by September 2015 the Care Quality Commission, Monitor and NHS England employed between them over 4 times more Grade 6 and 7 level civil servants than the Department of Health, and had 6 times more members of the Senior Civil Service at their disposal. In addition, as the Department of Health has experienced a 14% headcount reduction since 2010 it is clear that the capacity of the Department to direct the system had been 'hollowed out' over the Coalition's lifetime (Bouchal and Stephen, 2013).

This is clearly in line with what was intended by the Lansley White Paper. At first glance, it appears to show that the ability of Ministers

Table 5.1: Headcount comparison across the NHS system

Organisation	Grade 6/7		Senior civil service		Total employees	
	Head-count	Full time equivalent	Head-count	Full time equivalent	Head-count	Full time equivalent
Department of Health (excluding agencies)	698	664	170	164	2,011	1,927
NHS England	1,873	1,793	635	586	4,714	4,402
Monitor	279	252	68	60	523	485
Care Quality Commission	432	424	131	125	3,239	3,134

to interfere and steer the system was significantly and deliberately reduced with power passing to the tripartite structure of NHS England, Monitor and the CQC in quite a significant way. Looking beyond these figures, however, what became clear over the period of the coalition government was that despite this transfer of policy capacity to the tripartite structure, ministers still retained a number of key levers that enabled them to maintain their grip on NHS policy.

The levers still available to Ministers after the HSCA included the power of patronage (the ability to shape organisations through choosing or appointing the top team, a focus of critics, see Tallis and Davis, 2013), the power to set budgets for each of the tripartite organisations, and the ability to legislate to achieve Ministerial priorities. Being in command of those levers meant ministers would be powerful even when they did not pull them. As we shall see, the result was that ministers shaped the function and priorities of the three organisations to whom the running of the NHS had been entrusted and eventually took the NHS towards a different set of priorities and a different way of working to that envisaged by Lansley and his HSCA.

Monitor

Monitor had an extremely important but divided role in the HSCA. On one hand, it retained the role that it had been given by Labour, as the regulator for Foundation Trusts and the guarantor of their financial responsibility. In this role, Monitor was a sort of audit agency, monitoring the FTs' finances and suggesting changes that might improve financial performance. With the HSCA, it gained a second role, as a general public sector regulator responsible for competition and markets within the NHS. It was to enforce competition law and promoting market competition a role similar to that of OFGEM, the UK energy regulator or other sector-specific regulators found throughout UK governance. Its staffing reflected this dual role, with directors' backgrounds essentially split between management consultancy (especially McKinsey, but also PwC and KPMG), and antitrust enforcement including law firms and the Competition Commission (Greer et al, 2014).

Maintaining the role as an NHS competition authority as well as being an audit and improvement agency for the NHS was always going to be difficult. It is not hard to see conflicts between a mission to promote the financial stability and strategic direction of FTs, and a mission to promote market competition between FTs and other kinds of organisations such as private and third sector providers. Over time, we might reasonably expect one mission or the other to become dominant.

Monitor had begun its career as a competition regulator with a report, solicited by the Secretary of State, emphasising the importance of a 'fair playing field' in the health sector and Monitor's role in securing such fairness for, in particular, entrants to the new NHS markets (Monitor, 2013). Once Lansley had been replaced by Jeremy Hunt, ministers moved their rhetoric away from promoting the benefits of markets and competition and instead switched their focus to a new patient safety agenda in the light of the second Francis Report into care within the Mid Staffordshire NHS Foundation Trust (Francis, 2013, and see Chapter 16). The problem for the NHS under new Ministerial direction was not anti-competitive mergers between NHS Foundation Trusts or the denial of patient choice, but how to deliver a safe and sustainable service in the context of austerity.

This shift of emphasis affected the direction of Monitor. High cost investigations into hospital mergers dominated the headlines as did polemical transfers of services to private or social sector providers, increasing deficits, and highly visible problems with private providers such as Circle in Hinchingbrooke (Jarman and Greer, 2015). Critics of privatisation in the NHS, meanwhile, never let up (Tallis and Davis, 2013). In this climate, Monitor's efforts to enforce competition on the NHS became politically difficult. Indeed, so sensitive was Jeremy Hunt to the charges from Labour that the Conservatives were intent on privatising the NHS that he was reported to be 'relieved' at the decision to award the biggest contract for services to be put out to tender to an NHS consortium rather than to the private sector (Neville and Pimmer, 2014).

Without a Minister prepared to follow through on Lansley's ideological commitment to marketisation, Monitor's role as a competition authority was always likely to be compromised. Over the course of the Coalition, Monitor began to draw (or be drawn) back from any role as a competition authority, and started to once again resemble the Monitor of Labour – almost a sort of external finance director for FTs. The 2014 NAO report found that it had done a good job of monitoring trust finances and offering help, though (predictably) Monitor's help was less effective when the problems lay in the broader local health economy (National Audit Office, 2014). Meanwhile, within a year of its report on the fair playing field it found itself explaining how to promote integrated care through payment system reforms (Monitor, 2014) – not necessarily a sign of its wings being clipped, but certainly not the agenda the HSCA set out for it.

The June 2015 decision by the Department of Health to merge the position of Chief Executive of Monitor with the same position at the highly contentious Trust Development Authority into an organisation known as NHS Improvement was another marker of a shift back towards its Labour-era role as the guarantor of trust finances rather than a powerful market-creator.[1] Merging the TDA into Monitor can be expected to focus it still more on maintaining trust financial integrity, rather than promoting competition.

While hardly conclusive, it is also noteworthy that Monitor's board and executive directors changed composition on the margins toward the end of the Coalition, with three new board appointees who were long-time NHS professionals and managers rather than generalist management consultants or lawyers. This was a novelty in an organisation that had previously not been hiring top staff out of the NHS ranks.

Care Quality Commission (CQC)

In the effectively tripartite organisation of health care services in the HSCA, the CQC is responsible for guaranteeing the quality of health and social care. The CQC is an inspectorate, a kind of organisation long familiar in English public services, and often critiqued by those it inspects for excessive cost, heavy-handedness and arbitrariness.

The CQC's role in the tripartite structure was changed (and enhanced) with the ascension of Jeremy Hunt. Hunt diverted the conversation about the NHS from the unpopular HSCA by focusing on quality and safety. This striking political move appears to have worked, with attention lavished on NHS quality failures such as Mid-Staffordshire hospitals – particularly those experienced under the previous Labour government rather than the on-going effects of the

HSCA. In this project the CQC would play a major role, providing evidence of deficiencies in NHS quality and taking decisive actions.

The CQC's role at the start of the coalition reforms remained precarious, however. 2012 saw significant criticism of the regulator by the Public Accounts Committee, which also criticised the DH for not holding CQC to account (Public Accounts Committee, 2012) and a critical internal DH report authored by the Permanent Secretary. Amidst a general loss of faith – within the NHS and in the media – about the ability of the regulator to either identify or address major systemic failings such as those identified at the care home Winterbourne View, Chief Executive Cynthia Bower and much of the top team resigned.

This provided an opportunity for the DH and Ministers to reshape the CQC. They did so in a number of ways. First, the Secretary of State used the power of patronage and appointment to 'bolster' the executive team. David Behan, a former DH board member and Director General for Social Care, was brought in as Chief Inspector. Behan was soon followed by Sir Mike Richards as Chief Inspector of Hospitals and Professor Steve Field as Chief Inspector of Primary Care. Richards had previously been Director of the National Cancer Strategy at the Department of Health and Field was formerly Deputy Medical Director at NHSE and had been the Chair of the NHS Future Forum, the group set up to rescue the HSCA during the famous 'pause' imposed by Cameron (Timmins, 2012). As a further sign of the investment by the Secretary of State, the CQC board was re-engineered with a number of appointments seemingly in line with the Secretary's thinking. Most notably, David Prior (a former Conservative MP) became Chair of the organisation and after the 2015 election went on to become a Conservative Health Minister in the Lords. Camilla Cavendish, a *Times* journalist who subsequently became David Cameron's Head of Policy in Number 10, also became a CQC board member.

Second, unlike most NDPBS or DH quangos who survived the cull of the first years of the coalition government, the budget for CQC increased by more than 50%. Third, legislation in the form of the Care Act 2014 was also used to bolster the CQC's inspection regime in the light of the Francis Report recommendations (Francis, 2013). The Act covered a number of different issues, most notably the costs of long-term care, but it also created a category of 'fundamental duties' of health care providers such as respect, consent, and nutrition. The CQC gained powers to enforce these and other provisions, such as a duty of candour, with criminal proceedings. The CQC responded to these changes with a revised inspection framework and a new team of inspectors which would rate and more stringently enforce regulatory requirements.

Throwing significant political capital behind the CQC was a high risk strategy as it had the potential to identify failings and weaknesses in the NHS which would be seized upon by the media and the opposition. CQC's role would be contentious in any context, but it coincided with enough budgetary austerity to threaten quality and access in various parts of the NHS. In 2014, the CQC inspected 82 hospitals, found none 'outstanding,' 29 'good', 48 'need[ing] improvement' and 5 'inadequate' overall (Care Quality Commission, 2014). Even if CQC was focusing on problem sites, discomfort caused by those numbers might spill over from the NHS to its political masters.

Insofar as the objective was to turn attention from the failings of the HSCA and Coalition to the failings of the NHS, it seems Hunt's strategy worked. In the post-HSCA world, the media and the opposition were seemingly unsure where to pin blame. In fact, by backing the CQC against the NHS and professional bodies Hunt sought to demonstrate that his overarching commitment was to patients and their safety and that responsibility for failings of this nature lay with hospital managers, board members and ultimately individual professionals.

The basic question at the start of Cameron's second government is whether the CQC will be a credible actor in an NHS with an increasing number of trusts in deficit, particularly where safety concerns are said to be emerging because of financial constraints. Influential *Guardian* columnist Polly Toynbee was, in 2015, articulating the problems with its role and performance (Toynbee, 2015). Nursing staff numbers, for example, are a point of contention. In the light of the Francis Report and the push to reduce patient safety incidents (Chapter 16), Trusts sought to address the nurse–patient ratios that had been identified by Francis as a key weakness. Many trusts therefore became highly reliant on expensive agency nurses to address this shortfall, a factor which pushed them further into financial deficit and potentially worsened their performance in other areas – which could in turn lead to a poor CQC rating. If a hospital as prominent as Addenbrooke's in Cambridge can be put into special measures due to staffing problems, it is easy to see how almost any part of the NHS is at risk (Campbell and Elgot, 2015).

In an NHS whose budgets are dependent on central decisions and trade-offs made in the Treasury, a quality inspectorate will always face the accusation that it is promoting distorting, or impossible, objectives on incomplete data. If the Secretary of State uses CQC as a human shield deflecting attention from NHS organisation and finances to poor quality, then the CQC is not going to be popular with the rest of the NHS. Nor is the role likely to be sustainable should the Secretary of State, or government priorities, change.

NHS England (NHSE)

It was apparent from reading the initial White Paper preceding the HSCA that the Commissioning Board, now NHSE, would be a crucial actor in the system. To start, its volume of commissioning and national scope give it great powers to shape the Service. Furthermore, it clearly inherited a role that Lansley mostly tried to eliminate, namely the responsibility for managing disruptions in the system such as provider failure or gross financial imbalances across a local health economy. Finally, lacking the clear mandates and regulatory model of CQC and Monitor meant that it was the only national body with both a mandate to ensure the NHS functioned and a set of tools to do it. It was a natural home for the continuing central management of the NHS.

Its staffing suggests as much. In terms of staffing, its initial origins and orientation are as clear as Monitor's. Monitor was staffed to bring private sector competition and consultancy expertise into the NHS. NHSE, by contrast, was by 2013 a virtual DH in exile, with the bulk of senior staff from the DH who had been engaged in health care services and performance management moving over to NHSE (See Table 5.2).

In that capacity, it looked like the old Management Executive of the 1980s – a managerial unit dedicated to the NHS. When, in 2013, it hired Chief Executive Simon Stevens, who had been a very influential advisor to Tony Blair before a decade with the US private health insurer UnitedHealth, the links between the existing NHS management elites and NHSE became more visible and stronger. If people with past history, connections, and knowledge of NHS management were valuable, then it would be meaningful that NHSE abounded in them (Greer et al, 2014). NHSE also, unlike the old ME, housed Chief Professional Officers such as the Chief Nursing Officer and hired its own Medical Director.

Stevens', and NHSE's, most visible and strategic move was to articulate a 'Five Year Forward View' (FYFV) (NHS England, 2014). This was a bid to use the strategic flexibility, money, and managerial resources of NHSE to articulate an agenda that post-HSCA managers could adopt and use as a guide. It was couched in the kind of NHS

Table 5.2: NHS England in 2013–the Department of Health in exile?

Job in 2012	Name	Job in summer 2013
DH Chief Executive	David Nicholson	Chief Executive, NHSE
DH NHS Medical Director	Bruce Keogh	Medical Director, NHSE
DH Director-General NHS Operations	David Floyd	Deputy Chief Executive, NHSE
DH Chief Dental Officer	Barry Cockcroft	Chief Dental Officer, NHSE
DH Chief Pharmaceutical Officer	Keith Ridge	Chief Pharmaceutical Officer, NHSE
DH Chief Nursing Officer	Christine Beasley	Retired; replaced by new Chief Nursing Officer, NHSE
DH Director Financial Planning and Allocations, Strategy Finance and NHS Directorate	Richard Murray	Chief Analyst, NHSE

language that managers are accustomed to interpreting. Rather than enunciating more or less fleshed-out rules in the manner of regulators Monitor and CQC, it mapped out a direction and set of priorities that barely mentioned competition.

Notably, it placed the first really serious bet on an image that had been in the peripheral vision of many in the NHS for at least a decade: health systems. This is the basic idea that the old NHS structure, with a primary care sector dominated by GPs and a hierarchical hospital sector for acute episodes, was anachronistic. This is a popular idea in the United States, where it has been adopted by large health care companies that operate vertically integrated territorial monopolies. Foundation Trusts are obvious candidates to be the core of a similar set of integrated territorial monopolies. The FYFV did not prescribe precisely how to integrate care, but the idea of vertically integrating health care around existing hospitals clearly drove its proposals.

Such a model obviously was a poor fit with the HSCA and its disintegrating tendencies, and created obvious potential for a conflict with Monitor since such models threatened both market entry and competition. Its adoption probably marked the eclipse of both the HSCA's notion of competition, and Monitor's role as a powerful competition authority. The FYFV included some components that promised to test the HSCA's promise of a hands-off relationship between the government and NHSE. The FYFV did not just express strong views that might diverge from those of ministers; it also explicitly promised to advocate before government for policies and resources that the government had rejected. While we have anecdotal reports that the Secretary of State was in close contact with Stevens, the actual politics can only be guessed. It is easy to imagine that the NHSE's staffing and ability to shape both system architecture and priorities make it an appealing vehicle for the Secretary of State to make policy.

The Department of Health (DH)

NHSE, then, became the winner of the three organisations in an NHS focused on managing financial constraint and increasingly open to integration despite the HSCA. If the centre of the NHS has moved to NHSE, then what is the purpose of the Department of Health?

The relationship between the DH and the NHS has been unstable for a very long time (Greer and Jarman, 2007; Jarman and Greer, 2010). The problem is that the NHS dominates the attention of the DH, especially its ministers, and so power tends to flow to the organisation that deals with the NHS, but power also tends to stay with ministers, and they are in the DH. The sheer size of the NHS also tends to obscure the fact that the DH, without the NHS, is still a large department. Social care, public health, and health workforce and research are all large expenditure areas even if they usually lack the political salience and cachet of health care. The DH without the NHS is by no means a shell compared to the rest of Whitehall, but the DH without the NHS looks small and inconsequential in the context of English health care policy.

The post-HSCA DH was set up as a smaller department, shorn primarily of the NHS management staff, who mostly moved to NHSE. The remaining NHS management staff were housed in the TDA, which in theory was supposed to fade away as non–FT trusts were merged or graduated. In this, it resembled the DH at the start of the Management Executive's career in the 1980s, with staff and units for public health (the Chief Medical Officer and oversight of Public Health England), social care, research, and a miscellany of corporate functions such as communications. That left it with six Director-General level staff and a Permanent Secretary – much smaller than the old DH, but a reduction in departmental (if not quango) staff that was roughly proportionate to other Whitehall departments (Greer et al, 2015). Given that many of the key DH staff reappeared in NHSE, it is not clear that the senior levels of the NHS are much smaller.

The DH has, since then, been stable on paper. Everyday top-down NHS management and contention over control of the system has mostly been in the space of Monitor, CQC and the NHSE. Secretary of State Hunt, perhaps frustrated by the Rube Goldberg machine that his predecessor built, has been notorious for calling trust chief executives to account in the most literal way possible – on the telephone (Jarman and Greer, 2015). In other words, the DH seems to be in a phase in which it is side-lined by ministers relative to NHS bodies. This phase creates interesting questions and even opportunities. For example, the CMO in office, Sally Davies, seems to be focusing on research and very broad public health as a response to the existence of a Medical Director in NHSE and a whole agency, Public Health England, that does not report to her.

Discussion

In short, our evaluation of the HSCA's provisions for the central management of the NHS suggests that it has failed. It has not removed ministers from NHS management, as we see in both their direct actions and in the way organisations' agendas reflect ministerial preferences. It has not clarified organisational responsibilities, as the many conflicts at the start of HSCA implementation showed, and it has not evolved as intended – Monitor and competition enforcement lost out, CQC took on great prominence, and NHSE's central role constantly expanded despite the FYFV's lack of interest in competition.

Conclusion

We have seen this film before (Edwards and Fall, 2005; Klein, 2006, 2010). The stylised plot is a common one in NHS policy since 1980. Ministers at the centre, charged with responsibility for a health system that they cannot control, are willing consumers for organisational designs that promise them good outcomes, legibility to the centre, and a set of automatic incentives that harness competition through carefully constructed mimic markets (Greer, 2016). In practice, this means, first of all, the creation of a powerful management infrastructure that responds to ministerial policy designs, and second, intricate legislation setting up markets and a set of more or less autonomous regulatory agencies charged with enforcing those rules. The result is usually a market that, if it functions, does not do what ministers want, and a reversion over time to more direct use of the management structure to tell the system.

The NHS has already seen some full cycles. On the management side, Thatcher's Management Executive produced a management structure that responded to the ministerial team. By the time Alan

Milburn entered office, he was not clear what the DH was for and merged them, with the DH subsuming the ME in name and the ME subsuming the DH in reality. On the market side, regulatory agencies have three flaws: they are (by design) rigid in what they do and which rules they enforce, they lack policy tools to affirmatively do what ministers want (for example, enforce seven-day NHS services), and they cannot be tasked with the large residuum of powers that the centre exercises but are clearly unrelated to or conflict with their core mandates. As a result, they become irrelevant to, or obstacles to, ministerial objectives and tend to lose power.

The history of the NHS, and of the Coalition reforms so far, suggests some patterns in organisation at the top:

1. large management agencies such as NHSE will become the focus of ministerial attention and eventually be merged with the Department;
2. regulators will be side-lined in favour of that agency because their enforcement of rules impedes or distract ministers;
3. the more rigid the legislative framework for regulators, the less likely it is that they will be seen in a positive light by ministers; and
4. ministers will get their way (for example, there is no obvious reason why Monitor and the TDA should issue guidance about appropriate agency nurse policies, but they have, at a time when the Secretary of State is interested in the topic) (Monitor and Trust Development Authority, 2015).

This kind of instability and shifting use of central policy tools is not unique to the English NHS. Rail transport regulation has seen a similar instability since privatisation, and for many of the same reasons (Lodge, 2002; Wolmar, 2001, 2015). In the original design at the time of privatisation under John Major's Conservatives, an Office of the Rail Regulator (ORR, renamed the Office of Rail and Road in 2015), akin to Monitor, was charged with ensuring competition in a market while the Rail Safety and Standards Board, akin to CQC, was charged with ensuring safety. The bidding process would design the services. Blair's government, frustrated with its inability to direct the system but unwilling to cut out the mimic market, created a powerful commissioning body, the Strategic Rail Authority (SRA), akin to NHSE. It tried to use SRA commissioning to shape the system in pursuit of electorally popular objectives such as reliable timetabling that the ORR's regulatory tools could not force, and much energy was spent in conflict between the SRA and ORR. The role of the

Department for Transport was unclear in a system where ministerial attention focused on the SRA's policy areas and its frictions with the ORR, and so in 2004 Secretary of State Alistair Darling folded the SRA into the department. As with the HSCA reforms, the desire of the government to control the system for which it was held accountable led it to privilege a central commissioning body that could promise responsiveness and effectiveness over a rigid regulator. Once the SRA became the focus of ministerial attention, it was a matter of time before it was folded into a department on grounds of both savings and ministerial control.

It is unwise to predict specific legislative changes, and the experience of the HSCA seems to have left key players, including the Cameron government, with little desire for major new legislation. At the end of the Coalition government, the real, as against theoretical, roles of the different players were still stabilising. Nonetheless, it would not be surprising to see increasingly tight connections between ministers, DH and NHSE, continuing erosion of Monitor, especially its investment in competition, and serious conflict around CQC.

The first overall analytic point to make is that the Coalition government experience confirms two basic weaknesses of mimic markets. On one hand, they are never so intricately and accurately designed as to actually operate without central direction. They fail to work on some level, and the regulator looks too rigid to address the problem. On the other hand, even if the market 'sort of' works in the originally intended manner, it does not respond to political changes, and ministers prefer to work with and strengthen the agencies with the tools to affirmatively enunciate priorities and make changes across the system.

The second overall point is that all the organisations at the top of the NHS are very fragile. They depend on specific people and constellations of power. Changes in their top personnel can be highly informative but hard to read. For example, it is difficult by design to know who is in contact with ministers or what is happening in the boards of big agencies. Even if an agency does have strong leadership, a distinctive style, and a persuasive narrative of organisational purpose, that does not mean the political environment will sustain it.

The third point is that the NHS is a diverse, complex, and highly localised creature. Managing it from the centre is very hard. The HSCA finished a nearly forty-year process of eliminating self-governing professional bodies and autonomous regional or local bodies in favour of direct action by central bodies – Monitor, CQC, and NHSE. Older shock absorbers such as various Health Authorities, including appointed regions, had been whittled away since 1989, with more and more of the NHS organised into trusts with a direct relationship to central agencies. This is more or less automatically a formula for central overstretch and complaints about rigidity, as well as for de facto decentralisation such as NHSE's creation of internal regional management. Putting visible power in the hands of central agencies with a remit to enforce nationwide policies is nonetheless a recipe for massive, highly visible noncompliance (as quality and financial deficit data currently suggest) and an overstressed centre with too many competing poles of authority. The chimera of a perfectly designed market with effective, predictable regulators that permits the elimination of political intervention and central management is just that – a chimera. The central management of the NHS under the Coalition is simply confirmation of that.

Note

[1] The TDA was a small unit of the DH responsible for approximately two-fifths of trusts that had not, for whatever reason, become Foundation Trusts. Its stated mission was to support all trusts, but in practice it was engaged in performance managing non-FTs. It became extremely visible in the controversy about Lewisham hospital, a well-regarded and popular South London non-FT that was boxed in by troubled FTs with expensive PFIs. The DH's solution to the fiscal crisis of its FT neighbors was to start closing services at Lewisham. This decision steered patients and funds to the troubled FTs but lacked much other justification and outraged locals while making clear the advantages of FT status. The TDA, the instrument of this decision, became very prominent as a result.

References

Bouchal, P, Stephen, J, 2013, Whitehall Monitor 21: Analysis of Civil Service staff numbers, *Whitehall Monitor*, London: Institute for Government

Campbell, D, Elgot, J, 2015, Addenbrooke's hospital in special measures after 'serious staff shortages', *Guardian*, 22 September

CQC (Care Quality Commission), 2014, *The state of Health Care and Adult Social Care in England 2013/14*, London: CQC

Day, P, Klein, R, 1997, *Steering but not rowing? The transformation of the Department of Health: A case study*, Bristol: Policy Press

Edwards, B, Fall, M, 2005, *The executive years of the NHS: The England account 1985–2003*, London/Oxford: The Nuffield Trust/Radcliffe

Francis, R, QC, 2013, *Report of the Mid-Staffordshire NHS Foundation Trust Public Inquiry*, 3 volumes, London: Stationery Office

Greer, SL, 2006, A very English institution: Central and local in the English NHS, in R Hazell (ed.), *The English Question*, Manchester: Manchester University Press, pp 194-219

Greer, SL, 2016, Claiming authority over the NHS, in M Bevir and RAW Rhodes (eds), *Rethinking governance: Ruling, rationalities and resistance*, Abingdon: Routledge

Greer, SL, Jarman, H, 2007, *The Department of Health and the Civil Service: From Whitehall to Department of Delivery to where?* London: Nuffield Trust

Greer, SL, Jarman, H, 2010, What Whitehall? Definitions, demographics and the changing home Civil Service, *Public Policy and Administration* 25, 3, 251-70

Greer, SL, Jarman, H, Azorsky, A, 2014, *A reorganisation you can see from space: The architecture of power in the new NHS*, London: Centre for Health and the Public Interest

Greer, SL, Jarman, H, Azorsky, A, 2015, Devolution and the Civil Service: A biographical study, *Public Policy and Administration*, 30, 1, 31-50

Jarman, H, Greer, SL, 2010, In the eye of the storm: Civil servants and managers in the Department of Health, *Social Policy and Administration*, 44, 2, 172-92

Jarman, H, Greer, SL, 2015, The big bang: Health and social care reforms under the Coalition, in M Beech, S Lee (eds), *The Conservative-Liberal Coalition: Examining the Cameron-Clegg Government*, Basingstoke: Palgrave Macmillan, pp 50-67

Klein, R, 1998, Self-inventing institutions: Institutional design and the UK welfare state, in RE Goodin (ed.), *The theory of institutional design*, Cambridge: Cambridge University Press, pp 240-255

Klein, R, 2006, *The new politics of the NHS: From creation to reinvention*, Oxford: Radcliffe Medical

Klein, R, 2010, The eternal triangle: Sixty years of the Centre–periphery relationship in the National Health Service, *Social Policy and Administration*, 44, 3, 285-304

Lodge, M, 2002, The wrong type of regulation? Regulatory failure and the railways in Britain and Germany, *Journal of Public Policy*, 22, 3, 271-97

Monitor, 2013, *A fair playing field for the benefit of NHS patients: Monitor's independent review for the Secretary of State for Health*, London: Monitor

Monitor, 2014. Delivering better integrated care. 11 March. London: Monitor. Available at: https://www.gov.uk/guidance/enabling-integrated-care-in-the-nhs

Monitor and Trust Development Authority, 2015, *Nursing Agency Rules*, London: Monitor/TDA

National Audit Office, 2014, *Monitor: Regulating NHS Foundation Trusts*, London: NAO

Neville, S, Pimmer, G, 2014. 'NHS group wins biggest patient services tender' *Financial Times*, 1 October.

NHS England, 2014, Five year forward view, London: HM Government

Powell, M, 2015, Who killed the English National Health Service? *International Journal of Health Policy and Management* 4, 5 (May), 267-269

Public Accounts Committee, 2012, *The Care Quality Commission: Regulating the quality and safety of health and adult social care*, Seventy-eighth Report of Session 2010–12, London: House of Commons

Tallis, R, Davis, J, 2013, *NHS SOS: How the NHS was betrayed – and how we can save it*, London: Oneworld Publications

Timmins, N, 2012, *Never again? The story of the Health and Social Care Act 2012: A study in coalition government and policymaking*, London: Nuffield Trust

Toynbee, P, 2015, Jeremy Hunt's hit squad is a danger to our national health, *Guardian*, 22 September

Wolmar, C, 2001, *Broken rails: How privatisation wrecked Britain's railways*, London: Aurum Press

Wolmar, C, 2005, *On the wrong line: How ideology and incompetence wrecked Britain's Railways*, London: Aurum Press

An argument lost by both sides? The Parliamentary debate over the 2010 NHS White Paper

Ian Greener

This chapter examines the rhetoric of government and opposition in the Parliamentary debate over the 2010 NHS White Paper 'Equity and Excellence'. It treats the debate as a process of deliberative argument in which Secretary of State Andrew Lansley justifies his reorganisation, and explores the extent to which his policy argument was scrutinised by both the opposition and by members of his own coalition government. If representative democracy depends upon significant reorganisations being adequately explained, debated and examined, then it is important to consider the extent to which this happens, even while accepting that limitations in time and expertise in Parliament will always place limitations on this.

The chapter suggests that Lansley offered an unjustified reorganisation based on market-based governance (although presented as 'social enterprise'), and decentralised accountability, which would at the same time generate substantial savings in a time of financial austerity (see Chapter 2). This is contrasted with the often fragmented arguments offered by voices in the opposition. We ask questions about the extent to which Parliamentary debate is able to adequately scrutinise governmental proposals of the complexity of healthcare reorganisation, especially at the beginning of a new term in office.

Introduction

This chapter examines the 2010 Coalition Government's proposals to reorganise the National Health Service. This debate and policy discussion has been chosen because of being so contentious – with the government putting in place an unprecedented 'pause' in its passage through the legislature to address concerns from senior Liberal Democrats, medical representative groups and the general public. It is also the case that, despite the government struggling to get their legislation through Parliament, and perhaps losing the argument as to the necessity and form of their reorganisation, the legislation was still implemented in a heavily-modified form which led to significant disruption as Primary Care Trusts were abolished and GPs asked to lead the commissioning process (see Chapter 18).

The chapter examines the Parliamentary debate around the reorganisation's White Paper, examining the extent to which the reorganisation was scrutinised, and suggesting that many of the problems the government experienced in passing the legislation came from the government's inability to present a coherent argument in their favour. It presents an argument-driven, rhetorical analysis of the debate, while accepting that alternative forms of analysis are equally possible.

It is commonplace within social policy writing to contrast 'rhetoric' with 'reality', with the former representing what policymakers say they are doing, and the latter what they actually are up to (Packwood, 2002). 'Rhetoric' has become associated with language designed to conceal, with falsity and, in political arenas, with the growth of 'spin' or even with 'political lying' (Oborne, 2005). The language used by policymakers is certainly rhetorical, in that it will often be designed as much to persuade as to explain. This does not mean that we should dismiss it as being unimportant, however. There are good reasons to redouble our efforts in scrutinising policy, not only to hold policymakers to account for what they say (which is an essential part of a democratic political process), but also because a close examination of the rhetoric of policy allows us to unpack the arguments policymakers present to us, and to scrutinise the basis on which policy arguments are being made.

This chapter proceeds as follows: first, it locates its approach within the field of critical policy studies, before presenting its methods in more detail, and then explaining the context of the 2010 debate on NHS reorganisation in more depth. It then analyses the Parliamentary debate around the government's White Paper 'Equity and Excellence', before presenting a discussion and conclusion.

Discourse in policy studies

The 'discursive turn' in policy studies attempts to move the focus of research away from rationalistic approaches that treat the definition, diagnosis and remedies to social problems as technical issues that are based on law-like causes (Howarth and Griggs, 2012). Instead, taking a discursive approach suggests the importance of interpretation and critical evaluation in policy analysis. Discursively-based research adopts a range of positions. It can be a supplement to positivistic approaches, where discursive methods can be treated as 'frames' (Schon and Rein, 1995) or as a means of treating discourses as variables that can be subject to empirical testing (Torfing, 2005). More radical approaches to discourse theory, however, suggest that a break from such rationalism is required (Fischer, 2003) in which discourse is not only a feature of social relations, but is also constitutive of them (Gottwiess, 2006).

The approach taken here treats policy as an attempt to articulate practical action, and acknowledges that the language in which policy is communicated may express more than policy-makers might intend (Bacchi, 2009). It treats policy as constitutive of the world rather than descriptive, following the insights of poststructuralist writers who regard human subjects, objects, social formations and symbolic formations not as fixed, but as constantly moving, changing and shifting. It uses a method that examines policy rhetoric as argumentation (for practical action), based on scholarship from Fairclough and Fairclough (2012) and Bacchi (2009).

Political discourse analysis

The approach taken here links directly to the discussion above in that it is specifically geared to consider how political problems are conceptualised and argued in policy debates. Policy is treated as a set of proposals for practical action based on the partial representation of a particular problem. The diagnosis of social problems leads to problematisations that carry with them biases toward particular outcomes. For example a diagnosis of a service having a lack of responsiveness to public need has tended in recent years to lead to a market-based solution because of the assumption this will lead to that service becoming more dynamic as a result (Greener and Powell, 2009).

The language which is used to construct policy carries rhetorical effects that will often reveal a great deal about the assumptions that particular policies hold about the world. It is not an overstatement to claim that we live by our metaphors (Lakoff and Johnson, 2008), our representations of our own and others' subjectivities, and how we describe social problems and desirable outcomes.

The approach to political argument analysis closest to that described above is that of Fairclough and Fairclough (2012), who present a range of political debates using a framework that disaggregates political argumentation into a range of analytically linked categories: circumstances (the background and constructed problem being addressed); goal (what the proposal is meant to achieve); means–goal (how the mechanism proposed will achieve the goal specified); values (the values that underpin the diagnosis of circumstances, goal and mean–goal); and the over-riding claim for action (what the policymaker says must happen – usually the adoption of the policy proposal).

There may be several goals and several means–goal links made in a policy proposal, and at the same time those opposing or arguing against proposals often make counter-claims that question goals, means–goal linkages, the circumstances as defined by the policy proposals, and which question the underlying values of the policy being proposed. Those against a particular proposal may also point out negative consequences they envisage as likely to occur, and offer their own alternative counter proposals. Viewing policy proposals in this manner allows us to explore the elements of argumentation offered by policymakers in a clear framework that illuminates their proposals, while at the same time making clear the points of difference with opposition voices, and gives us a means of assessing the likelihood that the proposals will achieve the goals of policymakers, by assessing the strength of policymakers' arguments not only in rebutting opposition voices, but in relation to factual and evidence-based claims that they may be making in their proposals.

The Fairclough and Fairclough model (2012) presents us with a clear framework, but there are also some potential problems. For all its strengths, it does treat its 'circumstances' category fairly briefly, when it is often the case that the definition of a policy problem carries with it a clear steer as to the likely solution that will be proposed to deal with it. In the terms suggested by Bacchi (2009), we must pay close attention to policy 'problematisations' – the way that policies and policymakers construct problems so as to favour particular attempts at solutions or exclude others. It is therefore important to examine carefully the way that policy problems are represented and constructed in policy documents and debates, to assess the extent to which those representations and constructions seem chosen in order to favour particular policy solutions.

Incorporating insights from Bacchi in terms of problematisation allows us to examine the debate concerning the introduction of the UK coalition government's NHS White Paper 'Liberating the NHS' in 2010 (Secretary of State for Health, 2010) to explore why its proposals proved so contentious. The paper here examines the debate concerning the White Paper rather than the compromised Bill that ended up being voted into law later on. It does this to try and capture the values and ideas that the government wished to introduce, and which the Conservatives appeared to have spent some time in opposition preparing, as well as the reaction to the White Paper and the counter-claims made by its opponents. It is the job of another paper to track the extent to which these objections and counter-claims were eventually addressed by legislation later on.

The NHS in 2010

By 2010, after increasing healthcare budgets considerably during the 2000s, the governing Labour party had both imposed central performance management of the NHS in England to an extent not seen before, and reinstated a market for care, allowing greater involvement from non-public providers more extensively even than the Conservative 'internal market' of the 1990s (Greener, 2008).

In the 2010 election the Conservatives managed to outflank Labour in relation to healthcare by promising to protect the NHS budget if elected, a promise Labour did not feel it could match. This led to something of a stalemate in which Labour were reluctant to campaign around healthcare – despite the improvements that had been achieved during the 2000s – while the Conservatives appeared wary of discussing any plans they had formulated in relation to the service (Timmins, 2012). The NHS was largely conspicuous by its absence in the televised debates between party leaders.

After the election, and the formation of the Coalition Government, the NHS did not appear prominently in the published coalition agreement (HM Government, 2010). Six weeks later, however, a White Paper appeared putting far more radical change at its centre (Secretary of State for Health, 2010). The story of how this dramatic change happened has already been the subject of a short book by Timmins (2012) (see Chapter 2).

The 'Equity and Excellence' debate

The debate on the NHS White Paper 'Equity and Excellence: Liberating the NHS' was held in Parliament on its publication date, the 12th July 2010, mere weeks after the Coalition government had come to power, and was recorded in Hansard in columns 661–681.

What follows is not a description of the debate, which can be downloaded in full through Hansard. Instead, it will first attempt to present a summary, in the participants' own words, of that debate, followed by an analysis of it. First, however, it is worth giving a brief outline of the debate.

The debate began with the Secretary of State Andrew Lansley giving a statement 'on the future of the national health service' (c. 661) which outlined the government's commitment to the 'core principles of the NHS', but noted that the 'NHS today faces great challenges', also suggesting that 'For too long, processes have come before outcomes' and that the NHS needed to bring 'NHS resources and NHS decision making as close to the patient as possible' (c. 661).

Lansley went on claim that the reorganisation would bring 'real, local democratic accountability to health care for the first time' and that it would 'liberate the NHS from the old command-and-control regime' and allow 'any willing provider to deliver services to the NHS' to create the 'largest social enterprise sector in the world' under the remit of an 'efficient and effective' regulator and an 'independent and accountable NHS Commissioning Board' (c. 662)

The reorganisation would simplify 'the NHS landscape', 'rebalance the NHS, reducing management costs by 45%...and abolishing quangos that do not need to exist' and 'phase out the top-down management hierarchy, including both strategic health authorities and primary care trusts' (c. 663).

Following Lansley's statement, Andy Burnham (the former Secretary of State for Health, leading the opposition in the debate) answered, followed by Lansley's responses, before the debate was opened to generally supportive comments from members from the coalition government, and hostile comments from the opposition.

The circumstances of the reorganisation

The opening presentations in the debate, from Secretary of State Lansley and his Shadow, Burnham, presented a picture of the government claiming that significant change was necessary: because of existing bureaucracy obstructing staff from doing their jobs and holding them back from achieving the best health outcomes (a claim disputed by the opposition); and because the NHS was facing considerable future challenges (not challenged by the opposition). In turn, the opposition suggested that the NHS was 'working well' and challenged the legitimacy of the reorganisation because of it not being included in either the coalition agreement or election 'manifesto commitments' (c. 663).

In his opening statement, Lansley characterised the NHS as 'stifled by a culture of top-down bureaucracy which blocks its staff from achieving the best health outcomes' (c. 661). He used the particularly memorable phrase that '[t]he current situation is akin to a shopping trolley being pushed to the checkout while the primary care trust is standing there with a credit card, bleating about whether things should be taken out of the trolley' (c. 666). The result of this bureaucracy and ineffective purchasing of care was that 'survival rates are worse than our international neighbours with targets focused on processes not outcomes' (c. 661). Lansley acknowledged that the NHS had made some progress in the previous decade, but claimed that more should be done in giving local healthcare organisations greater 'freedom' (so the best can be built upon) (c. 662). At the same time the NHS was having to change to deal with the challenges of an ageing population, advances in medical technology and rising expectations (c. 661).

Burnham, speaking for the opposition in response, claimed that the NHS had made 'hard won' progress on objective measures and international rankings, and that the government's proposals represented a 'huge gamble with a national health service that is working well for patients' (c. 663). He suggested that the reorganisation represented a 'U-turn of epic proportions' as it had 'spectacularly ripped up' the coalition agreement. Burnham claimed that the 'spin operation of the government' had billed the reorganisation as 'the biggest revolution of the NHS since its foundation 60 years ago' even though the coalition agreement had promised 'we will stop top-down reorganisations of the NHS'. (c. 663).

This opening exchange is interesting in that it would normally be the government defending a public service, and the opposition demanding change. Coming soon after a general election, however, these positions were reversed. This gave the opposition a problem in having to defend a service they were no longer responsible for (as it was the result of their own policy decisions), and the government good reasons to want to change things (so any improvements could be held up as being as a result of the changes they were proposing).

In terms of whether the structural reorganisation Lansley proposed was necessary, one member of the opposition asked whether he had heard of the old adage, 'If it ain't broke, don't fix it'. Lansley replied 'It is broke, and we are fixing it. We are fixing it because primary care trusts have not succeeded in delivering the outcomes that we are looking for, and they have consumed an enormous amount of money' (c. 676). This presented Lansley's problematisation of the extant system as both a failure to deliver outcomes and of bureaucratic waste.

Finally, the issue of whether health inequalities would be made worse by the reorganisation was raised several times in the debate, leading Lansley to present a final factor which his reorganisation was meant to address: 'It would be a good idea if Labour Members at least acknowledged that over the last 13 years health inequalities have widened in this country' (c. 681, and see Chapter 12).

In all then, the problematisation presented by the government was that of a health service producing poor outcomes relative to comparable systems, stifled by wasteful bureaucracy and unable to deal with the challenges it now faced (including growing health inequalities). The opposition, in contrast, suggested that the NHS was working well, and emphasised how the proposals were a 'gamble' that risked losing ground on previous 'hard won' progress, emphasising also the lack of democratic legitimacy the proposals held having not been a central part of the government's manifesto commitments in the 2010 election.

The reorganisation's goals

The reorganisation of the NHS was presented by the Coalition as being radical, and so one might have expected it to have ambitious goals. The goals specified in the White Paper and its debate were certainly wide-ranging. The opposition's position was that the NHS was already working well, and so did not need reorganising again. Perhaps more significantly, however, some members of the opposition appear to have suggested that the real aims of the reorganisation were not those purported by the Coalition – that the reorganisation was really about the privatisation of care rather than about improving healthcare. Lansley presented the goals of his reorganisation in a fragmented fashion, across several answers in the debate. In full, he gave the following aims:

- To deliver 'health outcomes as good as any in the world' (c. 661)
- to respond to the demands of an ageing population, advances in medical technology and rising expectations (c. 661)
- to create an outcomes framework setting out what the service should achieve, leaving the professionals to develop how those outcomes should be achieved (c. 661)
- for patients to be assured that services are safe (c. 661)
- for decisions to be made as close to the patient as possible ('no decision about me, without me') c. 661

- that patients should be given real choices: the right to choose their GP practice, and to have greater access to health information including the right to control their patient record (c. 662)
- to introduce real, local democratic accountability by giving local authorities the power to agree local strategies to integrated care and control over local improvement budgets (c. 662)
- for GPs to lead commissioning to respond to the wishes and needs of their patients, informed by the NHS commissioning board guidelines and standards (c. 662)
- for NHS trusts to be liberated from the command and control regime and become Foundation Trusts, with power increasingly placed in the hands of their employees (c. 662)
- for management costs to be reduced by 45% in four years, unnecessary quangos abolished, £1bn moved from back office to front line, £20bn of efficiency savings made by 2014, all of which would be reinvested in patient care (c. 663).

The government thus promised not only to drive up quality (outcomes) at the same time as reducing costs, but also simultaneously to change a range of structures to give patients more choice, increase democratic accountability, give GPs more responsibilities and to change the way NHS trusts work. Given this level of ambition the next section of the paper, which explores the means by which government plans to achieve these end goals, is extremely important.

This opposition, in response, presented the case for change not occurring. They appeared rather out-flanked, offering little in the way of an alternative plan other than the status quo – and so were left in the odd situation of having to defend a public service they were no longer responsible for running.

Burnham suggested that the NHS needed 'stability, not upheaval. All its energy must be focused on the financial challenge ahead' (c. 663), and that the opposition would support the government 'where sensible reductions' can be made to bureaucracy, 'but what [Lansley] calls pointless bureaucracy, we call essential regulation' (c. 664).

Other members of the opposition also suggested that the 'real' goals of the reorganisation were being concealed. Burnham suggested that government was 'removing public accountability and opening the door to unchecked privatisation' (c. 665), and 'the handing of the public budget to independent contractors' is 'tantamount to the privatisation of the commissioning function in the NHS' (c. 664). Later, another member of the opposition suggested that 'the real motive behind the reforms is to enable US multinational corporations....to parcel out health care to the private sector on a vast scale' (c. 673). To the last point, Lansley simply answers 'No, that is completely wrong on all counts' (c. 673). This allegation of hidden privatisation is an important one to which we will return.

Linking means and goals

Given the ambitious range of goals, and the dispute between government and opposition as to whether the NHS is 'working well' or not, a narrative about how the reorganisation would meet the coalition government's goals is clearly important.

Lansley's claim was that by removing bureaucratic barriers, and by putting in place social enterprise and GP commissioning, the ambitious outcomes of the reorganisation could be achieved. The opposition, in contrast, claimed that the proposed reorganisation would undermine accountability (and even increase bureaucracy), require GPs to take on commissioning roles with which they were not equipped to deal, and pass public funds to GPs without adequate oversight over how that money would be spent.

The reorganisation proposed two main means of achieving its goals. The first is to remove barriers, and the second to put in place 'social enterprise'. The first strand links back to Lansley's problematisation in relation to the NHS being stifled by top-down bureaucracy, and aims therefore to 'remove unjustified targets and the bureaucracy that sustains them' (c. 661). At the same time, however, targets would be replaced by an 'outcomes framework' to make sure standards are maintained (with a key difference being made between 'targets' and 'outcomes'). Finally, £20bn of efficiency savings would be generated by 'dismantling' bureaucracy (c. 663).

The second means was the creation of 'the largest 'social enterprise sector in the world', with improved regulation, so as not to be a 'free for all', but within which, through a system of 'any willing provider' and within GP-led commissioning (c. 662), payments would be a driver 'not just for activity, but also for quality, efficiency and integrated care' (c. 661). Lansley suggested that GP commissioning was about 'ensuring that those people who incur the expenditure- the general practitioners, on behalf of their patients-and who decide about the referral of patients are the same people who, through the commissioning process, determine the shape of the services in their area. It is more accountable' (c. 665).

What Lansley proposed, therefore, appeared to be a market-based programme of reorganisation labelled as 'social enterprise' – perhaps as an attempt to avoid the charge of privatisation, in which GPs (as the doctors closest to patients), 'commission' (rather than purchase, again avoiding obviously market-based language), services on behalf of their patients.

The 'leap' Lansley's reorganisation requires us to make, linking together the problematisation to the goals via the means described above, is that a reorganisation that strengthens the role of market-based mechanisms in the NHS in England could both improve care and save money. He was trying to show that this reorganisation was both a break from the past in expanding freedoms and social enterprise, and a continuity of the previous government's NHS where it appears to be showing progress.

The opposition, in turn, claimed that, rather than increasing accountability, the reorganisation would decrease it – and even increase bureaucracy at the same time; that GPs are not ready to lead the commissioning of services (and so this would result in them passing on or even privatising their new duties), and that GPs might misuse their new budgets to pursue cheaper rather than better healthcare.

In terms of accountability, Burnham claimed that the reorganisation would lead to 'the wiping away of oversight and public accountability' (c. 664) while at the same time creating the 'biggest quango in the world' (the new NHS commissioning board) but without explaining how it would be 'accountable to this House and to Members of Parliament'. Other opposition figures asked how GP practices would be 'watched over' in their spending, and claimed that 'The Secretary of State has been asked about the accountability of the GPs, and he has not answered.' (c. 673).

The claim that GPs were not ready to lead the commissioning of services was made several times, with suggestions from Burnham that the reorganisation represented 'the handing over of £80bn of public money to GPs, whether they are ready or not....only 5% of GPs are ready to take over commissioning....even the best GP practice-based commissioners are "only about a three" out of 10 in terms of the quality of their commissioning.' (c. 664). This claim is linked to the suggestion that the reorganisation was 'tantamount to the privatisation of the commissioning function in the NHS' (c. 664) and that it would 'cause significant problems with the progress' GP consortiums had already made under the previous government (c. 677).

Finally, there is an opposition claim that GPs would misuse their budgets. This is most clear when Tony Lloyd (Manchester Central) asked Lansley, 'how will he guarantee that GPs will not look for cheaper medicine rather than better medicine?' (c. 675).

In response to these concerns, Lansley appeared to grow increasingly impatient. After expressing the view that he has explained the accountability structure several times he says 'At the risk of repetition, let me say that GPs will be accountable to patients, who will exercise more control and choice. They will be accountable to the NHS commissioning board, which will hold their contracts, for financial control and for their performance, through the quality and outcomes framework. They will be accountable to their local authority for their strategy and for the co-ordination of public health services and social care.' (c. 673).

In response to concerns about whether GPs were ready or had the capacity to commission services, Lansley claimed

> The honourable Lady and all her colleagues completely underestimate the capacity of general practitioners, who are responsible for the overwhelming majority of patient contact in the NHS, not only to take on the responsibility of deciding whether they should incur the expenditure for the referrals they make but to have a say in designing those services. (c. 681)

Finally, in response to concerns about GPs pursuing cheaper rather than better care, he suggested a further accountability measure (which he had already positioned himself as defending above) 'Because patients will have increased choice [Hon. Members: 'How?']. Because patients will make their choices on the quality of service they receive, because the service will be free to them' (c. 675).

Lansley's claim, them, was that the accountability structures avoid the problems the opposition claimed they would create, but in answering, those structures appear rather complex. Lansley also does not give a clear answer to the concerns raised about privatisation by the opposition.

The government presented their reorganisation as an extension of values often presented in NHS White papers – including free, comprehensive and equitable care – adding to those to include decisions being made jointly, and the right to choice. The opposition instead proposed supporting that 'loyal public servants' be treated more respectfully, suggesting that the proposals were about privatising healthcare, and would lead to chaos rather than order as they would abolish 'essential regulation' which Lansley had been couching as 'pointless bureaucracy'.

Values

In terms of values, the government's proposals faced a difficult balancing act, both attempting to show they were supportive of the NHS (in terms of its 'core values'), but at the same time also showing that their proposals were different from what had gone before. To try and achieve this, Lansley proposed 'A comprehensive service for all, free at the point of use, based on need, not ability to pay. The principle of equity will be maintained, but we need the NHS also consistently to provide excellent care' (c. 661). This is a particular definition of equity, based on providing equity of access to excellent care (through choice and social enterprise), rather than the same care for all (see Chapter 12).

In addition to linking to values invoked by previous governments, new values were also proposed by Lansley, including 'No decision about me, without me' (c. 661) and the 'right to choose' (c. 662) for patients. Despite the title of the White Paper ('Liberating the NHS') neither liberty nor freedom are mentioned extensively in the debate, with a slightly stronger emphasis on democratic accountability, which is mentioned three times.

The opposition stressed instead values of stability and the respectful treatment of 'loyal public servants' (c. 664), expressing concerns about the privatisation of healthcare (c. 664), and that the proposed reorganisation would lead to 'chaos' not 'order' (c.665) leading to services that will 'vary from street to street' (c. 665). Burnham counterposes 'essential regulation' with the 'pointless bureaucracy' suggested by the government (c. 664).

Government and opposition claims

In sum, then, the government's main claim is that NHS bureaucracy is stifling creativity and should be abolished, with commissioning being made GP-led using a payment system that would be a driver for activity, quality, efficiency and integrated care by bringing the management of resources and the management of care together. Care providers should be made NHS trusts which are free from bureaucratic control, based on a social enterprise model governed on the principle of 'any willing provider'. Care should be outcome-focused. Commissioners should be rewarded for delivering care in line with quality standards set in a regulatory regime designed to ensure that services are safe, but which also aims for efficiency, effectiveness and comprehensiveness. Patients would be given more choices and decisions made as closely as possible to them, with a new regulator, 'Healthwatch', championing their needs. Democratic accountability would be increased by giving local authorities the power to bring NHS, public health and social care together by giving them control over local improvement budgets and strategies.

The countering claim offered by the opposition was that the NHS was working well, having made 'hard won' progress and needed stability to meet the 'financial challenge ahead', as NHS reorganisations 'cost money and divert resources'. The opposition argue that the proposed reorganisation would demoralise staff, and that redundancies and the abolition of national pay bargaining are a poor 'way to treat loyal public servants'. They also argued that the privatisation of commissioning commissioning, and the introduction of market forces would create 'chaos' in a system where there would be less public or parliamentary accountability than the existing system. Finally there was the claim that the reorganisation would not reduce bureaucracy but increase it as the NHS commissioning board would create biggest quango in the world, as well as creating inequity, as the reorganisation would make services vary from 'street to street' (c. 665).

The overarching narrative of the reorganisation

Lansley portrayed the NHS as a moribund, stifling organisation from which the reorganisation would free staff. How would the NHS be organised instead in the future? Through 'the largest social enterprise sector in the world', though he was keen to insist it would 'not [be] a free-for-all' (c. 662).

How about Lansley was mindful of potential allegations against him privatising the NHS, but wanted to claim to have captured the dynamism of the market. He attempted to achieve this by making use of 'social enterprise' instead. He also wanted to balance this market-based dynamism with effective regulation, wanting services to be efficient, effective and comprehensive on the one hand, but without them being bureaucratic – as his critique of the present system was based on it stifling staff through those means.

If freedom from bureaucracy and 'social enterprise' were the first two elements of the reorganisation, the third was Lansley's claim to be putting in place 'a long-term vision for an NHS that is led by patients and professionals'. He claimed he would 'bring NHS resources and NHS decision making as close to the patient as possible' by introducing 'real, local democratic accountability to health care for the first time in almost 40 years by giving local authorities the power to agree local strategies to bring the NHS, public health and social care together.'

The appeal of Lansley's narrative for the public comes in giving them the 'right to choose', presenting healthcare as another consumer choice, and at the same driving up clinical standards as a result. Intuitively, who does not want more choice? Furthermore, if such choices would actually make the NHS better as a result, what grounds could there be for not wanting to agree with the reorganisation?

Lansley's narrative is an attempt to explain how his reorganisation would both abolish bureaucracy, and ensure there would be proper regulation and democratic accountability; it would put control of the NHS in the hands of patients and professionals, even while it is itself is designed by politicians; it will drive dynamism through 'social enterprise', but at the same time legislate for a 'stronger economic regulator'. The narrative, therefore, attempts to conceal or gloss over the multiple, long-standing problems the reorganisation faced. It misrepresented an oligopolistic market structure as having the dynamism of perfect competition through the label 'social enterprise', with no clear strategy for dealing with the financial failure of healthcare providers. It described no means through which patients were meant to make choices between different healthcare providers, and failed to take account for the fact that GPs would almost certainly lack the time or ability to make commissioning decisions. Last, it failed to demonstrate why and how the NHS should be put through significant reorganisation at a time when large budgetary savings were required.

Lansley's narrative locates GPs, the doctors closest to patients, as shoppers for care on behalf of patients (using a supermarket metaphor), but conceals the rationing for care that would result. 'Social enterprise' in turn concealed the antagonism of public and non-public providers attempting to compete within scarce resource limits for care contracts, in a situation where there was no real scope to allow large public care providers to financially fail because of their size and importance to the care 'market', and because they were crucial in guaranteeing continuity of care provision should non-public providers exit or financially fail – which they certainly subsequently did.

The picture presented by the opposition represents an alternative, but equally unviable narrative, that of the existing organisational form working 'well', and no reorganisation being necessary, at a time when health services across the world were facing significant challenges. Burnham appeared to be suggesting that the more limited use of the market that the previous government put in place had ameliorated the fundamental tensions in healthcare explored above, but which still did not address the antagonism between resources and need. The narrative offered here was based on stability and continuity – both of which are undoubtedly virtues – but hardly offering an inspiring alternative imaginary for the future of the National Health Service where the basic antagonisms underpinning healthcare remained unaddressed.

Discussion and conclusion

Did the debate hold the proposals adequately to account?

The debate ended up serving neither the government nor opposition well either in terms of scrutinising the ideas it offered, or of holding the government to account.

On the government side, the proposals seemed to have been subject to little detailed scrutiny, with Lansley not able to respond to criticisms about the privatisation of healthcare and lack of accountability in his proposed structures without some effort. This meant that suspicions from clinical representative groups and the public more generally were not allayed or responded to in detail. Discussion in the debate was often personalised and even rude. This suggests serious problems in the Parliamentary accountability process in that it left issues about privatisation and accountability in the Bill unexplored in depth. By not opening these issues to scrutiny, the end result is that health service reorganisation, regardless of whether it was needed or not, has become such a difficult and even politically toxic issue that no political party is likely to attempt it again soon (Timmins, 2012).

In sum, too little time was spent on considering the problematisation of the debate and there is a lack of a narrative to link the aims and means of reorganisation, with no clear sense of the main problem the reorganisation was meant to achieve. This also led to ample space for the opposition to develop conspiracy theories about privatisation and challenge government with those.

The voice of the opposition was remarkably muted – perhaps because the main opposition party had been in government too recently to criticise the service being offered, or to offer an alternative vision to that of the government. This suggests a significant problem for opposition to a new government making radical proposals – how is the opposition to counter? Equally, it may well be that old divisions in the Labour party over its health policy had yet to be resolved. Former Secretary of State Burnham appeared to change many of his the views he had formerly espoused in government when he was in opposition between 2010 and 2015. His apparent inconsistency on issues such as the role of the market in improving NHS care, made sustained criticisms of the coalition government on their proposals more difficult to credibly make.

The combination of a government without a reorganisation narrative and an opposition unable or unwilling to offer alternatives led to a process in which proposals were debated, but not tested as fully. If politics is meant to lead to practical action, then the politics of the debate was not a success.

What was the reorganisation for?

If we examine the debate, then the argument that the reorganisation is ideological appears to be arguably the strongest. In the debate (in contrast to the White Paper itself) the government gives a range of problems which the reorganisation was meant to address, but fails to answer the charges against it around stealth privatisation, and so it is hard to refute the alternative explanations that link Conservative business interests to private healthcare providers and their roles in lobbying for market-based healthcare reorganisation.

The government's articulation of the reorganisation failed to explain how the means it proposed would deal with the ambitious goals it specified. Equally, the failure of the Parliamentary process, the closeness to the election meaning the opposition perhaps did not scrutinise the proposals or offer a coherent alternative, do not offer an encouraging picture of Parliamentary debate or White Paper presentation.

The NHS Bill, eventually passed in 2012 after over two thousand amendments, appeared to satisfy no-one in that the market-based solution was blunted in the face of Liberal Democrat concerns about accountability, an online petition supported by the public sufficiently forcing an extra debate in Parliament and increasingly widespread clinical opposition. At the same time, opposition concerns about privatisation appear not to have been fully alleviated, in that the increased entry of non-public providers into NHS provision, and which the coalition government was so keen to encourage, seems to have occurred.

A final question (which comes from the analysis above) is to ask why it was that the marketisation of care in one form or another was so accepted by both government and opposition. Why was no alternative proposed?

One possible answer is that a consensus between both main political parties about market-based healthcare reorganisation appears to have been reached, with the only dispute being the extent of the privatisation associated with it. The market-based logic had dominated public reform in the US and UK since the 1980s, with the NHS initially appearing as a laggard (Klein, 1986). As barriers to change, such as the institutional power of the medical profession in blocking reorganisation and Conservative concerns about appearing to privatise care, were eroded (the latter not least as Labour appeared so keen to introduce non-public provision in the 2000s), then it began to seem that the only solutions under active consideration, by consecutive governments, were market-based. Combined with the easy appeal of presenting such proposals to the public as extending their choices, the proposals offer a narrative of harnessing the intrinsic antagonisms present in healthcare to creative ends through market-based solutions, while extending patient choice at the same time. This narrative, however, fails to get to grips with the intrinsic tensions present in providing healthcare, and so is somewhat chimerical.

In conclusion, it appeared then that the government's presentation of their reorganisation, both in the White Paper and in Parliament, contributed substantially to the problems they experienced in taking their Bill through the legislature. Their problematisation failed to adequately justify the reorganisation, and left the government open to a justifiable counter-claim that the reorganisation was ideologically grounded in expanding the use of market mechanisms into healthcare. The lack of alternatives imaginaries to this market-based model in the debate, however, suggests a failure of the opposition to articulate a genuine alternative to the reorganisation. While the Labour opposition were to later put forward proposals for reduced competition and reduced non-public involvement in provision and purchasing in the NHS, their failure to articulate this alternative and mobilise behind it (even while such an alternative existed in Scotland) at the time of the White Paper debate may have been a result of the coalition proposals appearing so close to the election, or as a result of such proposals running counter to Labour government policy before the election. In either case, without such a counter-narrative, the ability to mobilise opposition to the extent of blocking the Bill was always reduced. If the coalition government were guilty of pushing through badly-through-out and argued legislation, the opposition were guilty of failing to organise to prevent it.

References

Bacchi, C, 2009, Analysing policy: What's the problem represented to be? French's Forest: Pearson Australia

Dryzek, J, 1997, *The politics of the Earth: Environmental discourses*, Oxford: Oxford University Press

Fairclough, I, Fairclough, N, 2012, *Political discourse analysis*, London: Routledge

Fischer, F, 2003, *Reframing public policy: Discursive politics and deliberative practice*, Oxford: Oxford University Press

Gottweiss, H, 2006, Rhetoric in policy making: Between logos, ethos and pathos, in F Fischer, G Miller, M Sidney (eds), *Handbook of Public Policy*, Boca Raton, FL: CRC Press, 237–250

Greener, I, 2008, *Healthcare in the UK: Understanding continuity and change*, Bristol: Policy Press

Greener, I, Powell, M, 2009, The evolution of choice policies in UK housing, education and health policy, *Journal of Social Policy*, 38, 1, 63–81

HM Government, 2010, *The Coalition: Our programme for government*, London: Cabinet Office

Howarth, D, Griggs, S, 2012, Poststructuralist policy analysis: Discourse, hegemony and critical explanation, in F Fischer, H Gottweiss (eds), *The argumentative turn revisited: Public policy as communicative practice*, Durham, NC: Duke University Press

Klein, R, 1986, Why Britain's Conservatives support a socialist health care system, *Health Affairs*, 4, 1, 41–58

Lakoff, G, Johnson, M, 2008, *Metaphors we live by*, Chicago: University of Chicago Press

Oborne, P, 2005, *The rise of political lying*, London: Free Press

Packwood, A, 2002, Evidence-based policy: Rhetoric and Reality, *Social Policy and Society*, 1, 3, 267–72

Schön, D, Rein, M, 1995, *Frame reflection: Toward the resolution of intractable policy controversies*, London: Basic Books

Secretary of State for Health, 2010, *Equity and Excellence: Liberating the NHS*, London: The Stationery Office

Timmins, N, 2012, *Never again?* London: King's Fund and the Institute for Government

Torfing, J, 2005, Discourse theory: Achievements, Arguments and Challenges, in D Howarth, J Torfing (eds), *Discourse theory and European politics*, Basingstoke: Palgrave Macmillan

SEVEN

UK-wide health policy under the Coalition

David Hughes

Introduction

A volume on health reforms under the Coalition must necessarily expand its focus beyond Westminster to consider the larger UK policy context. Legislation enacted in 1998 established devolved assemblies in Scotland, Wales and Northern Ireland with powers to make law or issue executive orders in certain specified areas, including health services. This meant that an English NHS overseen by the Westminster Parliament now existed alongside separate NHS systems accountable to devolved governments in the other UK countries. While there had long been significant differences in the legislative frameworks shaping health care across the UK, with a distinctive Health and Social Care (HSC) service in Northern Ireland and separate Acts applying to England/Wales and Scotland, devolution accentuated policy divergence to the extent that it is now misleading to write of a unitary British NHS (Greer, 2004a).

The major Coalition health reforms heralded by the Health and Social Care Act 2012 thus applied in the main to England only. However, the acceleration of market reform in England posed urgent questions for the devolved administrations. They needed to formulate appropriate policy responses that either maintained differences or moved closer to the English policies. There were operational issues concerning interaction with the larger English system, such as the cross-border healthcare arrangements between England and Wales and Scotland, and the sharing of English services such as certain National Institute for Health and Clinical Excellence (NICE) products under agreements made by the devolved governments. Divergence intensified political controversy; increasingly the devolved NHS systems found themselves subjected to critical comparisons, with those lining up for or against the English market reforms searching for evidence that would support their arguments.

Clearly the four UK NHS systems are not equal. The English NHS, serving a population of 53.9 million and employing 1.4 million people, dwarfs the NHS systems of the other three countries. In Scotland 140,000 NHS staff serve a population of 5.3 million, while NHS Wales' 70,000 employees cater for 3.1 million residents, and Health and Social Care Northern Ireland employs 62,000 staff (including social care staff) to care for 1.8 million people. Yet although the English system dominates in terms of scale and supporting infrastructure, the other systems remain important as alternative NHS models that may yet influence future UK-wide health policy.

This chapter describes these divergent approaches, but also sheds light on the nature of coalition policy making. This volume as a whole discusses a rare period of coalition government in the first-past-the-post Westminster system, but proportional representation in the devolved legislatures has produced coalition governments as often as it has single-party rule (see Table 7.1). Looking at the experience of UK devolution may help us better understand how far electoral outcomes – and periods of coalition rule – affect the magnitude and pace of NHS change.

Big bang reforms such as the 1991 NHS internal market are often said to depend on strong Parliamentary majorities, as was the position with the later Thatcher and the Blair governments. Meanwhile devolution resulted in coalition governments in Scotland, Wales and Northern Ireland, which in the view of many observers resulted in a slower pace of change. Greer (2004b, 105) suggests that proportional representation in the devolved countries is part of the 'environment [that] shapes the

Table 7.1: UK and devolved governments 1997–2015

Westminster	Scotland	Wales	N. Ireland
1997–2010 Labour			
	1999–2003 Lab-Lib coalition	1999–2000 Labour	1999–2002 Multi-party coalition/ direct rule
		2000–03 Lab-Lib coalition	
			2002–07 Direct rule
	2003–07 Lab-Lib coalition	2003–07 Labour	
May 2010–2015 Con-Lib Coalition	2007–11 SNP	2007–11 Lab-Plaid coalition	2007–11 Multi-party coalition
	2011– SNP	2011– Labour	2011– Multi-party coalition
May 2015– Conservative			

ideology and strategy of UK governments' by encouraging 'shifting coalition politics'. In the early 2000s it appeared that divergent NHS policies in these countries could partly be explained by cross-party agreement that a period of stability was preferable to further reforms of the English kind.

Paradoxically the next big round of English reform, as represented by the Health and Social Care Act 2012, came under a Conservative/ Liberal Democrat coalition, and just at the time when the pendulum was swinging to single-party devolved administrations in Scotland and Wales. This reversed the earlier pattern of strong Westminster government and weak assembly coalitions. Nonetheless another round of English-style reforms remained unattractive to single-party SNP and Labour governments in Scotland and Wales, which along with Northern Ireland's coalition government preferred to maintain relative policy continuity.

Health policy before 2010

Although the Health and Social Care Act 2012 is resulting in transformative change of the English NHS, it was the Blair government's English NHS reforms after 2002 that had the greater influence on current health policy in the three devolved countries. The incoming Labour administration had promised to replace the internal market with an integrated NHS, but within five years it returned to policies favouring markets and competition. A series of related reforms concerned with autonomous foundation trust hospitals, independent-sector treatment centres, increased patient choice of provider, standard national tariffs for hospital treatments, and arms-length regulation through the Care Quality Commission and Monitor, created a provider market in which economic levers again played a central role (Hughes and Vincent-Jones, 2008).

Scotland, Wales and Northern Ireland had followed England's lead by strengthening system integration and encouraging cooperation rather than competition. They moved to 'soften' the internal market by de-emphasising contracting and encouraging 'partnership' working between purchasing authorities and NHS trusts. Just a few years later with the return to a market in England, they needed to decide whether or not to take a different path. Although a Labour Government had introduced the English reforms, Labour-led coalitions in Scotland and Wales were unenthusiastic and none of the three devolved countries adopted the English model. In 2004 Scotland abolished NHS trusts, which became operating divisions of the existing health boards, thus ending its internal market. Wales continued for a few years with a system in which Local Health Boards (LHBs) purchased from NHS trusts, before abolishing its internal market in 2009. Northern Ireland, under direct rule for most of this period, stayed closest to the pre-1997 model and retained a soft purchaser/provider split. We will consider the similarities and differences in approaches in this period, before considering further policy development under the Westminster coalition government.

Scotland pre-2010

The Scottish Labour–Liberal government that held power from 1999 to 2007 legislated to make Scotland the first devolved country to abolish its purchaser/provider split, thus illustrating that coalition governments do not necessarily limit themselves to incremental policy change. The end of the internal market was accompanied by the creation of community health partnerships within health boards to strengthen primary care, a statutory duty of cooperation for health boards, and a duty of NHS bodies to encourage public engagement contained in the NHS Reform (Scotland Act), 2004 (http://www.legislation.gov.uk/asp/2004/7/contents). Guthrie et al argue that, in contrast to English control via a mix of hierarchical command and market levers, the form of governance implemented in Scotland at this time was 'more a blend of mutuality (control through group processes) and oversight (although with less aggressive performance management by central government)' (2010, 11). Rather than English-style arms-length regulation through bodies like the Care Quality Commission and Monitor, Scotland created a more collaborative independent regulator in the form of NHS Quality Improvement Scotland. After 2006 a new Health Minister introduced a tougher performance management regime. A delivery group was established to agree delivery plans with each Board, linked to new HEAT (health, efficiency, access and treatment) targets, which were to become a distinctive feature of the Scottish system, more rigorous than the equivalent systems in Wales and Northern Ireland (Steel and Cylus, 2012, 114).

Mutuality was based largely on the central role given to managed clinical networks (MCNs) – linked groups of professionals able to operate across organisational boundaries to deliver effective services – a development that had first appeared at the end of the 1990s. The MCNs were a key mechanism in what Greer (2004a) called Scotland's bet on 'professionalism' – its attempt to harness professional commitment and collaboration combined with performance management – as an alternative to market incentives.

The return to strong single-party government with the Scottish National Party (SNP) election victory in 2007 resulted only in incremental change to the NHS structure its predecessor had established. There were pledges to reduce waiting times and increase accessibility and accountability, and a halting of restructuring plans that threatened the closure of emergency departments in some small district general hospitals. The SNP's plan for a more accountable 'mutual' NHS in which patients acted as co-owners and co-producers of better health was set out in the action plan, *Better Health, Better Care* (NHS Scotland, 2007). Among the proposals were a series of actions to strengthen patient influence on the design and delivery of services, the enactment of a *Patient Rights (Scotland)* Bill, an 18 week GP referral to specialist treatment guarantee, and directly-elected health boards.

Wales pre-2010

Wales started the 2000s with a Labour–Liberal government which pledged to oversee a period of stability in the NHS. Limited structural reform in 2003 to abolish the five health authorities and transfer commissioning responsibilities to 22 LHBs led to tension with Liberal coalition partners who argued that stability would be undermined by further reorganisation. Against this background Wales was content to follow the Blair government's early policy of softening the internal market. The language of NHS contracts gave way to that of 'long-term agreements' (LTAs), harder-edged contracting mechanisms such as penalty clauses and financial incentives were dropped, and attempts were made to develop 'collegiate' approaches to commissioning services. The move to smaller commissioning bodies, coterminous with local government, represented a form of administrative decentralisation designed to make the NHS more responsive to local communities and improve opportunities for joint working. Greer (2004a) argued that 'localism' marked out a distinctive Welsh approach emphasising the importance of better coordination of services and attention to the social determinants of health in particular localities.

This policy direction remained unchanged when England turned back to markets. Wales continued with soft commissioning in a purchaser/provider split system, and introduced regional commissioning groups to improve coordination between LHBs and hospital trusts. The first signs of significant policy divergence came in areas where English policy had moved and Wales declined to follow. The new Labour government in the Assembly after 2003 decided against foundation trust hospitals, national tariffs and use of independent-sector treatment centres. It was unsympathetic to the idea of an arms-length regulator, which policy makers believed reduced Ministerial accountability, and created a new body, Healthcare Inspectorate Wales (HIW) to take over the majority of the Healthcare Commission's functions. Patient choice of hospital provider, a central plank of reform in England, was rejected in Wales in favour of strengthening public engagement and patient voice.

The Welsh policy of localism was given additional impetus by the policy document *Making the Connections* (WAG, 2006a), which set out the case for an integrated, collaborative model of public sector service organisations, better suited to Welsh conditions. The 2006 *Beecham Report* (WAG, 2006b) suggested the creation of multi-agency, local service boards (LSBs) in each local government/LHB area which would facilitate coordinated action and strengthen engagement with communities. Waiting times became a major focus in the mid-2000s after a critical National Audit Office (Wales) report highlighted unfavourable comparisons with England, and this emerged as an issue in the run up to the 2005 UK general election.

Somewhat paradoxically it took a return to coalition government, in the form of a Labour/Plaid Cymru administration elected in 2007, before Wales followed Scotland by ending its internal market. Under Blair and Brown the political landscape had changed as nationalist parties in Wales and Scotland took up positions to the left of the Westminster Labour government, uniting in their opposition to market-based health reforms. In 2009 Wales abolished NHS trusts, which were now absorbed into unified health boards, and ended commissioning in favour of planning. Hierarchical command and performance management against national standards returned as the main governance mechanisms, though arguably less effectively than in Scotland.

Northern Ireland

Reform moved more slowly in Northern Ireland than in Wales or Scotland, mainly because political instability led to the suspension of the Stormont Parliament and a period of direct rule from Westminster. At a time when politicians across the Protestant/Catholic divide found power sharing difficult, responsibility for maintaining an effective service fell mainly on civil servants and senior managers. Greer (2004a, 4) characterises the approach that emerged as 'permissive managerialism', what he describes as 'a system that focuses on keeping services going in tough conditions and otherwise produces little overall policy'.

Actually it is incorrect to say there was no policy development. Irish policy makers were well aware of the need for modernisation and overhaul of public services, and in 2002 one of the final acts of the devolved Northern Ireland Executive had been to launch a major Review of Public Administration (RPA) that was to impact on health services by the end of the decade. The initiative was taken forward by the direct rule ministers from autumn 2002 and the RPA investigated almost 150 bodies, including the District Councils, the Health Boards and Trusts and the Education Boards, before reporting in 2005. The reform proposals that emerged included a reduction in the number of existing Trusts from 19 to 6, replacement of the old Health and Social Services Boards with a single authority overseeing local commissioning groups, and the formation of a Patient and Client Council to replace the four health and social services councils.

Devolved rule was re-established in 2007 with a multi-party coalition government, and a Draft Programme for Government was approved early the following year. The overall emphasis of the RPA report had been on cooperation within an integrated health and social care system, with an explicit rejection of competition as a driver for efficiency. However, an independent review undertaken by the economist John Appleby criticised the proposed re-configuration as representing a reinvented pre-1990 English NHS model. Appleby argued that

> while partnership and integration can generate good things for patients and users, there is a distinct danger that the performance model implied by the RPA's structural reform could fail to provide the necessary incentives and sanctions – or bite – to encourage providers of services to continually seek out new ways to improve their performance. (Appleby 2005, 171)

The Appleby report instead recommended a sharper separation of purchasers and providers, more use of penalties and incentives within contracts and reimbursement based on standard tariffs (closer to the English Payment by Results system). For a time movement towards English-style policies seemed possible, but in the event the Assembly government opted to maintain a direction of reform closer to the partnership policies emerging in Scotland and Wales, though with a soft internal market still in place.

Overview

By 2010 the three devolved assemblies were growing in confidence and capacity. The Scottish Parliament had had power to make law affecting healthcare since 1998, and was pushing for increased budgetary and fiscal autonomy. The Government of Wales Act 2006 (http://www. legislation.gov.uk/ukpga/2006/32/contents) gave the Assembly law-making powers in twenty designated subject areas, including heath, thus building on its authority to issue executive orders. Since establishment the Northern Ireland Assembly had had powers to legislate on 'transferred matters', including health and social services, and the more stable political climate meant that devolved policy making again became feasible. The multi-party coalition government in power from 2007 to 2011 was the first since devolution to run its full course without suspension.

By 2010 the four UK health care systems lay along a continuum that ranged from England's regulated market, through Northern Ireland's soft purchaser/provider split, to the integrated health boards found in Scotland and Wales. Policy divergence already extended into such domains as use of private providers for NHS services, patient choice (Peckham et al 2012), patient and public involvement (Hughes et al, 2009), and (to a lesser extent) approaches to health inequalities (Smith et al, 2009). Charges for prescription drugs still in place in England had been phased out in the devolved countries. Hospital car parking charges remained in England and Northern Ireland, but had been ended by most Scottish and Welsh hospitals. Scotland had broken rank with the other countries to offer free personal social care for the over 65s.

Devolved health policies under the UK Coalition Government 2010–15

The formation of the UK Conservative/Liberal Democrat Government in May 2010 coincided with a period of deepening austerity (see Chapter 3). Chancellor George Osborne's Spending Review in October foreshadowed average cuts in departmental spending of about 19% and a loss of over 400,000 public sector jobs. Arguably, policy development in the devolved countries had been facilitated by relatively generous block grants from the UK Parliament, which between 2002/03 and 2009/10 had allowed real-terms health spending per person to grow by 43% across the UK as a whole (Johnson and Phillips, 2014). Now there were to be substantial cuts in central funding of the devolved governments over the following four years – 6.8% for Scotland, 7.5% for Wales and 6.9% for Northern Ireland. While the UK Government pledged to protect the English NHS from a real-terms funding cut, only the Northern Ireland Executive – with its combined health and social care system – followed suit. The Scottish and Welsh governments committed only to maintain NHS spending in cash terms, so as to avoid the harsh cuts in other departmental budgets imposed in England. As a consequence health spending per head in all three devolved countries dipped after 2010, with Scotland and Wales seeing overall falls during the four-year period, and Northern Ireland then raising spending and seeing a slight overall rise by 2014/15 (see Figure 7.1).

Austerity brought renewed calls from governments for further performance improvement and cost savings, and raised questions about how far NHS systems that emphasised integration and cooperation could meet these challenges when compared with the more market-

Figure 7.1: Spending on health per head of population 2010–11 to 2014–15 (2014–15 prices)

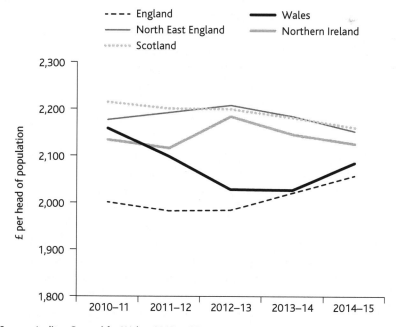

Source: Auditor General for Wales, 2015 p. 27

oriented English service. The Westminster Government's strategy was to seek further efficiency gains through a stronger dose of market medicine, harnessing competition and financial incentives. But strikingly there was no move in the devolved countries to cope with difficult economic conditions by following the English model; instead the devolved governments opted to stick to their integrated public NHS models, in each case seeking to fashion a distinctive approach appropriate to local conditions.

Scotland post-2010

As the SNP moved towards a second term in office, mutuality, partnership, and patient rights remained as central policy themes. Ministerial statements continued to be unsympathetic to market reform or increased private provision of NHS services. The proposed Patient Rights (Scotland) Act (http://www.legislation.gov.uk/asp/2011/5/contents) was duly enacted in 2011, giving patients the statutory right inter alia to have their needs and what would be of optimum benefit considered, to have access to an independent Patient Advice and Support Service, and recourse to an enhanced patient complaints and feedback system.

In 2011 the Scottish Government published its 20:20 Vision (NHS Scotland, 2011) – a strategic plan for the NHS up until 2020. The major innovation was a move towards integrated health and social care services based on close cooperation between Health Boards and Local Authorities. This strategy also emphasised the importance of health promotion and disease prevention, more use of day-case treatments as the norm in hospitals, more community-based treatments and rapid return home of patients after hospital treatment. There was to be a new quality strategy and the establishment of a Scottish Patient Safety Programme.

While seemingly the proposals for integration took Scotland closer to the Northern Ireland model of a single unified health and social service, in fact the approach was more incremental and permissive. The arrangements set out in the Public Bodies (Joint Working) (Scotland) Act 2014 (http://www.legislation.gov.uk/asp/2014/9/contents/enacted) allowed pairs of Health Boards and Local Authorities to choose between two implementation models. They could elect to delegate responsibility for planning and resourcing services to an 'Integration Joint Board', or alternatively empower the Health Board or Local Authority to act as the lead agency taking responsibility for organising integrated health and social care services.

Translating this policy blueprint into an operational reality proved difficult in a period of financial constraint. The funding pressures affecting NHS Scotland after 2010 were partly a result of a diminishing block grant from Westminster, but also reflected the Scottish Government's decision to limit protection of the NHS budget so as to soften cuts to other public services. Audit Scotland's figures show a real terms reduction in NHS spending of about 0.7% between 2008/09 and 2014/15 (Auditor General for Scotland, 2015, 9).

Tightening funding contributed to problems of rising waiting times and uneven staff recruitment. Arguably the HEAT target system – Scotland's performance management alternative to English market levers – allowed it to cope better with these pressures than the other devolved administrations (see Steel and Cylus, 2012, 113). However waiting times continued to be a problem until the end of the period. The Auditor General's 2015 report found that seven of nine key waiting times targets and service standards had been missed, suggesting a general decline in performance in recent years. The Auditor General concluded that financial pressures were threatening to derail long-term plans, and that the 'Scottish Government needs to increase the pace of change if it is to achieve its 2020 vision' (Auditor General for Scotland, 2015, 6).

The foregoing problems also put question marks against the Scottish Government's policy of phasing out use of the private sector for NHS work. SNP campaigning in the run-up to the 2015 Scotland independence referendum had made much of the threat posed by the agenda of privatisation represented by the ongoing English NHS reforms. Yet paradoxically the value of private sector services purchased by the NHS appeared to be rising during the period of SNP rule. Audit Scotland estimated that overall spending on the private sector by the NHS in Scotland has risen from £72.3m in 2009/10 to £85.2m in 2014/15, an 18% real terms increase (Auditor General for Scotland, 2015). This was mainly to meet waiting time targets and standards by increasing short-term capacity, but also for some specialist services not available in NHS hospitals.

Wales post-2010

The transition from the Labour/Plaid Cymru coalition to a Welsh Labour Government did not signal any major change in policy direction. Although an updated strategy document *Together for Health* was produced (Welsh Government, 2012), this continued the established policy themes of a service better attuned to Welsh needs and preferences, equitable healthcare for all, and improved quality (Riley, 2016). The major challenges recognised by policy makers remained those identified in the Wanless Report (WAG 2003): poor health arising from social disadvantage, shortcomings in NHS resource utilisation, ineffective joint working between health and social care services, weak public engagement, and the need to shift activity from acute hospitals to new services and plan better for an ageing population with more chronic illness. Generally the approach was to move incrementally forward to address these problems, at least as far as budgetary constraints and political controversy allowed. Alleged shortcomings in standards and outcomes in the Welsh NHS had figured in the 2010 election campaign and continued to feature in the policy debate over the Health and Social Care Bill, with pro-marketeers pointing to Wales as an example of what an old-style public NHS would deliver. The Welsh NHS remained in the firing line throughout the Coalition's term, as when PM Cameron stated at the 2014 Welsh Conservative conference that 'when Offa's Dyke becomes the line between life and death, we are witnessing a national scandal' (BBC, 2014). This made the NHS an area of vulnerability for Welsh Labour politicians and meant that performance against standards, particularly those relating to waiting times, ambulance response times, healthcare acquired infections, and care quality, stayed high on political agendas. The higher cross-border flows between England and Wales compared with the other devolved countries opened a space for controversy and criticism, whether in terms of just who was eligible for free prescriptions, access to high-cost cancer drugs in Wales, or Welsh Health Boards' continued use of English treatment centres to manage waiting times.

With the Welsh system still adjusting to the abolition of its internal market in 2009, NHS managers were working to re-establish an effective planning system and bed in the integrated LHBs. Under the coalition there had been a controversial attempt to rationalise acute services by concentrating some surgery in 'centres of excellence'. This policy had been largely halted in the face of campaigns to protect local hospitals, but was now considered again as a way of maximising value for money. Interestingly, the notion of commissioning reappeared around 2013, though in the context of the attempt to re-model the concept as a planning rather than a market instrument, and mainly in relation to emergency ambulance services, high-cost mental health placements, and joint commissioning with social services.

As elsewhere, policy makers were preoccupied with maintaining quality and performance standards under constrained NHS budgets.

The Assembly had voted to cap the NHS budget in order to give more protection to social care and schools than other parts of the UK. Consequently the Welsh NHS suffered a bigger financial squeeze than the services in the other devolved countries, although this was eased somewhat by an increase in funding in 2014/15.

The Welsh Government's big idea for improving services in a time of austerity is 'prudent healthcare'. This concept was developed by the Bevan Commission (2013, 3) , which advises the Health Minister, and has been defined as: 'healthcare which is conceived, managed and delivered in a cautious and wise way characterised by forethought, vigilance and careful budgeting which achieves tangible benefits and quality outcomes for patients'. Prudent healthcare is conceived as healthcare that is parsimonious but efficient; it seeks to get more for less by minimising waste and maximising clinical effectiveness. The initiative represents a re-packaging of several familiar components – co-production by professionals and patients, involving people in their care, prioritising according to clinical need (rather than targets), not over-treating, accelerating innovation, increased focus on patient safety and evidence-based treatments – and it remains to be seen whether it can achieve more than the sum of its parts. Certainly the initiative will face formidable obstacles in terms of re-jigging existing budgets, self-protective behaviour from the acute sector and opposition from some health professionals.

Riley (2016, 42), a recently-retired strategy advisor to the Department of Health and Social Services, has highlighted health inequalities as a key area for policy development during this period. Arguably, the Welsh Government moved more quickly than the other devolved administrations to take coordinated action across departments to address social disadvantage and the determinants of poor health. Better connections were made between policies targeting poverty reduction, community regeneration, early childhood support and more multi-faceted and integrated health policies (Public Health Wales, 2013). An important start had been made with the '1000 Lives' and '1000 Lives Plus' public health campaigns that sought to save lives and reduce preventable morbidity. This policy drive influenced the content of the Public Health (Wales) Bill that is before the Assembly at the time of writing, which inter alia will further discourage tobacco/nicotine use (one of the major drivers of health variations across social classes).

A balance sheet of achievement in Wales during this period shows a mixed picture. A recent Auditor General report concludes that

> Overall, the NHS has improved against some public health measures and against some of its key performance measures on quality. But against a context of rising demand and activity in some areas, notably cancer care, performance against measures of waiting times – for elective care, emergency care and cancer care – have deteriorated. (Auditor General for Wales, 2015, 11)

Problems in managing waiting times – especially in orthopaedics and ophthalmology – meant that several health boards increased the value of activity undertaken by private providers, causing politicians to backtrack from earlier promises to end use of the private sector for NHS work. Riley (2016, 41), suggests that while progress was made in many areas, there was a failure to achieve the cumulative policy development that should have been possible: 'Statements of strategic intention have not succeeded each other seamlessly or been followed through. Ministers can blame electoral and financial challenges, but it is difficult to see convincing drivers for success designed into the Welsh NHS'.

Northern Ireland post-2010

By 2010 Northern Ireland was moving ahead with the second phase of RPA reforms set out in the 2009 Health and Social Care (Reform) Act (NI) as the government simplified the structure of health and social services (O'Neill et al, 2012). The reforms created a single commissioning body, the *Health and Social Care Board* (HSCB), which set up subcommittees known as local commissioning groups (LCGs) to purchase services from five coterminous integrated care trusts. The HSCB was also responsible for managing contracts for primary health services provided by GPs, dentists, opticians and community pharmacists. Revenue resource limits (RRLs) were fixed for the individual trusts based on a weighted capitation formula, which took account of utilisation, age and gender structure and an 'economies of scale' component. Northern Ireland thus maintained a soft purchaser/provider split, which did not incorporate the building blocks of the English market such as clinical commissioning groups or foundation trusts, and (at least initially) made limited use of the private sector to control waiting times. National tariffs are not used for NHS work, although some contracts for private-sector work utilised tariff-based payments similar to those applying in England. As before the emphasis was on cooperation rather than competition.

At the May 2011 Northern Ireland election the Democratic Unionist Party and Sinn Féin remained the largest parties, and the Executive that resulted was again a five-party coalition with the Ulster Unionists losing one ministerial place compared with the previous administration. This left the policy direction set in 2007 broadly unchanged, although as in the other countries adjustments were needed to cope with worsening public finances. 2011 saw a second *Rapid Review* by Appleby (2011), which identified a potential £1 billion funding gap by 2014/15, and then a more substantial exercise undertaken by a panel led by John Compton, then Chief Executive of the HSCB. The resultant report, *Transforming Your Care* (DHSCS, 2011), still sets the policy direction for Northern Ireland at the time of writing. This was so despite a period of uncertainly when the coalition came under strain following allegations that Sinn Féin had continuing links with the Provisional IRA after the August 2014 McGuigan murder, and amidst wrangling about new welfare cuts proposed in the December 2014 Stormont House agreement.

Appleby (2011) had raised doubts about the sustainability of existing health and social care provision and *Transforming Your Care* aimed to identify a model of integrated services that could endure into the 21st century. The key themes resembled those found in the Scottish and Welsh plans, but were packaged to fit with the already unified HSC service. There were moves to reduce pressure on acute services by supporting people to live independently and to provide more care close to home. The report recommended an increased focus on patient safety and clinical effectiveness, and concentration of specialist services to maximise value for money. It suggested prioritising care for the most vulnerable. One innovative idea put forward was Integrated Care Partnerships – networks with representatives from general practice, pharmacy, acute medicine, nursing, allied health professions, social care and ambulance services who would work across organisational boundaries to develop new pathways and ways of working for particular client groups and conditions. As in Wales, initiatives to address inequalities in the healthcare domain were buttressed by cross-departmental actions to address poverty, sustainable communities, healthier behaviours, and early years of childhood interventions.

Like other parts of the UK, Northern Ireland used the private sector to control waiting times, but in September 2014 the HSC Board stopped renewing contracts with independent providers, which it said it could not afford to fund. This was a consequence of the worsening budgetary position, but also reflected the difficulty of arranging an emergency allocation during a period when cooperation between the governing parties in Stormont had broken down. However this appears to be a temporary situation as the HSCB's 2015/16 Commissioning Plan states that services will be purchased from the independent sector where appropriate.

Northern Ireland remained the only home country to combine a purchaser/provider split with integrated health and social services, but did not seek to emulate the changes occurring in England. Incremental development was hampered somewhat by the difficult financial climate and performance deteriorated in some areas as budgets became even less favourable after 2013. The latest Northern Ireland Audit Office Report cautions that

> the financial health of HSC bodies is weak and declining. Increasingly they have found it harder to balance their budgets in the face of rising inflationary cost pressures, demographic pressures from an increasing and ageing population and the pressures associated with new treatments and patient expectations, while at the same time delivering a challenging programme of efficiency savings. (Comptroller and Auditor General for Northern Ireland, 2015, 5)

The Audit Office found a deterioration in performance against several key targets in the preceding two years including the 13 week inpatient treatment target, the 18 week first outpatient appointment target, the 62 day urgent cancer referral to treatment target, and the 12 hour emergency care wait target (Comptroller and Auditor General for Northern Ireland, 2015, 16–19).

Discussion

There has been lively debate between commentators who detect a global trend towards convergence in health care systems (Wessen, 1999; Mechanic and Rochefort, 1996) and those who argue that political and ideological differences would ensure continuing divergence, in particular between planned and market systems (Powell, 1999; Stevens, 2009). The experience of the UK and other European countries suggests that divergent systems can indeed emerge and endure, even in societies with similar economic and cultural characteristics. In the decentralised Italian and Spanish national health systems, strikingly different policies have emerged at regional or provincial level, which mean that one 'system' can include different organisational variants with differing mixes of markets and planning (Del Pino and Pavolini,

2015). The UK experience supports the 'continuing divergence' side of the argument.

The English reforms introduced by Prime Minister Cameron's coalition government did not lead to immediate corresponding changes in the devolved countries, but they widened the gap between the market-oriented English system and the integrated public systems of the other three countries. Admittedly the English market remains a heavily managed one, and all the UK countries share a commitment to founding principles of the NHS such as universality, comprehensiveness and free services at the point of need, but a significant point of difference has opened in terms of utilisation of competition and non-NHS providers.

Scotland, Wales and Northern Ireland have each developed distinctive approaches which represent subtle variations on the integrated NHS model. Although the labels attached to programmes differ, they combine common building blocks such as partnership between professionals and service users, integrated working across organisations, public engagement, close to home treatments, and value for money (Prior et al, 2012). One might argue that what we are seeing here is similar to Freud's (1961, 78) 'narcissism of minor differences'; an attempt by devolved governments to over-emphasise small differences to underline national identity. Of course in the longer term there is the possibility that small differences become bigger ones. At present there is no sign that Scotland or Wales will draw nearer to the English market approach, and Northern Ireland, though retaining its soft purchaser/provider split, is edging closer to the other devolved countries.

Much has been made of the possibility that the 'natural experiment' created by the differing health policies of the four countries could yield valuable lessons, but comparative studies remain thin on the ground (Timmins, 2013). Policy and operational differences in areas like patient choice, patient and public involvement, and health inequalities have been investigated, but findings on system outcomes remain inconclusive. Systematic comparisons are hampered by lack of standardised definitions and comparable official data across the four countries, as well as differences in demography and morbidity. Given the problem of controlling for confounding variables and various concurrent reform initiatives occurring at a given time, it is unlikely that single studies can produce definitive findings on, say, whether the English market works more efficiently than the integrated Scottish system, or even which of the respective performance management systems works best. That is not to say that such questions are unanswerable, but it seems clear that we need to aggregate the findings of many studies conducted over a lengthy time period to be confident about the patterns emerging.

In a Foreword summarising the findings of the latest of the Nuffield Trust's comparative UK-wide studies, Jennifer Dixon and Andrew McKeon note that the

> different policies adopted by each country appear to have made little difference to long-term national trends on most of the indicators that the authors were able to compare. Individual countries can point to marginal differences in performance in one or more areas. This lack of clear-cut differences in performance may be surprising given the extent of debate about differences in structure, provider competition, patient choice and use of non-NHS providers across the four countries. (Bevan et al, 2014, 8)

This study suggests that in respect of performance on hospital waiting times England and Scotland do rather better than Wales and Northern Ireland, but does not answer the question of whether English-style market levers are necessarily better than performance management through Scotland's HEAT system.

The big question as the Westminster Coalition Government gave way to a Conservative one was whether, as the Health and Social Care Act began to take effect, divergence with the devolved countries would be accentuated, particularly in the area of privatisation. While NHS spending on non-NHS providers is edging up, and in 2014/15 stood at about £10.4 billion of £112 billion total NHS expenditure (Lafond, 2015), any mass transfer of core service provision away from NHS hospitals still lies in the future (see Chapters 3 and 11). Because of lack of directly comparable statistics it is difficult to be precise about the relative positions of the devolved countries. Perhaps surprisingly, spending on independent providers by health boards in Scotland and Wales is also rising, although it remains at close to 1% of total NHS spending (Auditor General for Scotland, 2015; Smith, 2015). Regarding capital expenditure too, all three of the devolved countries are continuing to use private finance initiative (PFI) contracts to build and run health and social care facilities, with numbers of projects lower than in England but not wildly out of line with relative populations (see table 2). This suggests that though NHS spending on the private sector is growing faster in England, there is also some continuing growth in the devolved countries.

Conclusion

As the period of Westminster coalition government ended, the policy gap between England and the three devolved countries continued to slowly widen. The English NHS reforms had not triggered major legislative changes elsewhere, but Scotland, Wales and Northern Ireland maintained their divergent paths with further incremental adjustments. Although Northern Ireland retained a purchaser/provider split, it showed no signs of convergence with the English policies. A new status quo was solidifying where the four systems retained a shared commitment to publicly funded, comprehensive healthcare, available to all permanent residents, while differing in their organisational characteristics and the benefits and entitlements provided (see Table 7.2).

The policy differences between England and the other home countries are seen by most commentators to reflect differing centres of political gravity and the greater acceptability of neo-liberal policies to the English electorate. However, political economy does not plausibly explain the differences between Scotland, Wales and Northern Ireland. Here we need to consider how healthcare systems are embedded within institutional frameworks shaped by different histories, policy legacies, interest groups and path dependent processes (see Hughes

Table 7.2: The NHS systems, their organisational characteristics, and charges and entitlements

	England	Scotland	Wales	N. Ireland
Population, 2015 (millions)	53.9	5.3	3.1	1.8
Spend per head, 2012/13	£1,912	£2,115	£1,954	£2,109
Organisational characteristics				
Purchaser/provider split	Yes	No	No	Yes
National tariffs	Yes	No	No	No
Integrated health and social care	No	Some projects	No	Yes
Current PFI projects, 2015	123	27	11	6
Charges and entitlements				
Free prescriptions	No	Yes	Yes	Yes
Free social care for over 65s	No	Yes	No	No
Free hospital car parking	No	Yes, except existing PFI contracts	Yes, except existing contracts	No

Adapted from Bevan et al, (2014, p 30). Spend per head data comes from same source. Source of PFI data: HM Treasury (includes social care provided by NHS authority) https://www.google.com/fusiontables/DataSource?docid =1a5elgg64bBjV9kFGbRyK78UQbWBOXjdbjrdX-d0L#rows:id=1 and Vincent-Jones, 2008; Quadagno, 2010). Greer (2004b, 7) argues that policy outcomes are inextricably tied to territories and their local history and institutions: 'policies have histories and contexts. They will be filtered through policy communities that are entrenched in their jurisdiction, and politicians whose sense of their own and their parties' situation shapes their behaviour'. These powerful institutional and micro-political forces are likely to keep the devolved governments on divergent policy trajectories well into the 21st century.

References

Appleby, J, 2005, *Independent review of health and social care services in Northern Ireland*, Belfast: Department of Health, Social Services and Public Safety of Northern Ireland

Appleby, J, 2011, *Rapid review of Northern Ireland Health and Social Care funding needs and the productivity challenge: 2011/12–2014/15*, Belfast: Department of Health, Social Services and Public Safety of Northern Ireland

Auditor General for Scotland, 2015, *NHS in Scotland 2015*, Edinburgh: Audit Scotland.

Auditor General for Wales, 2015, *A Picture of Public Services 2015*, Cardiff: Wales Audit Office, www.audit.wales/system/files/publications/POPS_2015_eng.pdf

BBC, 2014, David Cameron: Offa's Dyke is 'life and death' divider, www.bbc.co.uk/news/uk-wales-politics-26956254

Bevan, G, Karanikolos, M, Exley, J, Nolte, E, Connolly, S, Mays, N, 2014, *The Four Health Systems of the United Kingdom: How do they compare?* London: Nuffield Trust and The Health Foundation

Bevan Commission, 2013, *Simply Prudent Healthcare: achieving better care and value for money in Wales* www.bevancommission.org/sitesplus/documents/1101/Bevan%20Commission%20Simply%20Prudent%20Healthcare%20v1%2004122013.pdf

Comptroller and Auditor General for Northern Ireland, 2015, General Report on the Health and Social Care Sector2012/13 and 2013/14, Belfast: NIAO.

Del Pino, E, Pavolini, E, 2015, Decentralisation at a time of harsh austerity: multilevel governance and the welfare state in Spain and Italy facing the crisis, *European Journal of Social Security* 17, 2, 246–270

Department of Health, Social Care and Safety, 2011, *Transforming your care: A review of health and social care in Northern Ireland*, Belfast: DHSCS

Freud, S, 1961, *Civilization and its discontents*, London: WW Norton

Greer, S, 2004a, *Four-way bet: How devolution has led to four different models for the NHS*, London: UCL, The Constitution Unit

Greer, S, 2004b, *Territorial politics and health policy: UK health policy in comparative perspective*, Manchester: Manchester University Press

Guthrie, B, Davies, H, Greig, G, Rushmer, R, Walker, I, Duguid, A, Coyle, J, Sutton, M, Williams, B, Farrar, S, Connaghan, J, 2010, *Delivering health care through Managed Clinical Networks (MCNs): Lessons from the North. Report for the NIHR SDO Programme*. London: HMSO

Hughes, D, Vincent-Jones, P, 2008, Schisms in the church: NHS systems and institutional divergence in England and Wales, *Journal of Health and Social Behavior* 49, 4, 400–416.

Hughes, D, Mullen, C, Vincent-Jones, P, 2009, Choice versus voice? PPI policies and the re-positioning of the state in England and Wales, 12, 3, 237–250.

Johnson, P, Phillips, D, 2014, The *Scottish NHS: More financially secure outside the UK?* London: Institute of Financial Studies, www.ifs.org.uk/publications/7366

Lafond, S, 2015, Transparency: The cure to mistrust of the private sector in the NHS? *Public Finance*, August 14, www.publicfinance.co.uk/opinion/2015/08/transparency-cure-mistrust-private-sector-nhs

Mechanic, D, Rochefort, DA, 1996, Comparative medical systems, *Annual Review of Sociology* 22, 239–270

NHS Scotland, 2007, *Better health, better care: Action Plan*. Edinburgh: NHS Scotland

NHS Scotland, 2011, *Achieving sustainable quality in Scotland's healthcare: A '20:20' vision*. Edinburgh: NHS Scotland. Available at: http://www.gov.scot/Topics/Health/Policy/2020-Vision/Strategic-Narrative (accessed 15 April 2016)

O'Neill, C, McGregor, P, Merkur, S, 2012, *United Kingdom (Northern Ireland) health system review, Health Systems in Transition* 14, 10, 1–91, www.euro.who.int/__data/assets/pdf_file/0007/177136/Northern-Ireland-HiT.pdf

Peckham, S, Mays, N, Hughes, D, Sanderson, M, Allen, P, Prior, L, Entwistle, V, Thompson, A, Davies, H, 2012, Devolution and patient choice: Policy rhetoric versus experience in practice, *Social Policy and Administration* 46, 2, 199–218

Powell, FD, 1999, Patterns of health care system change, in FD Powell and AF Wessen, eds, *Health care systems in transition: an international perspective*, Thousand Oaks, CA: Sage, pp 393-413

Prior, L, Hughes, D, Peckham, S, 2012, The discursive turn in policy analysis and the validation of policy stories, *Journal of Social Policy* 41, 2, 271–289

Public Health Wales, 2013, Transforming health improvement in Wales: Working together to build a healthier, happier future. Available at: http://www.wales.nhs.uk/sitesplus/documents/986/PHW%20 Health%20Improvement%20Review%20Final%20Report%20-%20 260913.pdf (accessed 15 April 2016)

Quadagno, J, 2010, Institutions, interest groups, and ideology: An agenda for the sociology of health care reform, *Journal of Health and Social Behavior* 51, 2, 125–136

Riley, C, 2016, The challenge of creating a 'Welsh NHS', *Journal of Health Services Research Policy* 21: 40–42

Smith, KE, Hunter, DJ, Blackman, T, Elliott, E, 2009, Divergence or convergence? Health inequalities and policy in a devolved Britain, *Critical Social Policy* 29: 216–42

Smith, M, 2015, Welsh NHS spends £19m on private healthcare in just 12 months, *Wales Online*, October 12, www.walesonline.co.uk/ news/health/welsh-nhs-spends-19m-private-10237147

Steele, D, and Cylus, J, 2012, United Kingdom (Scotland): health system review. Health systems in transition, 14 (9). World Health Organization, 2012. Available at: http://eprints.lse.ac.uk/49652/1/ Cylus_Scotland_health%20_system_2012.pdf (accessed 15 April 2016)

Stevens, F, 2009, The convergence and divergence of modern health care systems, in WC Cockerham (ed.), *The New Blackwell Companion to Medical Sociology*, Oxford: Blackwell Publishers

Timmins, N, 2013, *The four UK health systems: Learning from each other*, London: The King's Fund

WAG (Welsh Assembly Government), 2003, *The review of health and social care in Wales*, The Report of the Project Team advised by Derek Wanless. Cardiff: WAG, www.wales.nhs.uk/documents/wanless-review-e.pdf

WAG, 2005, *Designed for life: Creating world class health and social care for Wales in the 21st century*, Cardiff: WAG

WAG, 2006a, *Making the connections, Delivering beyond boundaries: Transforming Public Services in Wales*, Cardiff: WAG

WAG, 2006b, *Beyond boundaries: Citizen-centred local services for Wales* (Beecham Report), Cardiff: WAG

Welsh Government, 2012, Together for health: A five year vision for the NHS in Wales, Cardiff: WAG

Wessen, AF, 1999, Structural differences and healthcare reform, in FD Powell and AF Wessen, eds, *Health care systems in transition: an international Perspective*. Thousand Oaks, CA: Sage, pp 369-348

Section C:
Commissioning and service provision

EIGHT

Clinically led commissioning: past, present and future?

*Kath Checkland, Anna Coleman, Imelda McDermott
and Stephen Peckham*

Introduction

One of the key elements of the Health and Social Care Act 2012 (HSCA 2012) was the transfer of responsibility for commissioning healthcare services from managerially led Primary Care Trusts (PCTs) to newly established Clinical Commissioning Groups (CCGs), led by General Practitioners (family doctors or primary care physicians, generally known as GPs). The 2010 White paper, 'Equity and Excellence' argued that:

> Commissioning by GP consortia [now known as CCGs] will mean that the redesign of patient pathways and local services is always clinically led and based on more effective dialogue and partnership with hospital specialists. It will bring together responsibility for clinical decisions and for the financial consequences of these decisions (Department of Health, 2010, paragraph 4.4).

The document goes on to acknowledge that this approach is not wholly new, arguing that, 'commissioning never became a real transfer of responsibility. So we will learn from the past, and offer a clear way forward for GP consortia' (Department of Health, 2010, paragraph 4.5).

In this chapter we examine that history, and explore what can be learnt from previous attempts to involve GPs in commissioning care. We will then apply that learning to the provisions of the HSCA 2012, highlighting the correspondences and discontinuities between what we know from history and what was proposed. We will then go on to present evidence from our research on CCGs, exploring what happened in practice when CCGs were established. Finally, we will discuss the continuing evolution of health policy in the UK in the light of both historical evidence and our current findings. Throughout this chapter, the focus is upon GP involvement in commissioning, rather than the wider concern of clinician involvement. This is because the explicit goal of the HSCA 2012 was to bring GPs back into the forefront of commissioning.

Clinically led commissioning: a brief history

This and the subsequent section draw on a comprehensive literature review carried out between 2011 and 2014 (Miller et al, 2012; Miller et al, 2015), where all the relevant references can be found. Clinical involvement in the commissioning of healthcare services started with the introduction of the quasi-market into the NHS in 1991. The function of *purchasing* services was separated out from their *provision*, with Health Authorities established as purchasing bodies, responsible for assessing population needs and purchasing care from semi-autonomous NHS Trusts. Needs assessment within Health Authorities was led by public health professionals, with managers responsible for agreeing and monitoring contracts (Flynn and Williams 1997). At the same time, GP practices were invited to take on budgets for some aspects of services, notably elective (planned) care and prescribing. This was known as GP 'fundholding' (GPFH), and over the next five years approximately 50% of GP practices took on GPFH. From 1991–2010, GP involvement in what came to be called 'commissioning' waxed and waned, with successive reorganisations increasing, diminishing and reintroducing GP involvement as governments wrestled with problems of efficiency, effectiveness and engagement.

Table 8.1 summarises the characteristics of the various GP-led commissioning initiatives.

Thus, the nature of GP involvement in commissioning has varied over time. In particular, the extent of GP involvement has oscillated between leadership (fundholding, Total Purchasing Pilots (TPPs), Primary Care Groups (PCGs), CCGs) and a more advisory role (Locality Commissioning, Primary Care Trusts (PCTs), Practice-based Commissioning (PBC)). Each iteration of policy was intended to remedy the problems of what went before. Throughout this period, however, the 'programme theories' underpinning clinical commissioning schemes remained the same: first, that engaged GPs would be more likely to be efficient and effective purchasers of services for this patients as they would have greater knowledge of patient needs; and second that incentivised GPs would be more likely to act

Table 8.1: History of GP-led Commissioning in England

Date	Innovation	Scope of scheme
1991–1995	Introduction of purchaser-provider split	Provision of care split from purchasing, with Health Authorities established as purchasers of care for geographical populations
	GP Fundholding (GPFH)	Volunteer GP practices provided with budgets to purchase care for their registered populations. Budgets covered **elective** care and **prescribing**
	Locality commissioning and GP commissioning	A variety of locally developed models of GP involvement, with varying degrees of power and responsibility
1995	Total purchasing pilots (TPP)	An extension of GP fundholding. Volunteer groups held a budget covering a range of services which was agreed with local Health Authority
1997	New Labour government elected – GPFH abolished, Primary Care Groups (PCGs) established	PCGs officially sub-committees of Health Authorities. Responsible for commissioning full range of services. GP majority on Board
2000	PCGs became Primary Care Trusts (PCTs)	Health Authorities abolished, PCTs given responsibility for commissioning full range of services and providing community services. GPs no longer in a majority, few GPs involved
2005	Practice-based Commissioning (PBC) introduced	Volunteer groups of GPs given indicative budgets covering variable range of services. Most covered elective services, prescribing and some also covered community and emergency services
2010–2012	Coalition government elected, announce abolition of PCTs and establishment of Clinical Commissioning Groups	GP-led organisations with full statutory responsibility for commissioning all services other than primary care and highly specialised services. Fully established by 2012.

Source: Miller, Peckham et al (2015), p 2

to constrain demand (Mannion 2008; Coleman et al, 2009b). In the next section we explore the evidence about how the various initiatives played out in practice.

Clinically led commissioning: research evidence

The largest body of evidence available focuses upon GPFH and its derivatives, including TPPs. The key research focus was on outcomes, with a tendency to focus on the easily measured – for example changes to GP prescribing. Few studies focused on how these were achieved and whether clinical engagement was an important factor, or explored the relationship between clinical leaders and the wider body of GPs. Only a small number of studies explore the leadership positions clinicians held and the degree of influence they exerted over commissioning decisions. Even fewer studies examined the influence of GP fundholders on other bodies with which they interacted, for example the Health Authority (HA) or provider organisations.

Motivations underlying GP involvement in the various types of clinically led commissioning vary, depending upon the nature of the scheme. Common to all, however, was a belief that GPs, as frontline clinicians, bring valuable clinical and patient-specific knowledge to the table, and a desire to innovate. Furthermore, evidence suggests that the extent to which GPs felt able to innovate was a key determinant of the extent of their engagement. Where autonomy is granted and 'success' experienced, engagement grows, but where perceived autonomy and control is less, GPs tend to disengage. Maintaining wider clinical engagement (beyond the leaders) was agreed to be a priority, but the extent to which this was achieved varied considerably. Engagement was easier in smaller schemes but these tended to be limited in scope, while more comprehensive schemes found it more difficult to engage with a wider GP community. Engagement was, notwithstanding, time-consuming and labour intensive.

In terms of outcomes related to clinically led commissioning, the evidence is not strong. The most detailed evidence comes from GPFH and TPP, focusing on easy to measure activity such as changes in referral patterns, prescribing costs and waiting times. There is some evidence that GPFH tended to reduce the rate of growth in both prescribing costs and referral rates, although causation cannot be assumed, as those practices which took up GPFH tended to differ systematically from those which did not. Despite these caveats, however, it seems likely that responsibility for a budget tends to make practitioners think more carefully about their prescribing and referral decisions, and to focus on improving quality of care within their practices, but this does depend upon good relationships with frontline GPs, who need to feel that the commissioning body has legitimacy and that the actions they are being asked to take are reasonable. Peer review by trusted peers seems to be an important mechanism underlying this (Coleman et al, 2009b). This is easier to achieve in smaller schemes, and can be enabled by relatively modest incentive schemes (Checkland et al, 2011). There is some evidence that clinically led commissioning of various types led to the establishment of a greater range of services in the community, such as physiotherapy services, and to the development of better liaison between primary and secondary care, via, for example, 'discharge liaison officers'. Such services were rarely critically assessed for quality or costeffectiveness, however, with their establishment alone often being claimed as a 'success'. Priorities for service development tended to be based upon individuals' areas of interest or perceived local need, rather than a more systematic assessment of needs or service gaps. Furthermore, secondary care services tended to resist attempts at disinvestment, meaning that many such 'out of hospital' services represented duplication rather than substitution. There is very little evidence of any clinically led commissioning schemes generating significant changes to secondary care services, although where schemes made this their main focus they were able to make some short term changes to the pattern of hospital use. There is no evidence to support the contention that clinically led commissioning of any kind led to an overall improvement in quality of care.

HSCA 2012: what was intended to happen?

The White Paper, 'Equity and Excellence' (Department of Health, 2010) was published early in the life of the new Coalition Government. Its contents were generally seen as a surprise, as the Coalition agreement had specifically ruled out any significant reorganisation of the NHS (Cabinet Office 2010). As has been discussed elsewhere in this volume, the White Paper proposed a wholesale reorganisation in which Primary Care Trusts would be abolished, with commissioning responsibilities split between newly constituted 'Clinical Commissioning Groups' (CCGs) and a new arms' length body, initially known as the 'NHS Commissioning Board' (later renamed NHS England). CCGs would be responsible for commissioning secondary care, community and urgent/emergency services, while NHS England commissioned primary care services (including general practice, dentistry, pharmacy, optometry and so on) and specialised services. The 'vision' underpinning the reorganisation was of an NHS that:

- is more transparent, with clearer accountabilities for quality and results;
- gives citizens a greater say in how the NHS is run;
- is less insular and fragmented, and works much better across boundaries, including with local authorities and between hospitals and practices;
- is more efficient and dynamic, with a radically smaller national, regional and local bureaucracy; and

- is put on a more stable and sustainable footing, free from frequent and arbitrary political meddling.

(Department of Health 2010, 9)

It was argued that CCGs would 'shift decision making as close as possible to patients', and 'build upon the pivotal and trusted role that primary care physicians already play' (Department of Health 2010, 27). The document sets out the perceived shortcomings of previous clinically led commissioning initiatives, and argues that the establishment of GP-led CCGs will avoid the problems associated with these previous initiatives. Membership of a CCG was to be compulsory for all practices, and an ambitious timetable was set out with CCGs established in shadow form in 2011, taking over full responsibility in April 2013. A series of further documents set out more details about the establishment, governance and responsibilities of CCGs (Department of Health 2011a; Department of Health 2011b; Department of Health 2011c; Department of Health 2011d; Department of Health 2011e; Department of Health 2011f). It was argued that CCGs would be different from their predecessors by virtue of their status as 'membership organisations':

> CCGs will be different from any predecessor NHS organisation. While statutory NHS bodies, they will be built on the GP practices that together make up the membership of a CCG. These member practices must decide, through developing their constitution, and within the framework of legislation, how the CCG will operate. They must ensure that they are led and governed in an open and transparent way which allows them to serve their patients and population effectively. (NHS Commissioning Board, 2012c, 4)

It was also argued that the 'added value' that GPs would bring to commissioning included:

- strengthened knowledge of the needs of individuals and local communities and the variation in the quality of local services, by harnessing the unique role of general practice to be in everyday contact with patients, their families, and carers;
- increased capability to lead clinical redesign and engage other clinicians based on the understanding of clinical risk and evidence of best practice;

- better involvement and engagement of local people to adopt improved services and move from familiar but outdated services based on the focus on quality and outcomes and the trusted positions held in communities;
- improved uptake of quality based referral options across practices based on greater involvement in priority setting and redesign;
- greater focus on improving the quality of primary medical care as a key part of clinically led redesign of care systems.

(NHS Commissioning Board 2012 paragraph 3.14)

It is instructive to test these claims against what is known from research. First, GPFH, TPP and PBC were all underpinned by the idea that GPs, as frontline clinicians, understood the needs of their patients. Evidence suggests that, in practice, while they were responsive to the needs of individuals, clinicians involved in commissioning were not necessarily better than their managerial counterparts in assessing wider need (Miller et al, 2012). Second, there is little evidence from previous clinically led commissioning schemes that GPs are more capable of leading large scale service redesign than PCTs. In terms of 'engagement of local people', those involved with PBC had aspirations to improve public engagement, but there is little evidence of significant success (Coleman et al, 2009a). The suggestion that the 'trusted position of GPs in the community' would enable them to persuade the public of the need to make significant changes to services such as significantly redesigning (or even shutting) hospital services is interesting, and yet the counterargument can be made that GPs' position in the front line might make them less likely to support radical service redesign, as they would potentially be exposed to any public anger in their day to day work. It is certainly true that evidence suggests that referral patterns can be influenced by clinician–led commissioning authorities who are perceived to have local legitimacy, and that such groups can support peer–led approaches to quality improvement, but neither of these necessarily requires the clinical commissioners to hold statutory authority.

Taken together, the evidence base underlying these claims to benefits associated with the development of CCGs would seem to be weak. On the other hand, there is clear evidence from the past that clinician engagement in commissioning is more likely to be sustained if they feel themselves to have autonomy and freedom to innovate. As statutory bodies, CCGs were established with the freedom to decide what they commissioned, at least in the area of secondary care and community services; the extent to which they had freedom to innovate therefore depended upon the accountability and management mechanisms established in practice.

CCGs: what do we know?

Since 2011 the Policy Research Unit in Commissioning and the Healthcare System (PRUComm) has undertaken three phases of research on CCGs. The first phase, from early 2011 through to December 2012, followed CCGs from their initial establishment in 'shadow' form, through to their preparations for 'authorisation' as full statutory bodies. The second phase of the study ran from April 2013 until March 2015, focusing upon the claims made by participants in the research about the 'added value' that GPs brought to commissioning. Research methods and results from both of these phases of the study have been published in academic papers (see above) and in a number of reports (Checkland et al, 2012, 2014; McDermott et al, 2014; Miller et al, 2012). The final phase of this research commenced in April 2015, focusing upon the devolution of additional commissioning responsibilities to CCGs. In autumn 2014, CCGs were invited to express interest in taking on responsibility for commissioning GP services. This means holding responsibility for GP practice contracts, and raises issues of conflicts of interest as GP-led organisations will be commissioning their own practices. Three 'levels' of involvement were offered: full delegation of responsibility; joint commissioning, with CCGs and NHSE (NHS England) working together; and 'greater involvement', in which CCGs would advise NHSE on aspects of primary care commissioning (NHS England, 2014b). There is a clear expectation that those CCGs which opt for a lower level of involvement will, over time, move to take on further responsibility, but no firm timescale has been set for this.

This section is an updated version of evidence previously published as a paper in the *British Journal of General Practice* (Checkland et al, 2013b). We are grateful to the journal for permission to reproduce this here.

CCG autonomy and decision making: structures and governance

On paper, CCGs have significantly more autonomy than any previous clinical commissioning organisations, in that they are the statutory body and will carry full budgetary responsibility. In this section we discuss the development of CCGs structures and governance procedures, in order to explore how far this autonomy and associated ability to make decisions is being realised in practice.

Guidance for CCGs about structures and governance was non-prescriptive, suggesting only that CCGs should have a 'Governing Body', which is responsible for ensuring 'that CCGs have appropriate arrangements in place to ensure they exercise their functions effectively, efficiently and economically and in accordance with any generally accepted principles of good governance that are relevant to it' (NHS Commissioning Board, 2012c, 32), and that they should set up relevant subcommittees as required. As a consequence, we found significant complexity and variety associated with emerging CCG structures and governance arrangements, with widely differing subcommittees and groups which were referred to using a bewildering variety of names. Terms used included: board or shadow board; executive or executive committee; clinical commissioning committee; council of members; forum; collaborative; locality; cluster; senate; and cabinet. Total governing body size as reported in the survey also varied considerably, as did membership, with some establishing a relatively small group, dominated by GPs, while others opened membership up to a variety of other professionals such as social service representatives and public health specialists. Smaller groups might find decision making easier to achieve, but at the expense of less engagement with the wider health community.

Over time, there was a developing consensus around use of the title of 'Governing Body' for the main statutory body, but considerable variety remained around the naming of other subcommittees. This made direct comparisons difficult, as it was not always clear how far bodies in different sites with different names corresponded to one another. In order to overcome these difficulties, we sought to identify groups by their functions rather than their names. Overall, we found the following functions represented in our study sites: an overarching 'Governing Body', holding statutory responsibility once authorisation was completed; a number of 'Operational' bodies, including a number of different committees or workstreams; a formally constituted operational group, often called an 'Executive', which undertakes day to day management of the group's activities; a 'Council of Members' (CoM), consisting of practice representatives; and 'Locality groups', consisting of smaller groups of representatives from a geographical area. Not all sites had Locality groups, and two had also convened a wider group of clinicians, managers and representatives from outside (for example, from the local authority or the local provider trust) to provide more general advice.

Even when it was possible to identify separate groups at each of these different levels, the distribution of functions in a given site was more fluid than this typology suggests with, for example, no clear separation between Governing Body functions and more operational work, and with considerable time spent in meetings discussing who should be responsible for which type of decisions. The extent of the complexity embodied in these different groups and subcommittees is illustrated by this quotation from a manager in one of the larger CCGs that we studied:

> Well, because we're a large CCG, if we have everybody...the meeting's going to be, ah, less than, um, efficient. So what I've done is created a proposal for two boards. One is the statutory board ... The governing body. And the other is more of a... subsidiary board. So you have the locality chairs on one subsidiary board comprised solely of GPs, you have a superior board – the oversight and governance board – comprised of some GP representatives from the lower board, and all those statutory appointees. [Manager, ID 60]

In addition to their complex internal governance processes, CCGs are also externally accountable to NHS England and, more indirectly, to the local Health and Wellbeing Board (HWB). Thus CCGs, although they have complete budgetary control, may be significantly constrained in their ability to make rapid decisions or act autonomously in practice.

Engagement with members

In a clinical commissioning organisation with decision-making power, active engagement of GPs increases the ability to achieve goals and to innovate, albeit at a cost of significantly increased administrative overheads (Miller et al, 2012). In this section we examine evidence from our study about GP engagement and involvement.

CCG 'ownership'

Official guidance stressed the importance of GP engagement, explaining that: 'CCGs are also membership organisations, accountable to constituent GP practices' (NHS Commissioning Board, 2012b, 3), and suggesting that member practices should be actively engaged with all key decisions (NHS Commissioning Board, 2012a). This implies that CCG members should see themselves as 'owners' of the CCG and of its plans. In practice, constitutions, strategic plans and commissioning plans were generally developed by an executive group of GPs (aided by managers), and then submitted to the wider membership for approval. It is not yet clear how far the GP members will see themselves as 'owning' these plans. The smaller CCGs in our study took this seriously, working hard to try to ensure that the wider body of members 'owned' the agenda. In one site, this issue was revisited in almost every meeting, and Council of Members meetings were actively used to engage the members. One GP described this process:

> *We also have a check and balance of the Council of Members......
> The purpose was one, to hold us to account, but also to feed us
> information about what's a problem. And you saw with the Mental
> Health Strategy. 'This is wrong'. People giving both specific
> examples and endorsing broad feelings about how it did ... And
> then go back to the provider of that service, and say 'This is what
> everybody is saying about it. What do you think you're going
> to do to change it?' So to be at that stage is actually really quite
> exciting because it's almost showing how we're going to operate in
> the future.* [GP ID 283]

Thus, this GP saw the Governing body as being 'held to account' by the membership. A manager from a different site sees it slightly differently, however, as quoted below, arguing that the Council of Members had given the Executive the power to make decisions, upon which the wider membership could then comment, rather than the wider membership owning the decisions. In other words, the Executive would be required to give an account to their membership, without necessarily being accountable in a more direct sense:

> *Yes, that... I suppose that really is they have given the exec team
> responsibility decide, you know, that direction and the plan, so
> your first signoff is with the exec team, but then you take it to
> the wider group to say this is what we're going to take forward
> .... so it's just really exposing it to the wider remit as a sort of
> communication exercise really, but also it's their then chance to say
> you're all barking up the wrong tree.* [Manager ID 42]

Engaging with members

All case study CCGs were in the process of deciding how they should engage with their members. Many different modes of communication and engagement were planned, such as circulated newsletters or briefings and intranet sites. We found three broad approaches represented in our sites. In some (usually smaller) sites, the key task was seen as getting grassroots members to engage with strategic planning, contributing ideas and 'owning' the strategy. In larger groups, the problem was more often formulated in terms of the need to disseminate information down, so that grassroots members were aware of what the CCG was doing. Finally, some fell between these two extremes, seeing the strategic role as falling to the Governing Body or executive group, but wishing to see a flow of 'frontline intelligence' up from the grassroots, in addition to the flow of information down.

To engage with members, five out of eight of the case study sites had established geographically-based 'locality' groups. In four of these, the Localities form the main forum through which members engage with the CCG, with wider membership meetings infrequent. In the fifth site, there is also an active Council of Members. Respondents across all these sites expressed a desire to have 'strong Localities'; however, it remained unclear what this meant or what a 'strong Locality' might do. The rationale appeared to be that 'strong Localities' were necessary to engage the membership, but their ongoing role in the wider organisation remained undefined and insecure. One of the key questions was how much responsibility could reasonably be delegated to Localities. In one of the larger sites it was stated categorically that Localities could not work autonomously. In another site, by contrast, Localities were given delegated authority to make significant commissioning decisions, commit specified amounts of the overall budget without Governing Body approval, and even manage contracts with their local providers. This approach generated significant local buy-in and enthusiasm; the downside was that it required a significant commitment of managerial resources at the local level.

These findings suggest that what it means to 'engage' grassroots' GPs in CCGs is yet to be clearly formulated. The meaning of 'membership', the extent to which grassroots' GPs are expected to 'own' the agenda, the purpose of 'communication' and the role of Locality groups all need to be more clearly defined. Furthermore, it seems that 'engagement' may mean different things in groups of different sizes, and that, as was seen in the Total Purchasing Pilots, larger groups may find particular difficulties, unless they are able to devolve meaningful power to their Localities.

Commissioning activity

Previous GP commissioners have tended to focus upon activity based upon their direct clinical experience, leading to a focus on such matters as hospital waiting times and the provision of additional community-based services, with limited engagement with a public health approach to population health. There is most direct evidence of GP commissioner impact on prescribing, improving services in primary care, and some limited impact on slowing the rate of increase in referrals and urgent or unscheduled care.

Commissioning responsibilities

At the time of the research, emerging CCGs were working as subcommittees of their local PCT Cluster, and were beginning to take over responsibility for leading commissioning, preparing to take over full responsibility from April 2013. Unlike all previous manifestations of clinically led commissioning, CCGs have statutory responsibility for virtually the entire commissioning budget. Respondents in our case study sites were very much aware of the implications of this, and of the challenges ahead:

> There is no longer going to be a PCT to pick up the pieces. We are going to have to hold each other to account (localities and GPs) and work hard at this. Localities need to own contracts. We have to look at financial credibility...We need to be on top of things from quarter one and decided how we are going to monitor things [Extract from fieldnotes executive meeting March 2012 M30]

Some Governing Body members appeared to recognise the need to take as broad a view as possible of the commissioning task, moving away from small scale, practice-level interventions:

> for me it's really amazing to watch these clinicians leading change on a really significant scale, and it's very different to, I guess, what I thought might happen, after seeing those early stages of practice based commissioning, which were, you know, doing a little bit of dermatology in your practice, for other practices, it was very small scale. [Manager ID 204]

We also found that, in general, meetings of Locality groups and Councils of Members tended to remain more focused upon more familiar topics such as small scale interventions to improve care for long term conditions in general practice.

Engaging with public health will be important if CCGs are to move beyond such small scale practice-level change. Under the new architecture of the NHS, responsibility for public health has moved to Local Government authorities. Our case study sites were aware of the need to work closely with public health, with, for example, some participants acknowledging the difference between 'formal' public health knowledge and 'informal' general practice knowledge about health needs. Some sites were keen to 'embed' public health at Governing Body level, whereas others saw it in terms of public health offering the CCG a service. Respondents in all sites expressed concerns about the ongoing relationship between CCGs and public health. In the face of this uncertainty, personal experience of working together was seen as important:

> ...at the moment, there's still quite a good link, historical...with the public health and the names and faces are still there, and as a consequence what we get is based on those relationships, isn't it; do we have a thorough understanding of what public health information we would want contract to be provided to us, I don't know about that, that's a difficult one. It's a relationship that, hopefully, will just continue. [GP ID 104]

Research suggests that interactions between CCGs and their public health colleagues can take a number of different forms, with some public health professionals seeing themselves as 'co-owners' of the CCG agenda, while others act as 'critical friends' or 'service providers' (Warwick-Giles et al, in press). The implications of these different approaches are not yet clear.

One of the key areas in which our case study CCGs told us that they felt that CCGs would add value and 'do things differently' from previous clinically led commissioning schemes was in the area of negotiating with providers:

> We're beginning to see some successes in terms of GPs' involvement in some of the, some of the contracting rounds, so...They actually go along to the Contracting meetings. And, you know, and giving clinical view and clinical input around some of those discussions and conversations. And that can add real value in terms, for both the providers and the commissioners, to really start driving forwards some of those tricky conversations. [Manager ID 54]

When we followed this up in phase two of our study, however, we found that, while interactions between commissioners and providers could be enhanced by the involvement of clinicians, this requires careful orchestration, with detailed planning, proactive chairing and a selective approach as to where to focus clinicians' attention. This is important, as GPs have limited time and are under considerable pressure. This GP highlighted the stress he was facing:

> *And I spent yesterday, six hours in a Joint Strategic Needs Assessment on the Health and Wellbeing Board, for which I have not been paid, and I won't get paid. That's why I am still catching up on my clinical work, and I came in at 7 o'clock this morning to do all my paperwork and spent till 8 o'clock last night doing that. So I spend hours and hours of unpaid work.... doing the work that needs to be done.* [GP ID 218]

Research by the Kings Fund/Nuffield Trust confirms these findings, and suggests that GP involvement in CCG Governing Bodies is declining (Holder et al, 2015). Defining clearly where GPs 'add value' will be important if CCGs are to be sustainable.

Quality of primary care

Previous manifestations of clinically led commissioning have had some success in improving care quality in general practice. The CCGs in our study had ambition in this regard. In particular, there was ambition to undertake some kind of performance management, including performance against commissioning budgets, referral behaviour and prescribing costs. While official documents refer to 'improving quality' in primary care, most of our respondents were happy to talk explicitly about 'performance management'. Box 8.1 sets out the approaches seen.

Box 8.1: Approaches to quality improvement in primary care adopted by case study sites

- Sharing of named referral performance data (all sites)
- Sharing of named prescribing performance data (all sites)
- Sharing of named data detailing performance against budgets (some sites)
- Incentive schemes designed to target and improve performance (some sites)
- Visits to individual practices to discuss performance (some sites)
- Discussions of audit data in all practice meetings (some sites)
- Creation of intranet (dashboard) where data can be shared between practices (some sites)
- Referral management centre scrutinising all GP referrals (one site)
- 'Buddying' poorly performing practices with those doing better for support and guidance (one site).

In all sites, performance management activities similar to these had been running under previous structures such as Practice-based Commissioning (Coleman et al, 2009b). Some respondents, however, said that they were concerned that such performance review and management would be more difficult in future as they had fewer staff to do the work; in particular, visiting practices individually is very labour intensive and may not be possible. In addition, there was some tension identified between the desire to be a 'bottom up' organisation led by members and the perceived need to performance-manage those members.

How these tensions play out as CCGs take over responsibility for commissioning primary care services will be an important determinant of success. CCGs must maintain the trust and support of their members, while actively managing their performance and, potentially, enforcing local contract changes. The third phase of our research will explore the experiences of CCGs as they take over these new responsibilities.

Conclusions

If the split between 'commissioning' and 'providing' services is to be maintained, it seems clear that GP involvement is important. GPs in the UK are 'gatekeepers' to secondary care services, and, via their registered lists, are closely in touch with the health needs of the public. How best to involve GPs, however, is a question to which successive governments have provided different answers. The HSCA 2012 sought to give GP-led organisations statutory responsibility for a significant proportion of the commissioning budget. The argument underlying the abolition of PCTs was that they were too managerially dominated and had failed to engage GPs effectively. The solution – a significant reorganisation – contained some elements that seemed in keeping with available evidence. In particular, the HSCA 2012 seemed to promise significant autonomy to CCGs, with GPs firmly in the lead. In practice, however, their room for manoeuvre has been constrained by the financial challenges affecting the NHS as a whole, and it is not yet clear the extent to which CCGs will be able to make the significant service changes necessary to meet those challenges.

Since 2014, policy has moved forward rapidly. Simon Stevens took over as Chief Executive of NHS England, and quickly published his 'Five Year Forward View' (FYFV) (NHS England, 2014a). This document set out the scale of the financial challenge facing the NHS, and suggested that this challenge could only be met if the NHS did things differently. In particular, the FYFV advocates the establishment of what have come to be called 'vanguards' to test out new models for services. These include: Multispeciality Community Providers, bringing together providers of a variety of types of care in community settings; Primary and Acute Care Systems, vertically integrating primary and secondary care; Urgent and Emergency Care networks, bringing together providers of different types of urgent care across a geographical area; and a variety of other models focusing upon specific care settings such as care homes, community hospitals and maternity services. In addition, as discussed earlier, Simon Stevens suggested that the commissioning of primary care services would be delegated to CCGs. Taken together, these developments suggest a future for commissioning in general and CCGs in particular that will look quite different. The new models of care under development suggest a situation in which, rather than assessing needs and procuring services, commissioners set agreed outcomes and hold large providers to account for meeting them. CCGs seem to be stimulating the development of provider 'federations' (Welikala, 2015), in which groups of general practices work together as providers across a larger footprint, and this brings potential conflicts of interest.

How these developments will play out in the longer term is currently unclear, with many questions remaining about the status of CCGs as membership organisations, the extent to which they can hold large providers to account and their management of conflicts of interest. The direction of travel – towards a greater focus on care provision in community settings – is supported by the evidence that we have presented here from the long history of GP involvement in commissioning.

Disclaimer

The research on which this chapter is based was carried out by the Department of Health-funded Policy Research Unit in Commissioning and the Healthcare System. The views are those of the authors, not the Department of Health.

Acknowledgements

This chapter is based upon research which has been published as a series of reports, accessible via the PRUComm website (www. prucomm.ac.uk) and in academic papers (Checkland et al, 2013a; Checkland et al, 2013b; Coleman et al, 2014; Perkins et al, 2014; Petsoulas et al, 2014; Segar et al, 2014; Coleman et al, 2015; Coleman and Glendinning, 2015; Miller et al, 2015). Part of the chapter was previously published as an article in the *British Journal of General Practice* (Checkland et al, 2013b), and we are grateful to them for permission to reproduce it here. Table 8.1 is reproduced from Miller et al (2015) with permission from the *Journal of Health Services Research and Policy*.

We would like to acknowledge with gratitude the significant contribution of the wider PRUComm research team in carrying out and writing up this research. These were complicated projects, carried out at speed, and would not have been possible without the hard work, responsiveness and intellectual engagement of the team. Andrew Wallace, Rosalind Miller, Christina Petsoulas, Dorota Osipovic, Neil Perkins, Michael Wright, Erica Gadsby and Julia Segar contributed to data collection, analysis and report writing. In addition, Stephen Harrison and Rosalind Miller co-authored the literature review, while Andrew Wallace, Julia Segar, Christina Petsoulas and Rosalind Miller co-authored the *British Journal of General Practice* paper on which this chapter draws.

References

Cabinet Office, 2010, The Coalition: Our programme for government, London: Cabinet Office

Checkland, K, Coleman, A, Harrison, S, 2011, When is a saving not a saving? The micro-politics of budgets and savings under Practice-based commissioning, *Public Money and Management* 31, 4, 241–248

Checkland, K, Coleman, A, Segar, J, McDermott, I, Miller, R, Wallace, A, Peckham, S, Harrison, S, 2012, *Exploring the early workings of emerging Clinical Commissioning Groups: Final report*. London: Policy Research Unit in Commissioning and the Healthcare System (PRUComm), http://blogs.lshtm.ac.uk/prucomm/files/2012/11/Pathfinder-project-final-report-revised-v10-combined-post-peer-review-FINAL-correct-date_titles.pdf.

Checkland, K, Allen, P, Coleman, A, Segar, J, McDermott, I, Harrison, S, Petsoulas, C, Peckham, S, 2013a, Accountable to whom, for what? An exploration of the early development of Clinical Commissioning Groups in the English NHS, *British Medical Journal Open* 3, 12

Checkland, K, Coleman, A, McDermott, I, Segar, J, Miller, R, Petsoulas, C, Wallace, A, Harrison, S, Peckham, S, 2013b, Primary care-led commissioning: Applying lessons from the past to the early development of clinical commissioning groups in England, *British Journal of General Practice* 63, 614, e611–e619

Checkland, K, Coleman, A, Perkins, N, McDermott, I, Petsoulas, C, Wright, M, Gadsby, E, Peckham, S, 2014, *Exploring the ongoing development and impact of Clinical Commissioning Groups*. London: Policy Research Unit in Commissioning and the Healthcare System (PRUComm).

Coleman, A, Checkland, K, Harrison, S, 2009a, Still puzzling: Patient and public involvement in commissioning, *Journal of Integrated Care* 17, 6, 23–30

Coleman, A, Checkland, K, Harrison, S, Dowswell, G, 2009b, *Practice-based commissioning: Theory, implementation and outcome: Final report*, Manchester: University of Manchester, National Primary Care Research and Development Centre

Coleman, A, Checkland, K, Segar, J, McDermott, I, Harrison, S, Peckham, S, 2014, Joining it up? Health and wellbeing boards in English local governance: Evidence from Clinical Commissioning Groups and shadow health and wellbeing boards, *Local Government Studies*, 40, 4, 560–580

Coleman, A, Checkland, K, Segar, J, McDermott, I, Harrison, S, Peckham, S, 2015, Leadership for health commissioning in the new NHS: Exploring the early development of Clinical Commissioning Groups in England, *Journal of Health Organization and Management* 29, 1, 75-91

Coleman, A, Glendinning, C, 2015, Going round in circles? Joint working between primary health and social care, *Journal of Integrated Care* 23, 2, 53–61

Department of Health, 2010, Equity and excellence: Liberating the NHS, London: The Stationery Office

Department of Health, 2011a, *Commissioning support: Clinical Commissioning Group running costs tool, a 'ready reckoner'*, London: The Stationery Office, Gateway Reference 16585

Department of Health, 2011b, *Developing Clinical Commissioning Groups: Towards authorisation*, London: The Stationery Office, Gateway Reference 16367

Department of Health, 2011c, *The functions of GP commissioning consortia: A working document*, London: The Stationery Office, Gateway Reference 15472

Department of Health, 2011d, *Healthy lives, healthy people: Update and way forward*, London: The Stationery Office, Gateway Reference 129334

Department of Health, 2011e, *Joint strategic needs assessment and joint health and wellbeing strategies explained: Commissioning for populations*, London: The Stationery Office, Gateway Reference 131733

Department of Health, 2011f, *Operational guidance to the NHS: Extending patient choice of provider*, London: The Stationery Office, Gateway Reference 16242

Flynn, R, Williams, G (eds), 1997, *Contracting for health: Quasi-markets and the NHS*. Oxford: Oxford University Press

Holder, H, Robertson, R, Ross, S, Bennett, L, Gosling, J, Curry, N, 2015, *Risk or Reward? The changing role of CCGs in general practice*, London: King's Fund/Nuffield Trust

Mannion, R, 2008, General practitioner commissioning in the English National Health Service: Continuity, change, and future challenges, *International Journal of Health Services* 38, 4, 717–730

McDermott, I, Coleman, A, Perkins, N, Osipovic, D, Petsoulas, C & Checkland, K, 2014, *Exploring the GP 'added value' in commissioning: What works, in what circumstances, and how?* London: Policy Research Unit in Commissioning and the Healthcare System (PRUComm), http://blogs.lshtm.ac.uk/prucomm/files/2015/10/CCG2-final-report-post-review-v3-final.pdf.

Miller, R, Peckham, S, Checkland, K, Coleman, A, McDermott, I, Harrison, S, Segar, J, 2012, *Clinical engagement in primary care-led commissioning: a review of the evidence*. London: Policy Research Unit in Commissioning and the Healthcare System (PRUComm).

Miller, R, Peckham, S, Checkland, K, Coleman, A, McDermott, I, Harrison, S, 2015, What happens when GPs engage in commissioning? Two decades of experience in the English NHS, *Journal of Health Services Research and Policy*, 21, 2, 126-133

NHS Commissioning Board, 2012a, Clinical commissioning group authorisation: Draft guide for applicants, April 2012, Leeds: NHS Commissioning Board

NHS Commissioning Board, 2012b, Clinical commissioning groups HR guide, May 2012

NHS Commissioning Board, 2012c, Towards establishment: Creating responsive and accountable Clinical Commissioning Groups, February 2012, Leeds: NHS Commissioning Board

NHS England, 2014a, *Five year forward view*, London: NHS England

NHS England, 2014b, *Next steps towards primary care co-commissioning*, London: NHS England

Perkins, N, Coleman, A, Wright, M, Gadsby, E, McDermott, I, Petsoulas, C, Checkland, K, 2014, Involving GPs in commissioning what 'added value' do they think they bring to clinical commissioning groups? *British Journal of General Practice* 64(628), e728–e784

Petsoulas, C, Allen, P, Checkland, K, Coleman, A, Segar, J, Peckham, S, McDermott, I, 2014, Views of NHS commissioners on commissioning support provision: Evidence from a qualitative study examining the early development of clinical commissioning groups in England, *British Medical Journal Open* 4, e005970

Segar, J, Checkland, K, Harrison, S, Coleman, A, McDermott, I, Peckham, S, 2014, Changing the ties that bind? The emerging roles and identities of general practitioners and managers in the new Clinical Commissioning Groups in the English NHS, *Sage Open* Oct–Dec, 1–12

Warwick-Giles, L, Coleman, A, Checkland, K, in press, Co-owner, service provider, critical friend? The role of public health in Clinical Commissioning Groups, *Journal of Public Health* (http://jpubhealth. oxfordjournals.org/content/early/2015/10/06/pubmed.fdv137. abstract?sid=587c1b31-a60b-4877-b0e7-73040c378524)

Welikala, J, 2015, Revealed: Which CCGs are paying GP practices to form federations. *Health Service Journal*, 30 June, 2015(http://www. hsj.co.uk/news/primary-care/revealed-which-ccgs-are-paying-gp-practices-to-form-federations/5087243.article)

NINE

'Much ado about nothing'? Pursuing the 'holy grail' of health and social care integration under the Coalition

Robin Miller and Jon Glasby

Seeking greater integration in the delivery of health and social care has been a longstanding aim of different governments over time, yet deep-seated and seemingly intractable barriers remain. While the Coalition has stressed the importance of integrated care and introduced a number of new initiatives, it remains open to question as to whether health and social care are more or less joined up than they were in 2010. Against this background, this chapter begins by summarising the state of play at the end of the New Labour governments of 1997–2010 and the main reforms introduced under the Coalition government of 2010–15. After this, the chapter considers the emerging evidence about the impact of the Coalition's policies, and offers some initial thoughts on how such developments might be interpreted. Given limited formal evidence and the fact that the two authors have been actively involved in some of the policy debates described, the chapter draws on both formal and informal sources of knowledge, and seeks to combine a review of the published data with some more personal reflections. In the process, a 'three stream multidimensional policy implementation framework' is used to critique the implementation of integration policy by the Coalition (Exworthy and Powell, 2004). As the title of this chapter implies, it is relatively easy to make a rhetorical commitment to greater integration (in one sense, who would argue for greater fragmentation?) – but delivering this in practice is much harder.

Health and social care prior to 2010

In 1998, an early New Labour discussion paper on joint working between health and social care set out a strongly worded critique of what happens when potential partners fail to work together effectively. Although this is now dated, we quote this diagnosis of the problems to be solved on a regular basis, as it seems to us to so accurately reflect the practice realities that we observed at the time and the negative impacts that can still occur when frontline agencies fail to collaborate:

> All too often when people have complex needs spanning both health and social care good quality services are sacrificed for sterile arguments about boundaries. When this happens people, often the most vulnerable in our society … and those who care for them find themselves in the no man's land between health and social services. This is not what people want or need. It places the needs of the organisation above the needs of the people they are there to serve. It is poor organisation, poor practice, poor use of taxpayers' money – it is unacceptable. (Department of Health, 1998, 3)

Around this time, the then Secretary of State for Health, Frank Dobson, described the relationship between health and social care as a form of 'Berlin Wall' (see, for example, Hansard, 1998) – and this metaphor of a physical barrier artificially separating two territories was picked up instantly by a broad range of policy makers, practitioners and policy commentators. This commitment to joint working was part of a broader 'modernisation' agenda or 'third way' which emphasised the perceived benefits of partnership working, collaboration and networks in place of the more competition-based approaches of previous Conservative governments (see, for example, Glendinning et al, 2002). Indeed, these UK developments were also mirrored in a number of other developed countries and have been viewed as a part of a broader attempt by national governments of all persuasions to respond to (Glasby and Dickinson 2009):

1. The impact of New Public Management and the need to create greater coordination following the fragmentation of previous reforms.
2. A recognition that partnership working is essential to respond to the challenges of individual organisations and the complexity of current social problems.
3. The need to respond to a series of social changes (including a rise in the number of people with chronic or long-term conditions, technological advances and changing public expectations).

4. Diversity of professional knowledge and skills is necessary to respond to the increasing complexity of needs but this diversity can result in clashes in perspective and culture.

Whatever the motivation, the New Labour mantra of 'joined-up solutions to joined-up problems' certainly led to a range of new cross-cutting initiatives, such as efforts to tackle health inequalities (via 'Health Action Zones'), improve the quality of life of children and families in deprived communities ('Sure Start') and regenerate run-down neighbourhoods ('the New Deal for Communities'). In health and social care, there were a series of new approaches pioneered (see Box 9.1), and services at various stages between 1997 and 2010 certainly felt much more joined-up in practice than they had prior to 1997. While evidence of tangible improvements in outcomes was hard to pinpoint and while many local areas found it hard to sustain meaningful joint working in a system not designed with integration in mind (see, for example, Wistow & Dickinson, 2012; Glasby and Dickinson, 2014; RAND Europe/Ernst and Young, 2012), our belief is that most areas of the country were working together in different ways and having different conversations about the shared nature of many of their challenges than had been the case previously. Many

Box 9.1: Key initiatives under New Labour

- Creation of Health Action Zones to tackle health inequalities in a series of deprived local communities.
- Passage of the Health Act 1999, enabling local health and social care partners to pool budgets, create integrated provider organisations and/ or delegate one partner as the lead commissioner for a particular user group (powers often known as the 'Health Act flexibilities').
- Creation of a small number of Care Trusts (fully integrated health and social care organisations) as well as a national network of Children's Trust (often more virtual in nature).
- The advent of health scrutiny, with local authority scrutiny committees having the power to comment on major changes in local health services and review different health-related topics locally.
- Establishing a legal duty of partnership.
- A series of 'integrated care pilots' to test new ways of integrating services locally.
- Requirement for local authorities and Primary Care Trusts to develop Joint Strategic Needs Assessments of the health and wellbeing of their local population

frontline practitioners and managers could have operated in relative isolation from each other in the mid-1990s. By 2010 however it was common for local health and social care partners to be taking collective stock of local needs, making joint appointments, pooling some of their resources, developing new shared approaches to commissioning, exploring scope for joint training and development, co-locating frontline staff and creating more integrated, multidisciplinary teams. Joint working, in short, was closer to becoming core business – even if it remained difficult to achieve in practice in a divided system.

The White Paper and the 'discovery' of integrated care

By the end of the Coalition government in 2015, the importance of 'integrated care' was widely recognised and almost endlessly discussed, both in national policy and local practice (see below for a series of more detailed examples). This was not the case at the start of the Coalition, however, with no explicit references to integrated care in the Coalition agreement (HM Government, 2010) and the 2010 White Paper, *Equity and Excellence* (Department of Health, 2010) almost entirely silent on the subject of integration. While earlier Liberal Democrat policy papers and the 2010 manifesto had pledged to seek greater local democratic control of NHS services via new elected Health Boards in place of more managerially led Primary Care Trusts (PCTs) (Liberal Democrats, 2010), the subsequent Coalition White Paper took a different tack by announcing:

- The abolition of PCTs and Strategic Health Authorities (SHAs)
- The creation of GP-led Clinical Commissioning Groups to commission health services on behalf of the local population
- The transfer of public health responsibilities to local government
- The announcement of new Health and Wellbeing Boards (HWBs) to bring together CCG and local government leads in order to boost local democratic oversight of the new system (see Chapter 14 for further discussion)

For many commentators and members of NHS staff, the White Paper felt as if it placed much greater emphasis on choice, competition and markets than it did on partnership and collaboration, and there were a series of increasingly vociferous protests (see Chapter 2). In response, the Coalition announced that it would 'pause' the passage of the White Paper in order to consult further on the proposed changes, creating an 'NHS Future Forum' to debate the key issues and come back with more detailed recommendations. While this was a national body established by the Prime Minister, it was made up of a wide range of individuals from across the health and social care system, many of whom had significant and longstanding experience of the realities of frontline services. As but one example, the Future Forum Chair, Steve Field, was a practising GP in a deprived inner-city area of Birmingham, and with lots of practical experience of the complexities of patient need. Fearing that the proposed reforms would create greater fragmentation, the Forum focused a specific strand of its work on 'integrated care' (NHS Future Forum, 2012a), emphasising that this was crucial to responding to the challenges facing both health and social care:

> Regardless of whether our discussions were focussed on the issue of public accountability and patient involvement, competition and choice or clinical advice and leadership, concerns around integration came up time and time again. The importance of collaboration and integration between different care sectors and care settings are, therefore, strong themes in each of the separate work stream reports (NHS Future Forum, 2012b, 20)

This language is similar in many respects to the diagnosis of New Labour in the late 1990s, with the Future Forum highlighting that health, social care and other services were not sufficiently joined up around individuals and communities. It can also be seen, however, to be a response to concerns over the additional fragmentation that might be prompted by the Coalition's emphasis on greater provider diversity and competition. Certainly this was the belief at some local levels, with the Chief Executive of one of the most integrated health and social care organisations criticising the 'unintended consequences' of government policy as his organisation was effectively abolished under the reforms (Farnsworth, 2012).

Whatever the motivations, following the Future Forum report, the integration 'cat' was most definitely 'out of the bag'. The Forum had made a number of detailed recommendations (see Box 9.2), which were broadly accepted by the Coalition. In particular, the subsequent Health and Social Care Act 2012 included a 'duty to integrate' placed on NHS England, Monitor, CCGs and Health and Wellbeing Boards, with similar provision for adult social care in the 2014 Care Act. The extent to which these differed from previous New Labour 'duties of partnership' is debatable, however they could at least be seen as having symbolic importance. One major departure from the Future Forum recommendations was in relation to the new outcome frameworks developed for health, social care and public health. Despite the Forum's advice to the contrary, these remained separate rather than integrated – albeit with some shared priorities across the three areas of policy. This continued fragmentation in performance management therefore continued rather than addressed similar failings identified in the New Labour period (Exworthy et al, 2002).

> **Box 9.2: Recommendations from the NHS Future Forum (2012a) around integrated care**
> * Integrate around the patient, not the system
> * Make it easier for patients and carers to co-ordinate and navigate
> * Information is key enabler of integration
> * You can only improve what you can measure
> * HWB must become the crucible of health and social care integration
> * Providers need to be able to work together to improve care
> * Clarify the rules on choice, competition and integration
> * Freedom and flexibility to 'get on and do'
> * Allow the funding to follow the patient
> * National level support for local leadership is essential
> * Sharing best practice and breaking down barriers

From this point on, integration seemed to take centre stage within Coalition health and social care policy (at least rhetorically). Three key developments that followed from the Future Forum are summarised below (Better Care Fund, Pioneers and Vanguards, Commissioning and Procurement Rules and Regulations), but there were also a myriad of other initiatives. These included: named general practitioners being responsible for coordinating the care for people aged 75 years or older, the further extension of the personalisation agenda into areas of traditional NHS provision and an aspiration that mental and physical health should have 'parity of esteem'. Perhaps most significant of all was the growing assumption that integrated care should be the norm rather than the exception, with all parts of the health and social care system expected to work proactively towards this end. Reflected in countless ministerial speeches and government announcements, this aspiration and expectation was perhaps most clearly articulated in the 'Our Shared Commitment' report. This was produced by a new National Collaboration for Integrated Care and Support (2013) comprising key central governmental bodies, the Associations of Directors of Children's Services and of Adult Social

Services, the Local Government Association and National Voices. The latter was a grouping of 130 health and social care charities which developed a 'person centred narrative' of integrated care on behalf of the government. Based on the views of patients, service users and carers this narrative provided a clear articulation of how integrated care would be experienced by individuals and their family: 'I can plan my care with people who work together to understand me and my carers, allow me control, and bring together services to achieve the outcomes important to me' (National Voices, 2013, 3).

While this is easy to say and much harder to achieve in practice, these 'I statements' (as they became known) did at least attempt to define what we mean by 'integrated care' from the perspective of service users (see Chapter 15). The initial plan was for these statements to be translated into a national indicator which would be used to track progress. Ultimately, whether or not care has been 'integrated' is less to do with formal structures, funding and governance arrangements than with the experiences of service users. Perhaps integrated care is best understood in terms of experiences: if it feels joined up to people on the receiving end of care, this is what is most important.

The Better Care Fund

The Better Care Fund (BCF), or the Integration Transformation Fund as it was initially known, was announced in the 2013 Spending Round. Its stated aim was to deliver 'better, more joined-up services to older and disabled people, to keep them out of hospital and to avoid long hospital stays' (HM Treasury, 2013, 22). While this was commonly perceived (and arguably portrayed) as additional funding, it was in fact a top slice of existing funding streams which could then be transferred from NHS funds to a joint health and social care budget. It was to be brought in fully in 2015–2016 to a value of nearly £3.5 billion, with local authorities also receiving £200 million in 2014–2015 to prepare for the full roll-out. To access the fund, local HWBs had to approve a plan that detailed how the money would enable them to meet the national conditions and locally set targets against six performance indicators (see also Chapter 14). This local plan would then be subjected to a 'robust national assessment process' (Department of Health/Department for Communities and Local Government, 2014, 8) which included a review of quality by technical experts and triangulation with NHS England area teams and local government peers, and an assessment of risk to delivery due to local context and challenges. While nearly two-and-a-half billion pounds would be provided upfront to local areas, £1 billion would be subject to a 'payment for performance' framework connected with achievement of national conditions and locally set targets.

Following comments on a draft plan submitted in February 2014 all local areas submitted a final plan by April 2014 (see National Audit Office for a summary of events and for all key data in this paragraph; NAO 2014). These proposed pooling £5.5 billion of health and social care funds (voluntarily exceeding the government's expected amount). Ninety percent of the plans were assessed as being satisfactory by NHS England area teams and local government representatives and these estimated that there would be savings of £731 million. This was someway short of the £1 billion savings that government had forecast through reducing admissions and delayed discharge. More worryingly, a subsequent review by NHS England and the Department of Health challenged the robustness of the planning behind the estimated savings and calculated that these would amount to only £55 million (NAO, 2014). There are also concerns about the potential negative impacts on local NHS budgets and their ability to invest in community health services, and that local NHS providers had not been sufficiently consulted in the process. As a consequence the pay-for-performance element of the fund was revised, with some elements to be ringfenced for NHS services only. A BCF taskforce was also established to provide general support through guides and webinars, and targeted support for the areas seen to be most in need. The resubmitted plans forecast £532 million of savings with £200 million less being pooled than the first submissions.

The 'Integrated Care Pioneers' and subsequent 'Vanguards'

In their 'shared commitment', the National Collaboration for Integrated Care and Support (2013) acknowledged that there were 'significant challenges' to be overcome in order to achieve the required 'culture of cooperation' between different sectors and professionals and so achieve improvements in patient care and wellbeing (2013, 1). To help understand how to overcome these challenges at 'pace and scale' the Collaboration announced that there would be a series of 'local integration Pioneers' who would be able to test out new approaches to delivery and commissioning. Expressions of interest to become a pioneer were sought in May 2013, with the selected Pioneers being expected to:

- "Articulate a clear vision of its own innovative approaches to integrated care and support, including how it will (i) utilise the Narrative developed by National Voices and Think Local Act Personal's Making it Real, (ii) deliver better outcomes and experiences for individuals in its locality, and (iii) realise any anticipated financial efficiencies."

- "Present fully developed plans for whole system integration, encompassing health, social care and public health, other public services and the community and voluntary sector, as appropriate" (National Collaboration for Integrated Care and Support, 2013, 41).

The fourteen successful candidates were announced in November 2013 and would be given access to expertise, support and constructive challenge from a range of national and international experts. In early 2015 a second wave of eleven Pioneers was also announced. In practice, the selection of Pioneers appears to have been consciously diverse – in terms of the context in which they are working, the range of integrated care interventions that they were seeking to explore and their previous progress regarding integration (NHS England, 2014a). To share the learning from the programme, the Department of Health produced information on their initial plans with an annual update of local progress and commissioned an interim report (after the first year) and a full evaluation (running from summer 2015 to the end of the programme). To date, the signs are that progress has been slow in many areas, with challenges experienced in terms of trying to deliver ambitious plans in rapid timescales, recognition of the need to develop relationships over the longer term, difficulties evidencing improved outcomes, a series of perceived policy barriers to greater integration, and frustration around the quality of national support/repeated national demands for information, updates and data (personal communications; see also Erens et al, 2015). This mirrors almost exactly the experience of New Labour's 'integrated care pilots' in the late 2000s (RAND Europe/Ernst and Young, 2012), and cynics might feel that this was almost entirely predictable as a result.

Another concern expressed about the 'pioneer' process (which again mirrors experiences under New Labour) is a tendency for national policy to announce a high profile national initiative, but for policy focus to shift rapidly to new ideas and for the previous pilots to feel under-supported and confused by subsequent ambiguity. Once again, this seemed a case of history repeating itself when NHS England and other national partners announced a series of 'Vanguards' as part of the Five Year Forward View (NHS England, 2014b). Focused more on the integration of health services rather than on joint working between health and social care, the Vanguards were identified through a national application and subsequent selection process, and in one sense seem to have stolen the Pioneers' thunder. Certainly it caused significant consternation when it became apparent that, unlike the Pioneers, the Vanguards would have access to a £200 million Transformation Fund. Some areas contain both a 'pioneer' and a 'vanguard', while others were felt to be insufficiently integrated to be a pioneer but were subsequently identified as a 'vanguard'. Of course, both are also operating in a policy context not designed with integration in mind, and like New Labour's Care Trusts and integrated care pilots, may well struggle over time (although, like the former, some may also make significant improvements (Miller et al 2011). While integrated care remains a stated aim of policy, it still feels as if we have struggled to move beyond demonstrator projects, pilots, pathfinders, trailblazers, Pioneers and/or Vanguards to get to a stage where new ways of working of working become part of the mainstream.

Commissioning and Procurement Rules and Regulations

As suggested above, the work of the NHS Future Forum appears to have been significant in promoting the importance of integrated care, with growing fears that other aspects of the Coalition's reforms could create greater fragmentation through an emphasis on competition and markets. While stressing the importance of integrated care, policy makers did not accept the argument that greater competition would lead to greater fragmentation, and instead promoted the view that competition and collaboration could coexist (or indeed that competition could even be a vehicle for achieving integration). In many ways, this mirrors similar debates under the later years of New Labour, when there was also growing perceived tension between reforms based on collaboration and approaches based on competition. In response to these debates, the role of Monitor was changed – from encouraging competition to guarding against anti-competitive behaviour and ensuring that commissioners and providers worked to support integrated care (Monitor 2013). Similarly commissioners were given a duty to encourage collaboration as part of their procurement processes:

> Regulation 3 of the Procurement, Patient Choice and Competition Regulations sets out general requirements that commissioners must comply with when procuring NHS

> health care services. These include a requirement: ... to consider appropriate ways of improving services (including through services being provided in a more integrated way, enabling providers to compete and allowing patients to choose their provider). (Monitor, 2013,10)

Although various elements of competition law also apply, providers of NHS-funded services were also required 'not to act or behave in a way that would be reasonably regarded as being ...detrimental to enabling integration' as part of their license conditions (Monitor, 2015b, Annexe A). While not accepting that there was an inherent conflict between competition and integration, the Coalition did recognise that fulfilling their duties in both regards was potentially complicated for commissioners. They therefore sought to clarify how these potential tensions (or at least uncertainties) should be addressed through a series of guidance documents. For example, the substantive guidance on procurement and choice suggests how commissioned services could be required to incorporate multidisciplinary working in their services, improve the flow of information between services and share information and care planning. Ultimately, the main message seems to be that local context is key, and that an integrated care model could be seen as acceptable in one area while viewed as unreasonably limiting competition in another:

> It is possible to design models of care for patients that enable competition between providers to provide services, allow patients a choice of a provider and deliver care to individual patients in an integrated way. In other cases, the effect of a model of care on choice, competition and integrated care will require careful consideration to establish what will achieve the best overall outcome for patients (Monitor, 2015a, para. 7.4).

This discretion could also be seen as an opportunity to pass the responsibility for sorting out the potential policy conflicts to local areas. Practical changes were introduced to support commissioners in achieving integration. For example, to address concerns regarding the barriers from the national tariff payment system commissioners and providers could agree local variations to prices and currencies, and it was possible to issue longer contracts than the one year default within the previous NHS standard contract. This latter point was important for the introduction of lead-provider or lead-contractor arrangements, as these can take several years to be developed and embedded (Billings and de Weger, 2015). Such 'outcome based' models were included within the pioneer and vanguard programmes, with common characteristics being that they commission a lead 'integrator' to achieve set outcomes for a defined population with flexibility regarding the care models that are deployed and the subcontractors that are engaged. The Integrated Personal Commissioning programme launched in 2014 was another initiative seeking to use purchasing, albeit it at a micro- rather than macro-level, to facilitate integrated care. This selected eight demonstrator sites to explore how combined health and social care budgets could be used to support individuals with complex needs to have greater power over how their allocated resources could be spent (NHS England, 2014c).

Taking stock of the Coalition's track record

In seeking to take stock of these developments, we have drawn upon the 'big and little window' policy stream model developed by Exworthy and Powell (2004). This built on the work of Kingdon (1995) and proposes three streams that should be considered when analysing implementation – *policy* (goals and objectives), *process* (including causal, technical and political feasibility) and *resources* (financial and human). To these streams are added three dimensions – *vertical* (the link between central government and local agencies), *central–horizontal* (links within and between central government departments and national bodies) and *peripheral–horizontal* (links within and between local implementation agencies). Thus, debates about implementation need to consider the 'big windows' at national level as well as 'little windows' at local level, and successful implementation is more likely when there is alignment between these different policy streams.

Vertical

The overall policy intention to facilitate integrated care was certainly loudly promoted following the work of the NHS Future Forum report, with the National Collaboration providing a symbolic statement of intent as well as providing a platform to announce subsequent integrated care initiatives. There were, though, some mixed messages regarding the priority objective to be achieved – while better outcomes for individuals as represented in the narrative for person-centred integrated care was present in some statements, for central government the key focus of the Better Care Fund was clearly on reducing hospital admissions and lengths of stay as a way of achieving substantial savings. There was also a failure to deliver the promised national indicator for integrated care, with an interim guidance document on existing cross-cutting measures highlighting their inadequacy rather than a collective strength. Additional resource to support integration in local areas was generally limited to good practice guidance and learning materials with some expert support for the Integrated Care Pioneers and latterly for Better Care Fund development. The Five Year Forward View Vanguards were treated somewhat differently, however, with access to a £200 million Transformation Fund.

In terms of governance, the Coalition arguably displayed a confusing mix of different approaches at different times/on different topics. On some occasions, there was very much a hands-off approach in which local areas were given considerable flexibility to develop local arrangements. Examples here would include the ability to decide membership of HWBs beyond the mandated core, no central assurance process for Health and Wellbeing Strategies, freedom to explore new forms of delivery in the pioneer and vanguard programmes, and a potential loosening of national contractual terms and tariffs. On the other hand, the Better Care Fund was subject to strong central control with drafts as well as final submissions requiring central government approval. Its basic premise, in which funding that was previously expected by local areas was diverted into a new national pot, also reflects increased central interference. There were also mixed messages regarding local freedom to use competition (or not) within commissioning. While guidance suggested that local areas were able to judge how best to secure local services, Monitor could also step in to investigate any decisions that it viewed as potentially anticompetitive.

Perhaps the most interesting change in relationships between the centre and localities came via the NHS Future Forum, which was a national body made up of a number of individuals with significant experience of frontline service delivery and local leadership. When faced with policy makers' apparent emphasis on competition and markets, it is perhaps unsurprising that some of those with practical experience of trying to integrate care in practice took a different line, stressing the importance of integrated care, local context and actions to remove perceived national barriers. Having got integrated care on the agenda, however, the Forum seems to have had less long term influence around the subsequent detail of Coalition policy.

Central–horizontal

Throughout this period, previous arrangements were broadly maintained, with health and adult social care policy the responsibility of the Department of Health, local government finance overseen by the Department for Communities and Local Government, and the Local Government Association and Association of Directors of Adult Social Services as the national voices of local government/adult social care. While the advent of new national bodies (such as NHS England, Public Health England and the Trust Development Authority) may have added greater complexity, regulation remained primarily the responsibility of the Care Quality Commission (for quality of care) and a strengthened Monitor (for market regulation of NHS services). Despite the creation of an Integrated Care and Support Steering Group and a more person-centred narrative around the aims of integrated care, the creation of separate outcomes frameworks for health, social care and public health remained problematic.

In terms of funding, responsibility for public health transferred to local government and the Better Care Fund sought to shift some NHS resources into a more joint pot. The treatment of health and social care budgets was markedly different at a national level, however, with NHS funding being maintained while adult social care was subject to major cuts. This was estimated to have resulted in local authority adult social care budgets making savings of 26 per cent or £3.53 billion between 2010 and 2014 (LGA/ADASS 2014). Over time, moreover, even initiatives such as the Better Care Fund became more prescriptive and more focused on core NHS priorities, thereby weakening attempts to protect the social care budget and leaving less scope for local discretion.

Peripheral–horizontal

On one level, the delegation of the local public health responsibilities, staffing and budget from former PCTs to Local Authorities was a major structural change which had the potential to build greater links between the technical expertise of public health colleagues with local authority functions such as prompting social and economic wellbeing, housing, transport, regeneration and economic development (see Chapter 10). Indeed in one survey over 80% of Directors of Public Health thought that public health was well placed within Local Authorities, and 99% believed it had a prominent place on the Health and Wellbeing Board (NAO 2014b). The early experience suggests that the arrangements are taking time to bed down, however, and for the nature of the relationship between national Public Health England, Local Authorities and CCGs to be understood. By their nature many public health impacts take many years to evaluate and it is therefore too early to tell if the potential benefits will be realised (see also Chapter 14). Despite the common acceptance that an integrated care system should be based on outcomes rather than inputs and activities, how to set and measure these remained elusive (Miller and Rees 2014). Our work with local areas also suggests that the long established rifts regarding which area of service should take priority in regards to achieving financial efficiencies and gaining from any savings also continue, and this was displayed in discussions around the BCF.

While Health and Wellbeing Boards have provided a forum for the discussion of joint health and social care priorities, many have found it difficult to influence the decisions taken elsewhere by individual CCGs and by Council Directorates. Early on there was significant enthusiasm, with 90 per cent of local authorities expressing interest in becoming early implementers (DH 2011). At the end of their shadow year, a national survey found that the majority were positive about the future opportunities presented by these new structures, and by the associated processes of needs assessment and joint strategy (Humphries et al 2012). Many stuck to the core membership suggested in national guidance (although 50% included a representative from the voluntary sector) and most were chaired by a lead local Councillor. A number of shadow Boards were also unsure how they would resource the work of Boards going forwards, and were not always clear about the extent to which they felt able to influence key decisions locally and to add value to existing structures. Many Boards also failed to include an NHS provider perspective, and many local areas struggled with growing tensions between providers and commissioners as to who was the 'expert' in terms of what might be needed next. The interim evaluation of the Pioneers found that NHS providers often felt excluded from local partnerships and that Clinical Commissioning Groups varied in their confidence that the Fund would facilitate diversion from acute hospitals (Erens et al, 2015). Procurement guidance and its emphasis on avoiding 'anti-competitive behaviour' was also seen as a disincentive for collaboration between providers (Erens et al, 2015).

Conclusion

Different governments have pursued health and social care integration for many years, and the Coalition certainly made integrated care a key feature of the policy rhetoric. Despite this (and perhaps slightly unkindly), the subtitle of this chapter is 'much ado about nothing?' After the controversy created by the 2010 White Paper, *Equity and Excellence*, the Coalition seemed an enthusiastic convert to 'integrated care' with an ongoing series of initiatives and a central place in policy rhetoric. Whether this was a genuine conversion or more of an attempt to reduce the political backlash they were facing remains unclear. In spite of this emphasis in national policy, our own experience is that local health and social care partners in 2015 were facing an extremely difficult policy and financial context – with local services in some circumstances arguably even less joined up than they had been in 2010. Using Exworthy and Powell's policy streams approach, this lack of genuine action/change is perhaps more understandable. Despite some new structures, funding pots and initiatives, the relationship between the centre and local areas has remained heavily skewed in favour of the former, and central government has sometimes seemed just as silo-based as the frontline services that policy makers have aimed to integrate. Ultimately, it is difficult to integrate care at the best of times – but doubly so if there is relatively little local discretion permitted in practice and if the bulk of policy still is not designed with integration in mind.

Reflecting back on Coalition's overall track record, it is hard to avoid the conclusion that the government may have devolved responsibility for developing locally appropriate responses when the issues at stake were difficult (if not impossible) to solve, but retained a firm central grip when it suited policy makers. We do have the legacies of an important person-centred narrative for integrated care, personal budgets across health and social care, and some potentially helpful new models of care. Health and Wellbeing Boards may ultimately lack the authority to pursue genuine integration, the Better Care Fund was something of a fudge and has become increasingly prescriptive, local learning from pilots could be difficult to spread more widely, and significant tensions remain between collaboration and competition. For the new Conservative government, the pressure continues to build on the positives while both health and social care face a challenging financial context. The 'holy grail' of integration must at times seem as far as away as ever.

References

Billings, J, de Weger, E, 2015, Contracting for integrated health and social care: A critical review of four models, *Journal of Integrated Care* 23, 3, 153–175

Department of Health, 1998, *Partnership in action: New opportunities for joint working between health and social services: A discussion document*, London: Stationery Office

Department of Health, 2010, *Equity and excellence: Liberating the NHS*, London: The Stationery Office

Department of Health, 2010, *Early implementers of health and wellbeing boards announced*, London: The Stationery Office, http://webarchive. nationalarchives.gov.uk/20130805112926/http://healthandcare. dh.gov.uk/early-implementers-of-health-and-wellbeing-boards-announced/

Department of Health/Department for Communities and Local Government, 2014, *Better Care Fund policy framework*, London: DH/ DCLG

Erens, B, Wistow, G, Mounier-Jack, S, Douglas, N, Jones, L, Manacorda, T, Mays, N, 2015, *Early evaluation of the Integrated Care and Support Pioneers Programme: Interim report*, London: Policy Innovation Research Unit

Exworthy, M, Powell, M, 2004, Big windows and little windows: Implementation in the 'congested state', *Public Administration* 82, 2, 263–281

Exworthy, M, Powell, M, 2004, Big windows and little windows: Implementation in the 'congested state', *Public Administration* 82, 2, 263–281

Exworthy, M, Berney, L, Powell, M, 2002, 'How great expectations in Westminster may be dashed locally': The local implementation of national policy on health inequalities, *Policy and Politics* 30, 1, 79–96

Farnsworth, A, 2012, Unintended consequences? The impact of NHS reforms upon Torbay Care Trust, *Journal of Integrated Care* 20, 3, 146–151

Glasby, J, Dickinson, H (eds), 2009, *International perspectives on health and social care: Partnership working in action*, Oxford: Blackwell-Wiley

Glasby, J, Dickinson, H, 2014, *Partnership working in health and social care: What is 'integrated care' and how can we deliver it?* (2nd edn), Bristol: The Policy Press

Glendinning, C, Powell, M, Rummery, K (eds), 2002, *Partnerships, New Labour and the governance of welfare*, Bristol: The Policy Press

Hansard, 1998, *Health and social services (co-operation)*, HC Deb 02 June 1998, 313, cc165–6

HM Government, 2010, *The Coalition: Our programme for government*, London: Cabinet Office

HM Treasury, 2013, *Spending round 2013*, London: the Stationery Office

Humphries R, Galea A, Sonola L, Mundle C, 2012, *Health and Wellbeing Boards: System leaders or talking shops?* London: The King's Fund

Kingdon, J, 1995, *Agendas, Alternatives and Public Policies* (2nd edn), Boston: Little, Brown & Co

Liberal Democrats, 2010, *Manifesto 2010*, London: Liberal Democrats

LGA/ADASS (Local Government Association and Association of Director of Adult Social Services), 2014, *Adult social care funding: 2014 state of the nation report,* London: LGA

Miller, R, Dickinson, H, Glasby, J, 2011, The care trust pilgrims, *Journal of Integrated Care* 19, 4, 14–21

Miller, R, Rees, J, 2014, Mental health commissioning: master or subject of change? *Mental Health Review Journal* 19, 3, 145–155

Monitor, 2013, *Substantive guidance on the Procurement, Patient Choice and Competition Regulations*, London: Monitor

Monitor, 2015a, *Complying with Monitor's integrated care requirements*, London: Monitor, www.gov.uk/government/publications/integrated-care-how-to-comply-with-monitors-requirements/complying-with-monitors-integrated-care-requirements

Monitor, 2015b, *Integrated care license conditions: Guidance for providers of NHS-funded services*, London: Monitor

NAO (National Audit Office), 2014, *Planning for the Better Care Fund*, London: National Audit Office

National Collaboration for Integrated Care and Support, 2013, *Integrated care and support: Our shared commitment*, www.gov.uk/government/uploads/system/uploads/attachment_data/file/287815/DEFINITIVE_FINAL_VERSION_Integrated_Care_and_Support_-_Our_Shared_Commitment_2013-05-13.pdf

National Voices, 2013, *A narrative for person-centred coordinated care*, www.england.nhs.uk/wp-content/uploads/2013/05/nv-narrative-cc.pdf

NHS England, 2013, *Annex to the NHS England planning guidance: Developing plans for the Better Care Fund (formerly the Integration Transformation Fund)*, www.england.nhs.uk/wp-content/uploads/2013/12/bcf-plann-guid.pdf

NHS England, 2014a, *Integrated care and support pioneer programme: Annual report 2014*, Leeds: NHS England

NHS England, 2014b, *Five year forward view*, Leeds: NHS England

NHS England, 2014c, *Integrated personal commissioning prospectus: making a reality of health and social care integration for individuals*, Leeds: NHS England

NHS Future Forum, 2012a, *Integration: A report from the NHS Future Forum*, London: NHS Future Forum

NHS Future Forum, 2012b, *NHS Future Forum: Summary report on proposed changes to the NHS*, London: NHS Future Forum

RAND Europe/Ernst and Young, 2012, *National evaluation of the Department of Health's integrated care pilots*, Cambridge: RAND Europe

Wistow, G, Dickinson, H, 2012, Integration: work still in progress, *Journal of Health Organization and Management*, 26, 6, 676-684

TEN

Public health: unchained or shackled?

David J Hunter

Introduction

As in the case of other parts of the UK wider health system, it has been a turbulent time for public health since 2010. Not only has the function undergone major structural and cultural change following its return to local government from the NHS, where it had been located since 1974, but it has had to confront new challenges in public health arising from lifestyle behaviours and a widening health gap between social groups. All of this has occurred during a period of unprecedented financial austerity affecting public services in general but local government in particular. This chapter reviews the state of public health in the lead up to the changes announced by the Coalition government in 2010. It then summarises the reforms before offering an interim assessment of their impact. Finally, it discusses the evidence to date concerning the reforms and speculates on likely prospects in the years ahead.

State of public health prior to 2010

Up until the passage of the Health and Social Care Act 2012, responsibility for public health in England lay with the NHS and in particular, at local level, with Primary Care Trusts (PCTs). Under the auspices of World Class Commissioning (WCC), introduced in 2007 to develop commissioning, PCTs' principal tasks included assessing the health needs of their communities and providing for them in regard to preventive and health care services. The purchaser–provider split was first introduced in 1991 with the aim of ensuring that purchasers assessed needs and provided for these in the most cost-effective way possible. From the outset, however, the real power continued to lie with the providers, and purchasing, or commissioning as it subsequently became known, largely failed to demonstrate its value. The WCC was a further attempt to revitalise the function.

For the most part, however, and despite WCC, public health remained a Cinderella sector within the NHS as, indeed, it had always tended to be since its transfer to the NHS from local government control in 1974. Spending on public health accounted for no more than 4% of the total health care budget. And even when budgets for public health had been agreed by PCTs, they were subject to frequent raids in order to maintain funding on acute care services or to fill gaps in spending on hospitals and beds. In his 2005 annual report, the then Chief Medical Officer for England, Liam Donaldson, lamented such tactics and criticised the lack of priority accorded public health by organisations ostensibly committed to its active pursuit. He wrote:

> This situation has not been created by any person or group of people. It is the result of many disparate factors, but at its heart is a set of attitudes that emphasises short-term thinking, holds too dear the idea of the hospital bed and regards the prevention of premature death, disease and disability as an option not as a duty. (Department of Health, 2006: 44)

Though the argument is a familiar one (having been made many times over the years by numerous commentators and advisors, including Charles Webster, the official NHS historian, Derek Wanless who advised the Labour government on the challenges facing the NHS over a 20 year period up until 2022, and this author) its articulation by a Chief Medical Officer lent it added weight (Webster, 2002; Wanless, 2002; Hunter, 2016).

It was not simply a case of insufficient resources being made available to public health, however, but also of the narrowness of the approach adopted. The focus on downstream individual lifestyle factors was seen to arise from the NHS's overriding preoccupation with disease and ill-health at an individual level. Insufficient attention has long been given to the myriad upstream influences on people's health, including the importance of housing and education among other public policy sectors (Hunter and Marks, 2016). The fact that unhealthy behaviours (smoking, drinking, lack of exercise and poor nutrition) seemed to cluster among certain deprived groups in society also suggested that an examination of the root causes of such behaviour was overdue (Buck and Frosini, 2012).

In recognition of the important role local government had in promoting health and wellbeing together with tackling health inequality, and inadvertently anticipating subsequent changes introduced by the Coalition government some years later, the Labour government introduced Director of Public Health (DPH) posts that were jointly appointed by PCTs and local authorities. While such posts did succeed to a degree in breaking down silos and in encouraging the adoption of a wider conception of public health, there were limits to their success given more general problems in regard to partnership working across the quite different cultures evident in the NHS and local government respectively (Hunter et al, 2010; Hunter and Perkins, 2014). Recounting his experiences as a jointly appointed DPH in Barnsley, Redgrave notes the considerable variety in arrangements and degrees of 'jointness' (Redgrave, 2007). For such posts to be successful, Redgrave insisted that a level of enthusiasm within the local authority to tackle health issues was essential but he also believed that PCTs must focus upstream on health as well as downstream on health care. He stressed the different skills DsPH needed to be effective, including having 'the political awareness and ability to operate outside their "comfort zone"' (2007, 228). For Redgrave, a pivotal factor in making joint posts work was the level of understanding in both local authorities and PCTs about the role and function of public health.

At around the same time as the growing appreciation of public health as being about more than what went on in the NHS, and after lengthy debate, there were advances in recognising the multidisciplinary public health workforce, including the establishment in 2003 of the UK voluntary register for public health specialists to accredit and quality-assure those who are non-medically qualified (Wright et al, 2014).

Towards the end of the Labour government's term of office, and despite its commitment to reduce them, a major review of health inequalities in England was commissioned. Known as the Marmot review after its chair, Michael Marmot, it documented the widening health gap in the UK and put forward six policy proposals embracing the life course to tackle the social gradient in health which required action across government at all levels (Marmot Review,, 2010). A commitment to tackling health inequalities was also a priority of the Coalition government in its public health white paper published within months of taking office (Secretary of State for Health, 2010). The white paper was offered as a response to Marmot's review and adopts a life course framework for tackling the wider social determinants of health. In his Foreword, the then Secretary of State for Health, Andrew Lansley, stated in the opening paragraphs that 'health inequalities between rich and poor have been getting progressively worse' and that 'we still live in a country where the wealthy can expect to live longer than the poor' (2010, 2). The promising start held out in the white paper, however, has not survived and the commitment has encountered severe difficulties with health inequalities widening in recent years (Smith et al, 2016).

Although unlikely given the systemic weakness of public health in the NHS coupled with the weakness of commissioning, had the WCC initiative been given sufficient time to prove itself, public health might just conceivably have assumed a higher priority. There were certainly a number of PCTs committed to such an outcome (McCafferty et al, 2012; Marks, 2014). As spending on the NHS began to level off around 2009–10, however, and as the prospects of further structural change loomed with the approaching general election of May 2010, PCTs became distracted and fearful for their future. Attention to, and investment in, public health stalled once again.

Summary of key public health reforms under the Coalition

Amidst general widespread opposition to the Coalition government's NHS reforms, those affecting public health received a warmer welcome in many, though not all, quarters. In an unexpected and unforeseen move, the government announced its intention to return public health to local government control by placing responsibility with upper tier or unitary authorities (Secretary of State for Health, 2010). Its thinking was shaped by the decision, also unexpected given that the Liberal Democrats had sought to make PCTs more democratic, to abolish PCTs and replace them with a larger number of Clinical Commissioning Groups (CCGs) in a move to empower GPs and give them control over real budgets and strategic plans for their communities. The move, however, was also in keeping with the new government's stated commitment to tackle the wider determinants of health and reduce health inequalities. In particular, it endorsed the Marmot agenda for change acknowledging that local authorities are well placed to adopt the life-course perspective articulated by Marmot. On the other hand, the decline in local authority control of key services, such as education with the arrival of academy and free schools, coupled with increased outsourcing of services to the private and third sectors, mean that 'place-based' approaches across the life course are becoming increasingly fragmented which adds to the difficulties of effective partnership working and of achieving whole of government action on health (Hunter, 2016).

Despite the various risks and suspicions in some quarters about the government's true intentions, the move to local government control of public health was widely welcomed by those who had long maintained that public health suffered from lurking in the shadows of the NHS (Elson, 1999; 2007). A key critic of government policy towards public health had been its advisor on the sustainability of the NHS, Derek Wanless (Wanless, 2002). In a hard-hitting report reviewing the state of public health, he argued that the NHS for all its pretence at being a health service was in fact little more than an ill-health service (Wanless, 2004). He feared for the future of the NHS and its financial sustainability if public health and prevention generally were not accorded higher priority. As things have turned out, his analysis and warnings have been proved prescient. Indeed, the NHS chief executive, Simon Stevens, endorsed Wanless's critique in his *NHS Five Year Forward View* and rounded on successive governments for having failed, despite signing up to Wanless's recommendations, to implement what he proposed in his 'fully engaged scenario' in which public health would have a core part to play in improving population health (NHS England, 2014).

Although Wanless did not advocate structural reform, since he believed the NHS had endured enough of it over the years, many working in public health and observing developments did not consider that real change was possible or likely as long as public health remained in the NHS's embrace. Just as the former CMO had opined, the urgent would always drive out the important. So when the Coalition government announced its plans for public health, there was a palpable sense that not only would the changes be good for public health but they would also reinvigorate and give new purpose to local government which had seen more and more powers removed from it. Partly reflecting public health's long history in local government during the era of Medical Officers of Health (MoHs) which was interrupted in 1974, many believed local authorities to be natural public health organisations so the coming home of public health was viewed with hope and optimism (Elson, 1999; 2004; Duggan, 2001). At last, it was believed, public health would be unchained. This is not to suggest that the era of the MoH was a golden age for public health but there were examples of inspired leadership which many believed were lost after 1974 (Gorsky, 2007).

Not surprisingly, most of the critics of the changes were those with clinical interests in public health who feared what would happen both to them personally and to the specialty of public health in a local government environment not known for its commitment to, or appreciation of, professional expertise. They foresaw the progressive downgrading and marginalisation of public health – something they had fought long and hard to resist in the NHS (Holland and Stewart

1998). While it is true that Directors of Public Health (DsPH) occupied senior management positions in both PCTs and in the higher tier Strategic Health Authorities (also abolished by the Coalition government), however, there was a widespread perception that many failed to punch above their weight and were content merely to proffer their advice in the form of an independent annual report rather than seek to fight for measures that would result in real public health improvements. It seemed that for many working in public health, remaining on the sidelines or in the shadows passed as a perfectly reasonable response to policies of which they disapproved and which they believed would harm the public's health. Part of the reason lay in many public health practitioners believing they lacked the political and advocacy skills to advance their interests (Hunter, 2007).

For others in public health, though, especially those who had come into the profession from a non-clinical background and who were seized by a sense of social injustice in the face of mounting evidence of growing health inequalities, they sought to challenge the accepted orthodoxy and above all wished to see tangible change resulting from their efforts. Such individuals also held to a different conception of public health and one that was much wider in its embrace of the social and structural determinants of health compared with the medical model. Indeed, the coming of age of the multidisciplinary public health workforce is one of the more interesting and positive developments in recent decades (Evans, 2003; Wright et al, 2014). It is now accepted that community development, education, health promotion, housing, social science, economics and other disciplines all have a part to play.

Of course, the traditional preoccupations of public health around health protection have remained important but these new entrants to the higher echelons of public health were more motivated by a sense of how best to promote health and wellbeing in their widest sense. They were imbued with the visionary thinking underlying WHO's Ottawa Charter published in 1986 (WHO, 1986) and more recent incarnations including WHO's Healthy Cities movement and the Finnish government's Health in All Policies (HiAP) initiative involving whole of government and whole of society approaches to improving health (Stahl et al, 2006). This was subsequently adopted by the European Commission and WHO and lies at the heart of WHO Europe's health policy framework, *Health 2020* (WHO, 2012). Those who ascribed to this wider view of public health felt the NHS was the wrong place for such an approach to take root. The move back to local government therefore offered real hope of a new dawn for public health.

The changes entailed DsPH and their public health teams moving to local government. Many had already established themselves in local authorities following the move to create joint posts noted earlier. In these cases, the dislocation and culture shock of moving out of the NHS was minimised. Nevertheless, while the intention was that public health would remain linked to the NHS via CCGs and providing them with public health advice, to all intents and purposes the move to local government and the future governance of public health required a separation from the NHS accompanied by a transfer of budgets based on previous spending on public health by PCTs. The budgets were also protected through a ring-fence for the first few years although this did not prevent unexpected cuts to overall funding levied by the Chancellor as part of his crusade to cut public spending and reduce the deficit, as discussed later in this chapter.

Health and Wellbeing Boards (HWBs) were introduced as the partnership of choice, bringing together all the interests in a local area with a commitment to health and wellbeing (see Chapter 14). The Boards' principal, and possibly only, power was to undertake a needs assessment and to produce joint Health and Wellbeing Strategies (HWSs) to which other bodies, notably CCGs, would sign up. The Boards possess no powers to require implementation of their priorities, however, which leaves open the question of how seriously committed local authorities and their partners truly are to action in public health. At the very least, the weaknesses surrounding HWBs provide the perfect excuse, if one were needed, for doing as little as possible in the face of other pressures, notably financial ones.

Since the changes were introduced in April 2013, a great deal of time and effort has been spent on securing public health's position within local government. Inevitably, given the diversity that characterises local government, there is no one or right model or accepted approach. Some local authorities have retained the DPH position and accorded it senior status within the officer team. Others have changed the title (to, for example, director of health improvement) or have merged the DPH post with the Director for Adult Social Services. In yet other places, the DPH role has been perceived to have been downgraded in terms of its repositioning under another directorate.

Then there have been the recent moves concerning devolution, specifically the so-called 'Northern Powerhouse' initiative which the Chancellor has taken a keen interest in pushing. At the outset, this referred to plans in Greater Manchester to devolve a range of powers, including over the health system, to a new combined authority (Association of Greater Manchester Authorities et al, 2015). In order not to be left out and to see devolution take effect more widely across England, however, the developments in Manchester have spawned a series of similar attempts to devolve powers to other local authorities, although not all involve health, or at least not for the time being. There remains in any case a large question mark over what form devolution in respect of the NHS might take given that the health service is 'national'. Retention of key powers by the Secretary of State for Health suggests that health system powers might in practice be delegated rather than devolved (Paine, 2015).

More generally, given all the other changes affecting local government, notably the public spending cuts affecting local services, devoting attention to public health has perhaps been less of a priority than it might otherwise have been in more 'normal' circumstances.

The changes in public health introduced by the Coalition government were not confined to the local level. Nationally, a new arm's length executive agency was created, Public Health England (PHE), to provide leadership for public health (see Chapter 5). Modelled largely on the Health Protection Agency which it replaced, PHE was given responsibility for two of the domains of public health: health protection, including emergency preparedness, and health improvement. The third domain, health service quality improvement, resides with NHS England and other agencies, notably the Care Quality Commission and, more recently, NHS Improvement. On public health matters affecting the NHS as well as local government, PHE and NHS England work closely together. PHE also provides public health information and evidence although its relationship with the National Institute for Health and Care Excellence (NICE), which is responsible for producing public health guidelines and quality standards, is still evolving. Despite the existence of PHE, there remains a sizeable public health group of civil servants located within the Department of Health which, inter alia, presumably exists to service the public health minister and Chief Medical Officer.

Evidence of the implementation and impact of the reforms

Given the policy churn noted above in regard to local government, at this stage it is hard to provide firm or convincing evidence concerning whether the changes are being implemented as planned or what their emerging impact has been. A lengthy transition period is one factor in the mix and the tough financial environment facing local government is another. Public health's funding position worsened following the

Chancellor's unexpected announcement in June 2015 that public health funding would be reduced by £200 million on a recurrent basis. Local authorities are disinvesting in areas such as prevention, addiction services, sexual health and weight management after a 6% cut in the public health grant for 2015/16, with more cuts planned for 2016/17 (Iacobucci, 2016). The decision to reduce public health funding is a curious and much criticised one that seems to fly in the face of government policy elsewhere, notably in NHS England's efforts, particularly through its chief executive, to raise the profile of, and priority attached to, public health and prevention.

The ring-fencing of the public health budget since 2013 has been one of the more controversial features of the reforms. The ring fence was expected to be lifted in 2016 but the Chancellor announced in November 2015 that it would remain in place until the end of 2017/18. Thereafter it is intended to fully fund local authorities' public health spending from their retained business rates receipts as part of the move towards 100% business rate retention. The unexpected retention of the ring fence for a further two years is also in order to afford a degree of stability following the transfer of services for 0–5s to local authorities.

Certainly the ring fence has accorded public health a degree of protection denied other local government services, but views are sharply divided over its merits. Supporters maintain it is essential to avoid budget raids which they say are already taking place in local authorities feeling the effects of the fiscal squeeze on their budgets (Iacobucci, 2014, 2016). The Public Accounts Committee (PAC), while acknowledging that the ring-fencing of grants to local authorities is unusual, also accepted that there was a risk that spending on public health will decline if the ring fence is lifted (House of Commons Committee of Public Accounts, 2015).

Critics of the ring-fence, however, maintain that it runs counter to the notion of ensuring that public health becomes the business of all local authority functions and that to single out one activity for such protection is both divisive and indefensible (Local Government Association, 2015). The Local Government Association (LGA) considers that the removal of the ring fence is important if full advantage is to be taken of the relocation of public health to local government. If public health funding continues to be treated separately from other grants with separate conditions, there is a danger that it will not properly integrate with all of the functions of local government. This brings alive all of the very real opportunities that exist within the transfer, for example working with schools to tackle childhood obesity.

Endorsing the LGA's view, and in contrast to the PAC, the Communities and Local Government Committee has expressed less sympathy with those who wish to retain the ring fence arguing that it is not in the spirit of the changes. Its preference is for the introduction of community or place-based budgeting (House of Commons Communities and Local Government Committee, 2013a).

For all the concern about the parlous levels of funding and the risks for public health associated with these, there are some early indications, together with more anecdotal evidence, that the changes are having a positive impact (Local Government Association, 2014). For instance, a survey of DsPH conducted in 2014 found that the relocation of public health to local government was 'achieving some of the outcomes and the direction of travel envisaged by policy makers' (Jenkins et al, 2015: 6). These gains were especially evident in those local authorities where good relationships had been established between elected members, local government officers and DsPH and their teams. Reinforcing these findings, a study of prioritisation in public health investment and disinvestment reported that the way in which evidence was conceived and used demonstrated the pivotal influence of context and values in public health priority-setting (Marks et al, 2015).

Potentially significant weaknesses lay in links with CCGs, however, which were reported as being weak and undeveloped (Jenkins et al, 2015). For their part, CCGs have been critical of the move of public health out of the NHS, regarding the changes as detrimental to the NHS's public health role which remains important but which is at risk of neglect. Whether the variable commitment of CCGs to HWBs reflects the traditionally weak engagement of GPs with public health may also be a factor.

HWBs have few powers and those they do have are not especially strong. One key power they do have, as noted, is the production of health and wellbeing strategies (HWSs) and if these achieve the buy-in from key stakeholders then there is the prospect of change being possible. The early evidence suggests that HWSs have some way to go before they are likely to have an impact, however. In an analysis of 47 HWSs, it was found that they were dominated by evidence of need and could profitably be strengthened by greater use of evidence of effectiveness for public health interventions (Beenstock et al, 2014). Perhaps not surprisingly, local authorities displayed varying interpretations of what should be contained in an HWS. Most timescales were short – three years or less. 'Evidence' was least often used to mean evidence of effectiveness or cost-effectiveness. It was not always obvious whether or how Joint Strategic Needs Assessments

(JSNAs) had been used to inform HWSs despite a clear requirement in the statutory guidance to do so. With public health now the responsibility of local government, however, the meaning of the term 'evidence' has come to the fore. Traditional notions of evidence include systematic reviews, peer reviewed journals and analysed data. In the majority of HWSs reviewed in the study mentioned above, however, these were not the sources of evidence referred to in most cases and JSNAs did not seem to refer to them either. A group of academics have proposed that a broad range of types of evidence, including case studies and local consultations, as well as more traditional types of evidence, might be used to inform local authority decisions (South et al, 2014). Moreover, political influences are now seen to be more significant drivers of public health decisions than the use of evidence in policy-making.

Another major plank of the public health reforms, Public Health England (PHE), has come in for varying degrees of criticism. While the House of Commons Public Accounts Committee concluded that PHE 'has made a good start in its efforts to protect and improve public health', it felt that the organisation lacked 'strong enough ways of influencing local authorities to ensure progress against all of its top public health priorities'. It also concluded that PHE needs to influence central government departments more effectively and 'translate its own passion into action across Whitehall' (House of Commons Committee of Public Accounts, 2015: 3). Achieving joined up government is, as many others have concluded, a perennial problem (Exworthy and Hunter, 2011). Furthermore, PHE, and indeed the Department of Health, cannot direct local authorities to act in accordance with their wishes as set out in their priorities and the public health outcomes framework. They can only persuade and influence what happens locally. Local authorities after all, and in contrast to the NHS, are democratically elected bodies accountable to their local communities. They do not answer to central government and if they did there would be little point in having locally elected bodies.

Neither has PHE escaped criticism for failing to provide national leadership for public health. Whereas NICE has been told by the government to steer clear of commenting on national policy, PHE, which has this remit, has been criticised for being too timid and for not 'speaking truth to power' (House of Commons Health Committee, 2014). The Health Committee considers that the relationship between the Department and PHE remains problematic and that PHE lacks the independence desired and expected of it (House of Commons Health Committee, 2014). In support of this claim, there is evidence to suggest that there has been political interference to suppress or delay the publication of PHE reports, most recently its review of the evidence concerning sugar consumption and the effects on obesity which proved to be critical of government policy or rather the lack of one (Tedstone et al, 2015).

PHE has the task of providing local authorities with evidence and decision support tools, although NICE, too, has responsibilities in these areas. Following a critical report from the National Audit Office (2014a), the Public Accounts Committee was dismissive of PHE's efforts so far in these areas and recommended improved responsiveness on the part of PHE to local authority requests for support, including help with understanding the evidence base and cost implications of different public health interventions (House of Commons Committee of Public Accounts, 2015). As noted earlier, however, in a study of prioritisation in public health spending which has involved academic researchers working with a few local authorities to determine what, if any, decision support tools they might wish to employ, providing such support in diverse and complex contexts which are often highly charged politically presents a series of challenges (Marks et al, 2015). Although DsPH might welcome more assistance with economic modelling and better advice on return on investment tools to forecast the financial impact of particular interventions, they are not the leaders in local authorities. That role rests with elected members who also need to be persuaded that such tools can help them realise their priorities and address their concerns.

Issues in regard to the workforce have also surfaced following the changes. An immediate concern has arisen over the recruitment and retention of DsPH. According to the Association of Directors of Public Health vacancies remain for around 20% of DsPH posts. Turnover is likely in the next few years given the age profile of DsPH. Part of the problem rests in the differing pay and conditions for staff moving from the NHS to local government. Of course, workforce issues are critical to the success of the reforms but it may be that the high turnover among senior level posts is not necessarily a bad thing in the longer term. Indeed, the move to local government allows for an overhaul of the workforce that is perhaps overdue. The next section returns to this issue.

Perhaps had the public health changes occurred at any other time, and possibly under a different government less opposed to public services, the optimism of those who had welcomed them would have been more fully justified and realised. For many working in public health, however, the changes occurred at precisely the wrong time if there was to be any serious chance of them succeeding. A number of reasons can be advanced for this state of affairs and the last section considers those.

Interpretation and discussion of emergent findings

While the prospects of a renaissance in public health occurring seem less certain than might have been the case when the changes were first announced, it remains early days in the overall scheme of things. Early findings from several studies indicate some encouraging signs that the advantages of a local government setting for adopting a wider public health perspective are being exploited. They also suggest anxiety over how far DsPH will be able to succeed and exert influence in a highly political context where traditional notions of evidence count for less when it comes to setting priorities and deciding which interventions to support or not. Such anxiety is evident in the significant number of vacant DPH posts.

Underlying these concerns are deeper issues relating to the very different cultural context prevailing in local government. Over time, this particular barrier can be expected to disappear as those working in public health will not have the NHS background which could be viewed as an impediment to progress. There is nonetheless also growing recognition, which preceded the recent public health changes but which has acquired added significance since, that much of the training public health practitioners have had is perhaps no longer 'fit for purpose' and that different skills and capabilities are needed to function successfully in a local government setting (Hunter, 2009). In addition to what might be regarded as more traditional technical expertise in public health, like epidemiology, such 'soft skills' would include political astuteness/awareness, communication, managing conflict, negotiating/influencing, and change management (Elson, 2008). Only by working across boundaries, and with and through others, is it likely that success will occur.

In this regard, HWBs are viewed as critically important although possibly not up to the job everywhere (Bentley, 2013). Some are seen as mere talking shops with no powers to effect change although this could change as a result of the devolved arrangements taking root in places like Greater Manchester. Under plans being developed there, HWBs might acquire a more central role, but there are also dangers in widening the remit of HWBs before they have established themselves as confident players in the new public health system and taken on board the lessons from previous efforts at partnership working (Perkins and

Hunter, 2014). For instance, many working in public health regard the government's focus on integrated care, including the introduction of the now discredited Better Care Fund (National Audit Office, 2014b), as having distracted HWBs and diverted them from their core business, namely, the promotion of health and wellbeing. While few dispute the importance of integrated care, there is a risk of HWBs being captured by this agenda to the exclusion of a proper focus on public health. The House of Commons Communities and Local Government Committee was sufficiently concerned about this danger to stress the need for HWBs 'to maintain a strategic and balanced outlook on their new responsibilities, focusing on promoting the health of their local population, rather than becoming exclusively preoccupied with the detail of health and social care commissioning and integration' (House of Commons Communities and Local Government Committee, 2013b: 16).

So far, much of the focus has been on ensuring that local authorities make good progress in improving the public's health. There is a key role for PHE here although it can only do its bidding through influence, not direction. Such a limitation, however, points to a tension at the heart of PHE's remit. On the one hand, it is accountable for securing improved public health outcomes. On the other hand, the levers available to it to ensure that such outcomes are realised are few and limited in their reach. It is true that some public health functions are prescribed and the Department of Health can attach conditions to the PHE grant given to local authorities. If the whole purpose and thrust of the changes is not to be rendered meaningless, however, it would not be appropriate to use such powers too often and become overly directive in regard to local government. Such a move would be fiercely resisted. Moreover, it is hardly in the spirit of devolving responsibilities which the government is keen to promote adopting the subsidiarity principle. Finally, PHE has emphasised its wish to be viewed as the friend of local government – ready to support and assist it when required. It can hardly appear in this guise while also wielding a big stick. How this tension gets resolved, if indeed it can be, and what has been termed 'sector-led improvement' assured, will be a key test for the new system in the months and years ahead.

PHE's remit includes public health at national level and, if necessary, at challenging government policy in areas where either there is none or where government has appeared reluctant to act. Although smoking is now regarded as an area of public policy where government is willing to act, most recently in respect of introducing plain packaging for cigarette packs, in other areas of concern to public health, notably a tax on sugar consumption and minimum unit pricing on alcohol, the UK government has resisted calls to act believing that it is not their job to meddle in people's lives but rather to provide them with the information to enable them to make healthy choices. Moreover, the government has resisted pressure to confront vested corporate interests via taxation and/or regulation opting instead for a voluntary approach as set out in the Public Health Responsibility Deal launched by the Coalition government in 2011. This aims to bring together public sector, academic, commercial and voluntary organisations to help meet public health goals and is being evaluated by the Department of Health funded Policy Innovation Research Unit. In contrast, the Scottish and Welsh governments have shown a greater determination to provide national leadership believing that in some areas of public health only government can act to create the conditions necessary for people to exercise healthy choices (Smith et al, 2015).

Changes in the public health workforce are also in hand, hastened by the return of public health to local government as well as by the financial pressures on public services. If public health is the business of the whole local authority, including those working in sectors like housing and education who may not consider themselves to be public health practitioners, then redefining the workforce to include such groups seems both desirable and inevitable. Indeed, the People in UK Public Health Group, set up under the auspices of the Royal Society for Public Health to advise the four health departments on future changes in the public health workforce, has a primary focus on shaping the vision and future priorities for a multi-disciplinary public health workforce fit for the 21st century, recognising that improving the public's health involves a broad range of people in a variety of professions, communities and settings (Royal Society for Public Health, 2015). The wider public health workforce is defined as 'any individual who is not a specialist or practitioner in public health, but has the opportunity or ability to positively impact health and wellbeing through their (paid or unpaid) work'.

There is clearly much work to be done and some urgency about making progress at scale. The NHS chief executive, Simon Stevens, has called for a 'radical upgrade in prevention and public health' and has committed the NHS to 'back hard-hitting national action on obesity, smoking, alcohol and other major health risks' in addition to advocating for 'stronger public-health related powers for local government and elected mayors' (NHS England, 2014: 3). Yet, in the face of such pressure, the UK government appears unmoved. The issue is also one for PHE to address especially following the Public Accounts

Committee's concern about PHE's influence across Whitehall, especially where a government department may develop a policy that cuts through a public health priority. The Department of Health works across government on public health, including through a cross-government group that includes relevant departments. PHE accepts that its work across government has not been as well co-ordinated or closely connected with its five priorities for health improvement as it should be, and that there should be a public health voice in major government departments. The agency plans to address this through attaching regional directors of public health to major government departments. It has to be said that previous efforts to adopt a whole of government approach have been underwhelming so in this case, as on so much else arising from the new public health system, the jury is out (Exworthy and Hunter, 2011).

Conclusion

While there is much to welcome in these changes within public health, it may be a case of the right policy at the wrong time. Long-term advocates of local government control over public health would not have chosen the current political circumstances for such a move and are therefore suspicious of what they perceive to be happening, that is, that local government is seemingly being set up to fail. Not only is there the government's fixation on austerity and a need, as it sees it, to reduce the deficit at all costs – which requires swingeing cuts to public services – but it is a policy fuelled by an unswerving neoliberal ideology. The resulting choices are entirely political, not economic, and the future fate of public health is not immune from their impact.

This larger programme of change, begun under the Coalition government and pursued with greater vigour since the election held in May 2015 which returned a Conservative government with a slender majority, has been well described by two political analysts who argue that the government's change programme is more than just a response to a large current account deficit. Rather, the deficit offers a convenient pretext, or mask, for what the real agenda is, namely, 'a restructuring of welfare benefits and public services that takes the country in a new direction, rolling back the state to a level of intervention below that in the United States – something which is unprecedented. Britain will abandon the goal of attaining a European level of public provision. The policies include substantial privatisation and a shift of responsibility from state to individual' (Taylor-Gooby and Stoker, 2011: 14). Some five years since those words were written, nothing that has happened suggests the analysis is fundamentally wrong. In such a climate, it is hard to predict what the prognosis for public health might be.

References

Association of Greater Manchester Authorities, NHS England, NHS Greater Manchester Association of Clinical Commissioning Groups, 2015, *Greater Manchester health and social care devolution: Memorandum of understanding*, Manchester: Association of Greater Manchester Authorities

Beenstock, J, Sowden, S, Hunter, DJ, White, M, 2014, Are health and well-being strategies in England fit for purpose? A thematic content analysis, *Journal of Public Health* 37, 3, 461–69

Bentley, C, 2013, Public health and local authorities, written submission in House of Commons Communities and Local Government Committee, *The role of local authorities in health issues,* Eight Report of Session 2012–13, HC694, Ev152–165, London: The Stationery Office

Buck, D, Frosini, G, 2012, *Clustering of unhealthy behaviours over time*, London: King's Fund

Department of Health, 2006, *The Chief Medical Officer on the state of public health*, Annual Report 2005, London: Department of Health

Duggan, M, 2001, *Healthy living: The role of modern local authorities in creating healthy communities*, Birmingham: SOLACE

Elson, T, 1999, Public health and local government, in S Griffiths, DJ Hunter (eds) *Perspectives in public health*, Oxford: Radcliffe Medical Press

Elson, T, 2004, Why public health must become a core part of council agendas, in K Skinner (ed) *Community leadership and public health: The role of local authorities*, London: The Smith Institute

Elson, T, 2007, Local government and the health improvement agenda, in S Griffiths, DJ Hunter (eds) *New perspectives in public health*, 2nd edition, Oxford: Radcliffe Publishing

Elson, T, 2008, Joint Director of Public Health Appointments: 6 Models of Practice, in DJ Hunter (ed) *Perspectives on Joint Director of Public Health appointments*, London: Durham University and the Improvement and Development Agency, Local Government Association

Evans, D, 2003, 'Taking public health out of the ghetto': The policy and practice of multi-disciplinary public health in the United Kingdom, *Social Science and Medicine* 57: 959–67

Exworthy, M, Hunter, DJ, 2011, The challenge of joined-up government in tackling health inequalities, *International Journal of Public Administration* 34, 4, 201–12

Gorsky, M, 2007, Local leadership in public health: The role of the medical officer of health in Britain, 1872–1974, *Journal of Epidemiology and Community Health* 61, 6, 468–72

Holland, WW, Stewart, S, 1998, *Public health, the vision and the challenge*, London: Nuffield Trust

House of Commons Committee of Public Accounts, 2015, *Public Health England's grant to Local Authorities*, Forty-third Report of Session 2014–15, HC 893, London: The Stationery Office

House of Commons Communities and Local Government Committee, 2013a, *Community budgets*, Third Report of Session 2013–14, HC 163, London: The Stationery Office

House of Commons Communities and Local Government Committee, 2013b, *The Role of local authorities in health issues*, Eighth Report of Session 2012–13, HC 694, London: The Stationery Office

House of Commons Health Committee, 2014, *Public Health England*, Eighth Report of Session 2013–14, HC 840, London: The Stationery Office

Hunter, DJ, 2007, *Exploring managing for health*, in DJ Hunter (ed) Managing for Health, London: Routledge

Hunter, DJ, 2009, Leading for health and wellbeing: the need for a new paradigm, *Journal of Public Health* 31, 2, 2002–4

Hunter, DJ, 2016, *The health debate*, 2nd edition, Bristol: Policy Press

Hunter, DJ, Marks, L, Smith, KE, 2010, *The public health system in England*, Bristol: Policy Press

Hunter, DJ, Perkins, N, 2014, *Partnership working in public health*, Bristol: Policy Press

Hunter, DJ, Marks, L, 2016, Health inequalities in England's changing public health system, in KE Smith, S Hill, C Bambra (eds) *Health inequalities: Critical perspectives*, Oxford: Oxford University Press

Iacobucci, G, 2014, Raiding the public health budget, *British Medical Journal* 348, g2274

Iacobucci, G, 2016, Public health: The frontline cuts begin, *British Medical Journal* 352, i272

Jenkins, LM, Bramwell, D, Coleman, A, Gadsby, EW, Peckham, S, Perkins, N, Segar, J, 2015, Integration, influence and change in public health: Findings from a survey of Directors of Public Health in England, *Journal of Public Health* Advance Access, doi:10.1093/pubmed/fdv139

Local Government Association, 2014, *Public health in local government: One year on*, London: Local Government Association

Local Government Association, 2015, *Spending review and autumn statement 2015*, On the Day Briefing, 25 November, www.local.gov.uk/documents/10180/6869714/On+the+Day+Briefing+SR+2015.pdf/fadcf449-c787-43c0-8648-1ccf403a9275

Marks, L, 2014, *Governance, commissioning and public health*, Bristol: Policy Press

Marks, L, Hunter, DJ, Scalabrini, S, Gray, J, McCafferty, S, Payne, N, Peckham, S, Salway, S, Thokola, P, 2015, The return of public health to local government in England: Changing the parameters of the public health prioritisation debate? *Public Health* 129, 1194–1203

Marmot Review, 2010, *Fair society, healthy lives: Strategic review of health inequalities in England post-2010*, London: The Marmot Review

McCafferty, S, Williams, I, Hunter, D, Robinson, S, Donaldson, C, Bate, A, 2012, Implementing world class commissioning competencies, *Journal of Health Services Research and Policy* 17, 40–8

National Audit Office, 2014a, *Public Health England's grant to local authorities*, Report by the Comptroller and Auditor General, HC 888 Session 2014–15, London: National Audit Office

National Audit Office, 2014b, *Planning for the Better Care Fund*, Report by the Comptroller and Auditor General, HC 781 Session 2014–15, London: National Audit Office

NHS England, 2014, *NHS five year forward view*, London: NHS England

Paine, D, 2015, Health secretary could overturn devolved decisions, *Health Service Journal*, 26 June

Perkins, N, Hunter, DJ, 2014, Health and Wellbeing Boards: a new dawn for public health partnerships? *Journal of Integrated Care*, 22, 5/6, 220–29

Redgrave, P, 2007, Making joint director of public health posts work, in S Griffiths, DJ Hunter (eds) *New Perspectives in Public Health*, 2nd edition, Oxford: Radcliffe Publishing

Royal Society for Public Health, 2015, *Rethinking the public health workforce*, London: RSPH

Secretary of State for Health, 2010, *Healthy lives, healthy people: Our strategy for public health in England*, Cm 7985, London: The Stationery Office

Smith, KE, Hill, S, Bambra, C (eds), 2016, *Health inequalities: Critical perspectives*, Oxford: Oxford University Press

South, J, Hunter, DJ, Gamsu, M, 2014, *What local government needs to know about public health*, A local government navigator evidence review, Local Government Association, www.solace.org.uk/knowledge/reports_guides/LGKN_NTK_PUBLIC_HEALTH_18-03-14.pdf

Stahl, T, Wismar, M, Ollila, E, Lahtinen, E, Leppo, K (eds), 2006, *Health in all policies: Prospects and potentials*, Helsinki: Finnish Ministry of Social Affairs and Health and European Observatory on Health Systems and Policies

Taylor-Gooby, P, Stoker, G, 2011, The coalition programme: A new vision for Britain or politics as usual? *The Political Quarterly* 82, 1, 4–15

Tedstone, A, Targett, C, Allen, R, 2015, *Sugar reduction: The evidence for action,* London: Public Health England

Webster, C, 2002, *The National Health Service: A political history*, Oxford: Oxford University Press

Wanless, D, 2002, *Securing our future health: Taking a long-term view*, Final report, London: HM Treasury

Wanless, D, 2004, *Securing good health for the whole population*, Final report, London: HM Treasury

WHO (World Health Organisation), 1986, *Ottawa charter for health promotion*, Geneva: WHO

WHO, 2012, *Health 2020: A European policy framework and strategy for the 21st Century*, Copenhagen: WHO Regional Office for Europe

Wright, J, Sim, F, Wright, K, 2014, *Multidisciplinary public health: Understanding the development of the modern workforce*, Bristol: Policy Press

ELEVEN

Provider plurality and supply-side reform

Rod Sheaff and Pauline Allen

Polymorphous plural providers

Not only healthcare financing but also its provision was nationalised when the NHS was founded. Besides guaranteeing access to healthcare, Bevan and the other founders also intended to – and eventually largely did – ' level up' a supply side comprised of diversely-owned providers which provided correspondingly diverse levels of service access, quality and responsiveness to healthcare needs. Since 1979 neo-liberal 'reforms' of the NHS have had a supply side component, that of introducing 'provider plurality' under which a range of differently-owned organisations provide NHS-funded services:

1. public firms, that is, state-owned providers (for example, NHS trusts) with a degree of financial autonomy and discretion in their use of resources.
2. professional partnerships (for example, most general practices), which a group of professionals jointly own and manage, and which employ other staff.
3. shareholder-owned, dividend-maximising firms including:
   a) private equity firms, whose shares are not publicly traded.
   b) corporations, whose shares are publicly traded.
4. proprietary (that is, owner-managed firms), whose shares are not usually publicly traded.
5. social enterprises, an ill-defined category ranging from not-for-profit providers which differ from corporations mainly in not distributing profits to shareholders to organisations whose workforce and/or consumers have a voice in controlling the organisation (Allen et al, 2011).
6. charitable, voluntary and self-help organisations which depend heavily on volunteer labour.

7. co-operatives and mutuals, democratically controlled by their workforce, consumers or subscribers.

In the circumstances that most NHS services have hitherto been provided by public organisations and professional partnerships, proposals for greater provider diversity mean shifting the proportion towards types (3) to (7) above. Whatever the effect on healthcare supply, such a contentious policy has already greatly increased the supply of euphemism, confusion and obfuscation in health policy debates. This chapter attempts to give an overview of the empirical patterns of development, and unpick some of the conceptual confusions.

Provider plurality and supply side reform before 2010

Until the late 1970s, the most salient English health policy debates were electoral bidding competitions about spending on the NHS and about the effect of private medical practice on NHS waiting lists. Parliament occasionally heard proposals to retract public funding and provider ownership at the margins of the NHS, raise prescription and other NHS charges, retain 'amenity' beds in NHS hospitals (for a fee patients could obtain better 'hotel' services), and allow consultants greater private practice. Mostly these policies had little practical impact but served, rather, a symbolic function of preserving the idea of the normality and legitimacy of plural provision and private payment for healthcare, not least for parts of the Conservative Party and like-minded pressure groups who were still sceptical about an NHS whose efficiency, popularity and indeed existence were living disproof of some of their policy, economic and moral principles.

Version 1: Provider plurality

With the Thatcher government (1979) their moment came, but also a dilemma. Financially and ideologically (Bacon and Eltis, 1976; Letwin, 1988), such governments disliked living with the welfare state, but electorally they could not live without it (Offe, 1982); Its 'flagship', the NHS, was too popular for direct attack. As their main intellectual foundation, NHS 'reform' policies since 1979, including provider plurality, have what some orthodox economists call the 'doctrine of the second best': if one cannot establish a conventional market, the next best thing is to establish institutions whose market 'distortions', taken together, minimise the overall deviation from perfect competition (Lipsey and Lancaster, 1956). This doctrine suggests the construction of quasi-markets (Enthoven, 1985; Bartlett and Le Grand, 1993) in which the state, social insurer or similar body purchases services on behalf of the consumer (Allen 2013) and in which plural providers of healthcare compete by stimulating innovation, improving healthcare quality and/or reducing of healthcare costs. For the NHS, the UK government envisaged District Health Authorities (DHAs) and GP fundholders purchasing healthcare on behalf of patients, with providers competing for contracts and thus for income (Department of Health, 1989).

From 1991 both these purchasers were allowed to commission non-NHS providers. Using Waiting List Initiative funds, DHAs could purchase private hospital treatment for patients who had been more than a year on NHS waiting lists, although these purchases remained only a small proportion of NHS in-patient work (see Chapter 12). Few GP fundholders commissioned private care for their patients. Economists often assume that in order to compete successfully in a quasi-market, providers need to take on certain more corporate characteristics: greater managerial discretion, provider retention of profits and losses, and governance through a Board of Directors (Harding and Preker 2000). Except for general practices, NHS providers were therefore reconstituted as NHS trusts partly on these lines but, importantly, not (yet) in respect of profit retention. From 1993 the Department of Health also encouraged private–public joint ventures, removing the requirement to assess them against a fully NHS-funded alternative (NHS internal *Executive Letter EL(93)37*, issued by the Department of Health in London in 1993). Soon after, the Private Finance Initiative (PFI) followed. NHS trusts made turnkey contracts with consortia of corporations and private equity firms to plan, finance, build and hospitals, and to provide the ancillary services, on-site shops and car parking. The trust paid the consortia for these but retained clinical budgets, income and management. To financially justify PFI hospital schemes sometimes required trusts to under-estimate future caseload and over-estimate clinicians' future productivity, so as to under-estimate the required beds (Pollock et al, 1999). The 1996 NHS (Residual Liabilities) Act made the Secretary of State for Health guarantor of PFI schemes in the NHS (Hellowell, 2014).

When the GPs' contract with the NHS was revised in 1990, general practices were no longer obliged to do their own out-of-hours (OOH) work: they could arrange, or pay, for another doctor to do so. Corporate deputising services developed as a result, but still more did GP cooperatives, some of which later diversified into providing medical call-centres and walk-in treatment centres (Sheaff et al,

2012). The 1997 Personal Medical Services (PMS) scheme opened up primary medical care to nurse-led providers, corporate and proprietary provision. Initially there were few such providers (for instance, there were probably fewer than 50 nurse-led general practices) but provider plurality had been extended into primary medical care.

Version 2: the Third Way

By 1997 the Labour Party had essentially accepted provider plurality, indeed the whole principle of an NHS quasi-market. Labour presented its 'Third Way' health policies as departing both from some aspects of Conservative 'reforms' (especially GP fundholding) but also – and more significantly for provider plurality – from Bevan's reliance upon nationalised healthcare providers. Nevertheless the Third Way was a mixed blessing for provider plurality. PFI 'Unitary charges' (management fees which an NHS trust paid the PFI consortium) were set at 2.5% pa of the project's capital cost or the rate of inflation if higher. From 2004, one change to the NHS contract with GPs (the General Medical Services (GMS) contract) was to make general practices, not named GPs, the contract signatories so that practices could change ownership without jeopardising their NHS contract. General practices were also permitted to opt out of OOH work: a death-sentence for many cooperatives. Some closed, others converted to proprietary or social enterprise status.

Version 3: or rather, version 1 recycled

By 2001 English health 'reforms' had become more overtly similar to pre-1997 policies, but New Labour took provider plurality further. New Labour's post-2001 reforms were their response to what they perceived as the failure of hierarchically-structured NHS providers during 1997–2001; and to what they perceived as the specific deficiencies of the Conservatives' internal market of the 1990s, particularly regarding motivation and incentives on the supply side. Indeed New Labour re-articulated the Conservatives' objectives for the first NHS quasi-market of the 1990s, and the principle of an NHS quasi-market itself, as 'four inter-related pillars of reform ... designed to embed incentives for continuous and self sustaining improvement' and produce 'better quality, better patient experience, better value for money and reduced inequality' (Department of Health, 2007b). These pillars were: demand side reform; transactional reform; system management and regulation; and supply side reform, including 'more diverse providers with more freedom to innovate and improve services' (Department of Health, 2007b).

Since the coalition and Conservative governments have continued most of them, it is worth describing these policies more fully.

1. **Demand side reform**: Under the 'Patient Choice' policy NHS patients could select from a range of hospitals, one of which had to be independent (Department of Health, 2007a). Under the 'Any Willing Provider' principle, patients could choose *any* hospital provider accredited by the NHS. Patients were thought likely to avoid under-performing hospitals, for whom the prospect of losing funding under the cost-per-case Payment by Results pricing system (see below) would create incentives to improve quality and access times. Real choice, New Labour assumed, would require an expansion of provider types and capacity. A similar 'Any Qualified Provider' policy for community health services (CHS) followed, with the aim of improving access to CHS and to allow the entry of new providers. Again, patients could choose from a national list of approved providers (Jones and Mays, 2013).

2. **Transactional reform**: a DRG-based system (the 'health resource groups' (HRG) or 'tariff') of fixed prices for procedures, for paying both public and independent hospitals was introduced (Department of Health, 2007b). Although this cost-per-case system is called 'payment-by-results' (PbR) it is actually payment by activity. The idea was to sharpen incentives and competition, with each episode of care being reimbursed – if it was not lost to another provider – at the national tariff rate, based on average costs. PbR was initially designed to cover acute hospitals' work and has not been expanded to community or mental health services, which are still paid for on block contracts, in effect fixed budgets (Allen et al, 2014).

3. **System management and regulation**: Alongside continuing hierarchical control by the Department of Health (and since 2013, NHS England), the NHS quasi-market was regulated at arm's length by the Cooperation and Competition Panel (CCP) which advised the Department of Health in accordance with the *Principles and rules for cooperation and competition* (Department of Health, 2010b). These principles required 'providers and commissioners to cooperate to deliver seamless and sustainable care to patients' and not to make 'agreements which restrict commissioner or patient choice against patients' or taxpayers' interests'. The Care Quality Commission

(CQC: formerly the Commission for Health Improvement and then the Healthcare Commission) was responsible for inspecting both public and independent providers; registering independent providers and publishing annual performance ratings for all NHS organisations. The other important regulator was (and remains) Monitor, the independent regulator of Foundation Trusts. It authorised Foundation Trusts and specified borrowing limits, ceilings on income from private treatments, the range of goods and services that could be supplied, and required financial and statistical information (Allen, 2006).

4. **Supply side reform**: New Labour's version of the 'public firm' idea was NHS Foundation Trusts (FTs). Being still state-owned, FTs are not independent providers, but are designed to mimic aspects of third sector providers by involving local people in their governance, and have a degree of managerial autonomy. From 2004 they were allowed to carry any operating surplus forward to the next financial year.

Commissioners were also encouraged to engage with new providers from the 'third sector' (social economy) including local voluntary groups, registered charities, foundations, trusts, non-profit social enterprises, and cooperatives (Department of Health, 2006). Finally, for profit providers were also encouraged to enter the NHS quasi-market on a larger scale. A 'Concordat' with the private hospital sector signalled that the NHS would continue purchasing private hospital treatments. Independent sector treatment centres (ISTCs), one per PCT, were set up specifically to carry out elective outpatient, day-patient and low-complexity in-patient surgery on NHS patients (House of Commons Health Select Committee, 2006). Initially the main providers were corporations: Capio (at least eight contracts), Carillon (trading as Clinicenta), Interhealth Canada, Mercury, Nations Healthcare, Netcare Healthcare, Partnership Health Group, Ramsay, Spire and Health Care UK. Some (but not all) ISTCs were subcontracted to their local NHS trust, thereby removing competition between those two providers. ISTCs were initially contracted nationally but the amount of patients treated has declined in recent years (Allen and Jones, 2011). The government also invited United Health, a major US health insurer, to pilot nurse-led case management of frail older people with frequent unplanned hospital admissions. This resulted in the 'Community Matron' system, but without further corporate involvement.

Liberating the supply side

The current NHS reforms, designed yet again to increase the market-like behaviour of providers of care (Department of Health, 2010a), span the Coalition and current Conservative government. The coalition's Health and Social Care Act (HSCA, 2012) took effect in April 2013. It applied competition law explicitly to the NHS quasi-market (den Exter and Guy, 2014). As the new economic regulator for the whole of the NHS (not only FTs) Monitor acquired some functions of the former CCP and, along with the national competition authorities (since April 2014, the Competition and Markets Authority, or CMA), powers to enforce competition law to prevent anti-competitive behaviour and to produce a level playing field which places neither public nor private providers at any substantial advantage in competing for NHS-funded contracts. *The NHS Procurement, Choice and Competition Regulations No. 2 2013* made elements of existing guidance matters for statutory regulation, including the PRCC and NHS procurement guidelines, and indicated that competitive procurement was to be preferred.

NHS Foundation Trusts were now permitted to obtain up to 49% of their income from non-NHS sources (this does not mean to have 49% private patients). They could reinvest profits from non-NHS income generation to benefit NHS patients (Monitor, n.d.). Each PCT was required to make at least three AQP contracts in 2012 (Allen and Jones, 2011), and more subsequently. Many of the PFI schemes were becoming ruinous for the NHS trusts involved, leading to attempts to buy some of the PFI schemes out. The courts ruled, however, that the government was exceeding its powers under the 2012 HSCA when it tried to spread the costs of the South London Healthcare Trust's PFI schemes (16% of its budget; Hodge, 2013) over nearby NHS trusts who had not been party to the schemes.

There have been two important qualifications to these policies. Monitor, firstly, is also responsible for promoting co-operation (see Chapter 5). It is for NHS commissioners (including Clinical Commissioning Groups, or CCGs), however, to ensure that the appropriate levels of both competition and cooperation exist in their local health economies (HSCA, 2012). Second, NHS England's *Five Year Forward View* (5YFV), did not mention competition between organisations and instead focussed on how organisations in the NHS need to cooperate with each other, indeed sometimes merge, for example to bring together a range of non-hospital services including GPs and CHS, or to integrate acute inpatient with primary care services. In November 2014, the Secretary of State for Health (Jeremy Hunt) indicated that he did not think that patient choice (that is, competition) was the best way to improve many services (West, 2014). Against this, Monitor's director of cooperation and competition argued that competition still had an important role in the NHS (*HSJ*, 28th November, 2014). There having been no relevant legislative changes, the HSCA remains in force.

Who was liberated, and what they did when they were

Data on how many non-NHS providers are entering the NHS quasi-market or their market shares are scarce. The picture – including the one below – therefore has to assembled from various discrepant sources, reporting different kinds of data (for example, numbers of contracts *versus* numbers of providers *versus* NHS expenditure on different contracts or different kinds of contractor).

With that proviso, it appears that the mix of NHS funded providers continued to shift towards non-NHS provision in acute (but non-emergency) hospital care, out-of-hours primary care, community health services and general practice. The providers of mental health services and social care were already very diverse. Of the 195 major contracts let competitively in 2013/14, 80 went to corporations and 48 to social enterprises, but the social enterprises' share was larger in cash terms (£690m, versus £490m to corporations) (Iacobucci, 2013). In 2015 CCGs held an estimated 15166 contracts with 'non-NHS' providers (Centre for Health and the Public Interest, 2015), on average about 90 per CCG, although many will be contracts with small providers such as small local businesses, charities or individual practitioners. The total value was £9.3bn, about 16% of CCG budgets, in addition to £0.6bn worth of such contracts made by NHS trusts (that is, to private providers as subcontractors to these trusts). These figures however must include private sector providers of all kinds, many of which are small local providers (for example, local charities, proprietary care homes) and all services (not just hospitals, but out-of-hours services, community health services, mental health provision, and so on). From 2006/7 to 2014/15, NHS patients treated by non-NHS providers rose from around 0.5% (73 000) to 2.6% (471 000) of all inpatient episodes (over 18 million in total in 2013/14). In 2014 corporations were an estimated 59% of the private providers contracted to CCGs. Private equity firms backed or owned 58% of those (Centre for Health and the Public Interest, 2015).

Hospitals

Private acute hospitals saw a slow rise (to 6%) in their share of NHS-funded hospital care, although that 6% represented about a quarter of their total income (Davis et al, 2015). The private hospitals receiving NHS contracts are mostly corporations, and private provision is concentrated in certain specialties. The private proportion is about a 12.5% share in trauma and orthopaedics (Appleby, 2015), (within this, 20% is for hip and knee replacements; see Competition Commission, 2013), rising to 34% in audiology, a very small care group. In outpatient care the proportion of non-NHS providers rose from 0.2% (123 000) to 5.5% (4.5 million) (Appleby, 2015). These are net increases, though, and some ISTCs have closed while others have been absorbed into the NHS. Accusations that ISTCs have 'cherry-picked' their case-loads appear unsubstantiated (Chard et al, 2011). Rather, 'lemon-dumping' takes the indirect form of transferring patients who develop complications or become unexpectedly ill back to an NHS hospital. Since private hospitals generally lack the facilities to treat such patients there is an obvious clinical rationale for these transfers. Any 'cherry picking' occurs by default when hospitals are designed – as ISTCs were – only for treating less complex or acutely ill patients: a very different service profile to 'full-service' NHS hospitals. In an earlier period, though, BUPA was alleged (Davis et al, 2015) to have offered some categories of cancer, cardiology and gynaecology patients a cash payment to seek treatment at NHS rather than BUPA hospitals.

Circle abandoned their management-only contract to run Hinchingbrook Hospital as it became unprofitable for them (Scourfield, 2016). PFI schemes also became increasingly financially problematic for NHS Trusts, on average costing about seven times their capital value over the schemes' lifespan (Davis et al, 2015) and, in the meantime, causing unsustainable over-spending in QE Hospital Woolwich, Princess Royal Hospital Orpington, Derby Hospitals and elsewhere. These problems have arisen when inflation has been low, and interest rates exceptionally low, by historical standards.

Evidence about service quality under plural provision is mixed. Two scientific and one 'grey' study each suggest little difference in the outcomes of NHS and ISTC treatment of NHS patients for cataract extraction, inguinal hernia repair, hip replacement, knee replacement and varicose vein surgery (Chard et al, 2011; Competition Commission, 2013). Earlier, Oussedik and Haddad (2009) found that ISTCs had higher rates of post-operative problems for hip and knee replacements, although the difference may partly reflect treatment away from the patient's locality of residence rather than provider ownership. Allowing for patients' pre-operative characteristics, ISTCs produced a slightly greater restoration of function after cataract extraction or hip replacement patients than NHS providers did, slightly less for hernia repairs, and no difference for two other treatments. ISTC patients also tended to be healthier, younger and thinner (Browne et al, 2008), however, and tended to be referred for less severe conditions (Chard et al, 2011). An explanation of these mixed findings appears to be that hospital ownership does not in itself affect the level of quality of the average NHS-funded patient's reported experience. The differences are instead entirely attributable to patient characteristics, case-mix differences and unobserved characteristics particular to individual hospitals (Perotin et al, 2013). At least two NHS contracts with corporate providers have been terminated for patient safety reasons (Clinicenta, Lister Hospital Stevenage, 2013; mobile ophthalmology services at Musgrove Park, Taunton, 2014. See Dyer, 2014). A study by Cooper et al, (2011), sometimes irrelevantly cited in this context, reports the effects of competition on in-patient mortality, and not the effects of diverse, still less corporate, hospital ownership.

Community Health and Out-of-Hours Services

Data by which to compare NHS and non-NHS providers are even more lacking for community health services (CHS). Attempts to convert NHS trusts to social enterprises have been concentrated in mental and community health services. NHS pay and conditions were guaranteed for existing staff but not for new staff, making NHS staff reluctant to exercise their 'right to request' the transfer (Sheaff et al, 2012). Corporate provision of CHS increased from almost nothing in 2010 to a position where corporations, especially Virgin Care, have won some large NHS contracts. In contrast SERCO withdrew altogether from providing NHS-funded clinical services after making multimillion pound losses on them. Similarly, non-NHS providers withdrew from bidding for CHS services in Cambridge, BUPA pulled out of contract negotiations for West Sussex MSK services (Ryan, 2015), and Peninsula Community Interest Company (a social enterprise) refused to re-bid for the mental health services in Cornwall which it had previously provided. By no means universal to begin with, CCGs' use of AQP contracts stagnated from 2013 (Williams, 2014) at about 130 registered providers, usually small to medium sized firms (BMA, 2013), with the largest numbers providing diagnostic and adult hearing services. By 2014 the NHS was also spending about

£3 billion a year to buy (mostly) CHS or health-related social care from local authorities and charities (Iacobucci, 2014).

In out of hours (OOH) services, by 2015 about 51% of the non general practice providers (44/86) were social enterprises (not for profit organisations), 24% (21/86) corporate and the same number NHS providers (Warren et al, 2015).

Without bespoke research it is difficult to ascertain the consequences of plural provision for CHS. Existing published data are nugatory and the fuller data-sets, promised for 2015, have yet to be published. The available evidence therefore comes mostly from media reports: a probably biased sample.

Two widely-known reports paint contrasting pictures. The CQC investigation of staff abusing residents with learning difficulties at Winterbourne View (then owned by Castlebeck Care) attributed these problems to inadequate staffing levels and poor care planning. NHS England subsequently announced 'closure or reform of up to 49 private hospitals that provide long-term accommodation for people with learning disabilities or autism whose behaviour is considered challenging' (Anon, 2016) and a reduction of referrals to private providers. The last large-scale NHS provider of such services (with no allegations of criminal abuse) also closed (Brindle, 2015). In contrast Circle, coordinating some local general practices (but not Bedford Hospital Trust, which refused Circle's contract offer) in providing 'integrated' MSK services in Bedfordshire, were claiming to be triaging all patients within 24 hours of referral, to have diverted about a fifth of GP referrals to 'more appropriate' clinicians, and reduced diagnostic and physiotherapy waits: 'All of this for a flat fee, instead of ever rising spending' (MSK spokesman, reported in Smith (2015)).

Patient informants for the 2012 GP survey evaluated NHS and social enterprise out-of-hours services providers similarly in respect of timeliness of care, confidence in the clinician they saw, and overall experience of the service. Corporate providers were evaluated lower ('moderate' to 'large' differences) on all three outcomes (Warren et al, 2015). Commercial providers saw fewer OOH cases per head of population than other providers (NAO, 2014). A CQC investigation into a patient's death in 2008 revealed that the company responsible, Take Care Now, was prone to under-staffing and had weak arrangements for managing patient safety, especially considering its heavy use of locum doctors from other European countries. Similar complaints – although no patient deaths – were also reported for SERCO's out-of-hours services in Cornwall, and sharp practice in reporting monitoring data (Comptroller and Auditor General, 2013).

General Practice

Under the Alternative Provider Medical Services (APMS) scheme, new general practice providers included companies, social enterprises, mutuals, 'groups of existing GPs' (Coleman et al, 2013) and joint bids from Foundation Trusts with out-of-hours care providers, and from private companies with local general practices. Many private primary medical care companies have developed, often partly or wholly GP-owned. A FOI enquiry showed that 23% of GP members of CCGs had a financial stake in a company providing services (though not always primary medical services) to that same CCG (Kaffash, 2013). Virgin ended its partnerships with GPs to prevent this apparent conflict of interest. Often badged as GP-led, the more expansive GP-owned companies (for example, Chilvers McCrea Healthcare, DMC Healthcare) had initially won contracts in their local area, and from that basis began winning contracts elsewhere.

Recently large federations of general practices have formed in Northamptonshire, Birmingham, London and elsewhere. Some have added a social enterprise or a looser confederal body as network coordinating body. The federating general practices usually seek economies of scale in management, and some economies of scope in their more specialised clinical services, sharing resources without changing GPs' ownership and management of the practices. A few professional partnership general practices have been taken over by NHS trusts, however (for example, in southern Hampshire; Bostock, 2015).

Doctors' everyday work practices under the APMS contractors appear similar to those in traditional professional partnerships in terms of the division of clinical labour and focus on meeting QOF targets (Coleman et al, 2013). Competition also stimulated at least some 'bad behaviour' on the part of existing providers:

'In Site 1 there were allegations by APPCs that other practices had removed signage and misdirected patients. In Site 2 there were suggestions that staff at a minor injuries service which shared premises with an APPC practice had deliberately misdirected patients away from the APPC' (Coleman et al, 2013).

Again, corporate and proprietary providers would relinquish unprofitable contracts. UHE withdrew from providing NHS-funded primary medical care altogether, and The Practice withdrew from particular contracts (for example, Woking, Leicester, Nottingham). NHS England selected 21 providers to take over at need struggling general practices in southern England. The 21 include NHS

Foundation Trusts, large merged general practices ('super-practices'), GP federations, out-of-hours co-operatives, Virgin Care, social enterprises and smaller private companies (*Pulse* 10th July, 2015).

An unstable quasi-market

The set of NHS contracts which private providers hold is in constant flux, often over short periods. Contracts for, say, OOH services or planned orthopaedic surgery have shifted between GP cooperatives, NHS trusts and corporate providers (and occasionally back again). Also, the ownership of corporate and proprietary and, to a lesser extent, social enterprise providers has been a succession of mergers, closures, acquisitions and re-naming. For example Virgin acquired and re-named Assura Medical 2010 (except for its property management business, but including Assura's 50% share in a number of general practices) and, in effect, took over a social enterprise providing CHS. Ramsay acquired Capio UK and its hospitals, day surgery providers and two neurological rehabilitation homes (2007). The Practice took over 30 GP surgeries from Chilvers McCrea, six from United Health and two secure immigration centre clinics from Drummond; and so on.

Despite the aims of competition policy, the NHS quasi-market is not a completely level playing field. On balance, private (especially corporate and proprietary) providers have in certain respects enjoyed less scrutiny and greater freedom of action than NHS providers. Freedom of Information requirements do not apply to non-NHS providers. Private providers can (and do) withdraw from financially damaging contracts, and transfer complex patients away. NHS trusts cannot. Private providers often structure themselves into separate operating and property-holding companies, as a means of converting profits from NHS contracts into interest payments or other ostensible 'costs' which they can then transfer more readily to other recipients (for example, holding companies), and may use off-shore status to reduce their tax payments. The playing-field has also been 'levelled' by limiting NHS providers' access to capital, so that NHS providers can only raise capital through PFI schemes (but see above) or from retained profits, open financial markets or Department of Health loans which follow 'generally accepted principles used by financial institutions' (Department of Health, 2014).

Against this, NHS providers are *electorally* 'too big to fail'. Monitor has allowed a number of NHS trusts and foundation trusts to continue operating despite being in evident financial difficulty (den Exter and Guy, 2014) (the combined deficits of all NHS trusts and NHS foundation trusts being above £500m at the end of 2015). Department of Health loans also cover these circumstances.

Trial, error and exit

For non-NHS providers the coalition government was a period of uncertainty, trial and error as they learned by experience which NHS-funded services they could and could not provide profitably. When it is easier for firms to leave a market than for new ones to enter it (for example, because of investment, 'first mover' or regulatory barriers to entry), a common effect of competition is market concentration on the supply side. Despite what competition legislation (which now applies to the NHS) may intend, seven private providers now have 88% of the independent provider market for NHS-funded inpatient work (Appleby, 2015).

Certain private providers found it hard to undercut NHS providers' costs and still turn a profit, as noted above. Since about two-thirds of the cost of healthcare is labour (see Chapters 3 and 13), reducing the use of expensive, that is, clinicians', labour is the main way of reducing costs (hence extracting profits) once the level of income from a contract is determined. This may explain the pattern of low staffing levels in some corporate and proprietary providers, of which Serco's out-of-hours service in Cornwall was the most publicised example (Comptroller and Auditor General, 2013). Facing the same cost patterns, however, NHS services are also understaffed at times (Mid Stafford Hospital being the notorious NHS example, see Healthcare Commission, 2009).

The fog of policy

The above patterns highlight several conceptual distinctions with policy implications.

Corporate versus private

Occasionally policy-makers themselves distinguish the different kinds of 'private' provision, although sometimes only to advocate one kind of private provider by appeal to another kind (for example, 'GPs are private providers so what is wrong with corporations providing hospital services to the NHS?'). Failure to distinguish leads to overlooking an important health policy scenario somewhat different from that of the NHS purchasing from healthcare corporations. The alternative scenario is one of competing public providers, social enterprises, charities and professional partnerships, but without corporate or proprietary providers. It raises the theoretical question of whether competition between public firms (or between social enterprises, or between professional partnerships) would have different loci (for example, speed of access rather than service quality) and consequences than competition between corporations. It also raises the policy question of whether the alleged adverse effects of corporate provision (Davis et al, 2015) can be avoided whilst retaining an element of private provision enabling the introduction of new models of care for NHS patients (for example, hospice care, which originated in the charitable sector).

Competition versus privatisation:

Advocates and opponents of provider plurality both usually equate 'competition' with privatisation, demonstrating euphemistic or lax thinking respectively. This failure to distinguish leads to overlooking another important health policy scenario, in which only public providers would compete for patient referrals and NHS contracts. Then provider competition would occur, without any provider plurality. There is some (Cooper et al, 2011; Gaynor et al, 2012) – though contested (Pollock et al, 2011) – evidence that competition between predominantly NHS providers may reduce hospital mortality for acute myocardial infarction patients. If so, competition between NHS providers produces at least some of the benefits of competition whilst non-NHS providers play a marginal role. US evidence also suggests that it is competition, not ownership, which affects provider behaviour (Allen, 2009).

The NHS contains two different structures for provider competition.

1. Competition for patients ('competition *in* the market'), that is, to attract self- and GP referrals, each referral triggering a payment to the provider. In this structure, plural providers can permanently coexist and compete in each local health economy.
2. Competition for contracts, ('competition *for* the market', 'managed competition'; Saltman and von Otter, 1992) under which providers compete for a usually time limited local monopoly to provide a service or groups of services. If a private provider wins, the result may be private provision without further competition.

Even if plural provision were necessary (which it is not: see above), it is also insufficient to stimulate provider competition for patients.

Supposing GPs abandoned their professional dislike of competing for patients, they would still have neither need nor reason to compete wherever the demand for general practice services exceeds the supply (that is, almost everywhere). The price of provider competition is an excess of supply over demand, or for the NHS over healthcare needs, irrespective of provider ownership (Dawson, 1994).

Policy messes

'Policy messes' arise when implementing one policy obstructs implementation of another (Winetrobe, 1992). Provider plurality seems to cause at least three.

Plural Provision versus Austerity:

Both Labour and the Coalition government responded to the 2008 financial market crash by cutting public expenditure, including NHS spending in real-terms, if not cash. At present (early 2016) NHS England and Monitor are proposing to reduce tariff prices by 7% overall and more than 10% for some orthopaedics work, a change predicted (Anon, 2015) to reduce private orthopaedics hospitals' income by 7% in 2016/17. As also noted above, private providers tend to withdraw from bidding for, or even keeping, unprofitable NHS contracts. Austerity seems to force governments to choose between cost containment and provider plurality.

Plural Provision versus Integrated Care:

Treating patients with multiple chronic conditions effectively requires combining separate clinical or therapeutic activities, often undertaken by different providers, into a coherent 'integrated' sequence of activities across often different settings (see Chapter 9). The more providers are involved, the more organisational interfaces these patients' care has to be coordinated across, and the harder it becomes to achieve the continuities of care (Sheaff et al, 2015). This is an argument for of having general practice, community health services and perhaps community hospital services provided by a single organisation rather than having a greater *plurality* of providers in each locality. The Five Year Forward View tacitly takes the point and opts for integrated care.

Plural Provision versus Political Accountability:

Supporters and opponents of plural provision respectively tend to assume that provider plurality will markedly improve or worsen the accessibility, provision, development or cost of NHS-funded services. Central regulation and mandated local commissioning practices may so tightly constrain all providers, however, that their ownership makes little difference to these policy outcomes. Evidence based medicine and professional bodies' disciplinary influence are equally agnostic about provider ownership (Andersen, 2009). In those circumstances the only coherent rationales for plural provision would be ideological or to satisfy vested interests outside the health sector. (Davis et al, 2015, report the numbers of Conservative – and other parties' – MPs with financial interests in private healthcare provision.)

Dismantling the NHS?

Current English health policy is therefore rather ambivalent, even incoherent, about plural provision. Plural provision would reinstate a contemporary version of pre-NHS healthcare supply patterns, as persist in many Bismarckian health systems (particularly Germany) and – more problematically – the USA. The logical conclusion, perhaps in some minds also the aim, of the policy is to reduce the NHS itself to a financing and quality-certification, strategic planning and service coordination ('commissioning') agency exercising governance over mostly independent providers. A standard riposte is that the NHS was established to guarantee patients' access to needed healthcare free of charge; provider ownership doesn't matter if the quality and cost of NHS services are good (Appleby, 2015). Provider plurality might make a difference in precisely these terms, though, and it remains to be shown whether it is for the better. Otherwise, what is the health gain from provider plurality?

References

Allen, P, 2006, New localism in the English NHS: what is it for? *Health Policy*, 79(2-3), 244–52

Allen, P, 2009, Restructuring the NHS again: supply side reform in recent English Healthcare policy, *Financial Accountability and Management*, 25, 4, 343–89

Allen, P, 2013, An economic analysis of the limits of market based reforms in the English NHS, *BMC Health Services Research*, 13(Suppl. 1), S1

Allen, P, Jones, L, 2011, Increasing the diversity of health care providers, in N Mays, L Jones, A Dixon (eds), *Understanding New Labour's market reforms of the English NHS,* London: Kings Fund

Allen, P, Bartlett, W, Zamora, B, Turner, S, 2011, New forms of provider in the English National Health Service, *Annals of Public and Cooperative Economics,* 82, 1, 77–95

Allen, P, Petsoulas, C, Ritchie, B, 2014, *Final report from study of the use of contractual mechanisms in commissioning,* Canterbury: Policy Research Unit on Commissioning and the Healthcare System.

Andersen, LB, 2009, What determines the behaviour and performance of health professionals? Public service motivation, professional norms and/or economic incentives, *International Review of Administrative Sciences,* 75, 1, 79–97

Anon, 2015, Prices for private providers to drop by 7% under new NHS price structure, *National Health Executive,* 16 December

Anon, 2016, Responses to the abuse of people with learning disabilities and autism and Winterbourne View, British Institute of Learning Disabilities (BILD) News and What's On web-page, http://www.bild.org.uk/news-and-whats-on/winterbourne-view, accessed 15 April 2016

Appleby, J, 2015, Paid for by the NHS, treated privately, *British Medical Journal* 350, ph3109

Bacon, R, Eltis, W, 1976, *Britain's economic problem: Too few producers,* London: Macmillan

Bartlett, W, Le Grand, J, 1993, *Quasi-markets and Social Policy,* London: Palgrave Macmillan

BMA, 2013, *Understanding the reforms…Choice and any qualified provider.* London: BMA Health Policy and Economic Research Unit

Bostock, N, 2015, Vanguard GPs open shared branch surgery to deliver seven-day access for 70,000 patients, *GPonline,* 2 September

Brindle, D, 2015, NHS to shut many residential hospitals for people with learning disabilities, *The Guardian,* 10 February.

Browne, J, Jamieson, L, Lewsey, J, Meulen, J van der, Copley, L, Black, N, 2008, Case-mix and patients' reports of outcome in Independent Sector Treatment Centres: Comparison with NHS providers, *BMC Health Services Research,* 8, 1, 78

Centre for Health and the Public Interest, 2015, *The contracting NHS: Can the NHS handle the outsourcing of clinical services?* London: Centre of Health and the Public Interest

Chard, J, Kuczawski, M, Black, N, van der Meulen, J, on behalf of the POiS Audit Steering Committee, 2011, Outcomes of elective surgery undertaken in independent sector treatment centres and NHS providers in England: Audit of patient outcomes in surgery. *BMJ* 343, d6404

Coleman, A, Checkland, K, McDermott, I, Harrison, S, 2013, The limits of market-based reforms in the NHS: The case of alternative providers in primary care, *BMC Health Services Research*, 13(Suppl 1), S3

Competition Commission, 2013, *Private Healthcare Market Investigation*, London: Competition Commission

Comptroller and Auditor General, 2013, *Memorandum on the provision of the outofhours GP service in Cornwall*, London: National Audit Office.

Cooper, Z, Gibbons, S, Jones, S, McGuire, A, 2011, Does hospital competition save lives? Evidence from the English NHS patient choice reforms, *The Economic Journal*, 121, 554, F228–60

Davis, J, Lister, J, Wrigley, D, 2015, *NHS for sale: Myths, lies and deception*, London: Merlin

Dawson, D, 1994, *Costs and prices in the internal market: Markets vs the NHS management executive guidelines*, York: CHE, University of York.

Department of Health, 2010a, *Equity and excellence: Liberating the NHS*, London: Department of Health.

Department of Health, 2014, Guidance on financing available to NHS trusts and Foundation Trusts, www.gov.uk/government/publications/guidance-on-financing-available-to-nhs-trusts-and-foundation-trusts

Department of Health, 2006, *Health reform in England: update and commissioning framework*, London: Department of Health, http://webarchive.nationalarchives.gov.uk/20130107105354/http://www.dh.gov.uk/en/Publicationsandstatistics/Publications/PublicationsPolicyAndGuidance/DH_4137226

Department of Health, 2007a, Health reform in England: Update and next steps, http://webarchive.nationalarchives.gov.uk/+/www.dh.gov.uk/en/Publicationsandstatistics/Publications/PublicationsPolicyAndGuidance/Browsable/DH_4125573

Department of Health, 2007b, *Options for the future of Payment by Results 2008/9 to 2010/1*, London: Department of Health

Department of Health, 2010b, *Principles and rules for cooperation and competition (revised edition)*, London: Department of Health

Department of Health, 1989, *Working for Patients*, London: HMSO

Dyer, C, 2014, Private provider's contract is terminated after half of cataract patients experience complications, *BMJ*, 349, g5241

Enthoven, A, 1985, *Reflections on the management of the National Health Service*, London: Nuffield Provincial Hospitals Trust.

den Exter, A, Guy, M, 2014, Market competition in health care markets in the Netherlands: Some lessons for England? *Medical Law Review*, 22, 2, 255–73

Gaynor, M, Moreno-Serra, R, Propper, C, 2012, Can competition improve outcomes in UK health care? Lessons from the past two decades, *Journal of Health Services Research and Policy*, 17(Suppl 1), 49–54

Harding, A, Preker, A, 2000, Understanding organizational reforms: The corporatization of public hospitals

Healthcare Commission, 2009, *Investigation into Mid Staffordshire NHS Foundation Trust*, London: Healthcare Commission.

Hellowell, M, 2014, *The return of PFI: Will the NHS pay a higher price for new hospitals?* London: Centre of Health and the Public Interest

Hodge, K, 2013, In-debt South London Healthcare NHS Trust 'should be broken up' *The Independent*, 8 January.

House of Commons Health Select Committee, 2006, *Independent Sector Treatment Centres*, London: House of Commons

Iacobucci, G, 2014, A third of NHS contracts awarded since health act have gone to private sector, BMJ investigation shows. *BMJ*, 349, g7606

Iacobucci, G, 2013. More than a third of GPs on commissioning groups have conflicts of interest, BMJ investigation shows. *BMJ*, 346, f1569

Jones, L, Mays, N, 2013, Early experiences of any qualified provider, *British Journal of Healthcare Management*, 19, 5, 217–24

Kaffash, J, 2013, Revealed: One in five GPs on CCG boards has financial interest in a current provider, *Pulse Today*, www.pulsetoday. co.uk/news/commissioning/commissioning-topics/ccgs/revealed-one-in-five-gps-on-ccg-boards-has-financial-interest-in-a-current-provider/20004369.fullarticle

Letwin, O, 1988, *Privatising the world: A study of international privatisation in theory and practice*, Cassell

Lipsey, RG, Lancaster, K, 1956, The general theory of the second best, *The Review of Economic Studies*, 24, 1, 11–32

Monitor, NHS foundation trust directory, www.gov.uk/government/publications/nhs-foundation-trust-directory/nhs-foundation-trust-directory#what-are-foundation-trusts

NAO (National Audit Office), 2014, *Out-of-hours GP services in England*, London: National Audit Office, www.nao.org.uk/report/hours-gp-services-england-2/

Offe, C, 1982, Some contradictions of the modern welfare state, *Critical Social Policy* 2, 5, 7–16

Oussedik, S, Haddad, F, 2009, Further doubts over the performance of treatment centres in providing elective orthopaedic surgery, *Journal of Bone and Joint Surgery, British Volume*, 91-B, 9, 1125–6

Perotin, V, Zamora, B, Reeves, R, Bartlett, W, Allen, P, 2013, Does hospital ownership affect patient experience? An investigation into public–private sector differences in England, *Journal of Health Economics*, 32, 3, 633–46

Pollock, AM, Dunnigan, MG, Gaffney, D, Price, D, Shaoul, J, 1999, Planning the 'new' NHS: Downsizing for the 21st Century, *BMJ* 319(7203), 179–84

Pollock, A, Macfarlane, A, Kirkwood, G, Majeed, FA, Greener, I, Morelli, C, et al, 2011, No evidence that patient choice in the NHS saves lives, *The Lancet*, 378(9809), 2057–60

Ryan, S, 2015, 'Bupa CSH pulls out of West Sussex MSK contract negotiations', *The Argus*, 26 January

Saltman, RB, von Otter, C, 1992, *Planned Markets and Public Competition*, Buckingham: Open University Press

Scourfield, P, 2016, Squaring the Circle: What lessons can be learned from the Hinchingbrooke franchise fiasco? *Critical Social Policy*, 36, 1, 142–52

Sheaff, R, Halliday J, Øvretveit, J, Byng, R, Exworthy, M, Peckham, S, 2015, Integration and Continuity of Primary Care: Polyclinics and Alternatives, an Organisational Analysis, *Health Services and Delivery Research*, 3(35)

Sheaff, R, Child, S, Schofield, J, Pickard, S, Mannion, R 2012, *Understanding professional partnerships and non-hierarchical organisations*, London: NIHR-SDO

Smith, W, 2015, What Circle has learned from its Bedford MSK contract, *Health Services Journal*, 7 October.

Warren, C, Abel, G, Lyratzopoulos, G, Elliott, M, Richards, S, Barry, H, Roland, R, Campbell, J, 2015, Characteristics of service users and provider organisations associated with experience of out of hours general practitioner care in England: Population based cross sectional postal questionnaire survey, *BMJ*, 350, h2040

West, D, 2014, Exclusive: Patient choice is not key to improving performance, says Hunt, *Health Services Journal*, 26 November

Williams, D, 2014, CCG interest in 'any qualified provider' scheme dwindles, *Health Services Journal*, 11 September.

Winetrobe, BK, 1992, A tax by any other name: The Poll Tax and the Community Charge, *Parliamentary Affairs*, 45, 3, 420–7

TWELVE

Achieving equity in health service commissioning

Martin Wenzl and Elias Mossialos

Introduction

Although the term *equity* did not feature in early policy documents related to the English National Health Service (NHS), equity was one of the main policy goals at its inception in 1948 (Delamothe, 2008). A particular concept of equity remains one of the central NHS principles, which state that, 'it meet the needs of everyone, […] be free at the point of delivery [and] […] be based on clinical need, not ability to pay' (NHS England, 2015a).

The current literature on equity in healthcare distinguishes between horizontal equity, requiring that *equals* be treated equally, and vertical equity, requiring that *unequals* be treated unequally (Mossialos and Dixon, 2002). For a healthcare system to be equitable, both concepts of equity need to be respected in financing and the distribution of services in the population. This requires that contributions be levied based on ability to pay and access to services be based on need.

In the context of an equitable distribution of services, frequently discussed notions of equity include equality in utilisation of care by those in equal need or equality in health outcomes (Powell and Exworthy, 2003). However, such policy goals may be undesirable or, at best, difficult for a health system to achieve. They would require public policy to impinge heavily on personal choices and life styles (Oliver and Mossialos, 2004). Also, the determinants of health have been shown to lie largely outside the realm of healthcare (Marmot, 2010). As a result, there is now a relatively broad consensus among researchers that equity of access is a more appropriate policy goal for healthcare. As Oliver and Mossialos (2004) have concluded, this is because equity of access

(1) [is] specific to healthcare and does not require that we discriminate between people who are already ill purely

> on the basis of factors that are exogenous to their health, and (2) [..] respects acceptable reasons for differentials in healthcare utilisation by those in equal need. (2004, 656)

To the extent that the combination of taxes from which healthcare is funded remains progressive overall, funding from general taxation ensures equity of financing in the English NHS. For various reasons, ensuring equity of access is more difficult. It requires policy to make value judgements in determining the characteristics, such as social class, income or ethnicity, according to which the population should be stratified and in who to consider *equal* vs. *unequal*. While need and access are relatively straight-forward theoretical concepts, their measurement in practice is difficult.

Covering notions of physical availability of services, the ability to access them as well as the cost of access (see Mooney, 1983) Goddard and Smith (2001) have defined access as 'the ability to secure a specified set of healthcare services, at a specified level of quality, subject to a specified maximum level of personal inconvenience and cost, while in possession of a specified amount of information' (2001, 1151). Utilisation has frequently been used as a proxy measure of access (Gulliford et al, 2003), which, however, implies acceptance of equal utilisation as an equity concept and fails to account for unmet need.

Unmet need might account for a significant proportion of need for care in a population but, by not leading to utilisation, it is by definition not observed. Although self-reported measures provide a possible solution, these are not without limitations and may be subject to biases by survey respondents (Allin et al, 2010). Differences in culture or personal illness behaviour are examples of acceptable reasons as to why felt need may not lead to demand. Even if demand is expressed, the more objective concept of normative need as defined by healthcare professionals or other agents of the healthcare system implies that not all demand leads to utilisation. There are further legitimate reasons, such as the absence of an effective intervention, trade-offs between risk and benefit in clinical judgement or other (for example, health economic) rationing mechanisms, for why felt need for health does not necessarily imply need for healthcare. Such rationing, however, is contrary to the principle of equity of access when demand does not lead to utilisation despite the general availability of an effective intervention, due to factors such as geography or socioeconomic status. Figure 12.1 provides a conceptual model of need, demand and use.

In addition to using utilisation as a surrogate measure of access, health status or other indicators associated with need have commonly

Figure 12.1: Relationships between need, demand and use

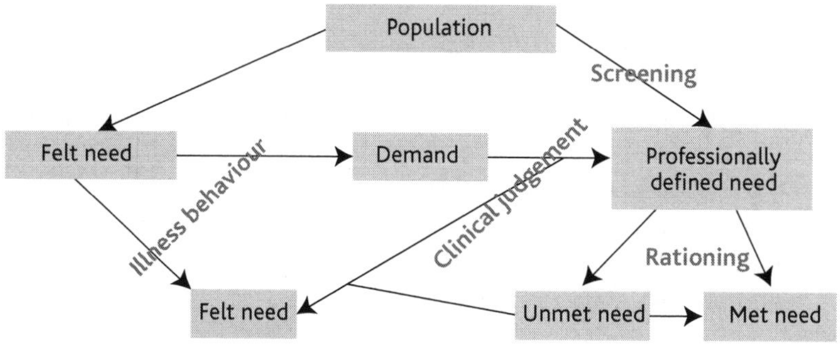

Source: Black and Grün (2005, 80)

been used as a proxy for need (Gulliford, 2003). Despite significant limitations against a principle of equal access for equal need (see, for example, Allin et al, 2010), equality in needs-adjusted utilisation (or, more accurately, health status-adjusted utilisation) across groups of the population for which equity is to be achieved is a common and indirect measure of equity.

Equity in the NHS prior to 2010

In what he termed the 'Inverse Care Law', Tudor Hart (1971) observed that people in areas with higher burden of disease and morbidity had access to fewer and lower-quality health services. Explicit methods of resource allocation from the funding source to regions and local areas have existed in England before the 1970s. Since that time, however, needs-based distribution of resources across the country has been considered one of the main mechanisms to achieve equity of access in the NHS. This has included, for example, policies to increase the availability of general practitioner (GP) services in areas with greater need (Goddard et al, 2010). More prominently, however, since the establishment of the Resource Allocation Working Party (RAWP) in 1976, efforts have revolved around the needs-adjusted allocation of the NHS budget to geographic areas. Although achievement of equity of access was the overarching goal of RAWP and remains the goal of geographic resources allocation in the NHS until today, this focus effectively delivers equal financing for equal need across areas while neglecting elements of access that are not related to financial input (Powell and Exworthy, 2003).

The purchaser–provider split and quasi-market introduced in 1991 endured reorganisations of the NHS through the 2000s, with devolved purchasers retaining significant discretion as to how to set priorities within their budget allocation (see Chapters 1 and 2). Health authorities and Primary Care Trusts, as purchasers, were responsible for needs assessment. For example, a Department of Health (2001) document on service delivery stated that, in their role as commissioners, Primary Care Trusts (PCTs) 'will become the lead NHS organisation in assessing need, planning and securing all health services and improving health' (2001, 5). Table 12.1 summarises the sequence of purchasing organisations created in the 1990s and 2000s and implications of their characteristics for equity (see Chapters 8 and 11).

After the report on health inequalities by Acheson (1998) reiterated many of the findings pointed out previously by Black (1980), policy under Labour in the late 1990s also saw an increased focus on the reduction of health inequalities, a new policy goal for the NHS that featured prominently in the 1997 White Paper and subsequent documents (see Chapter 10). The 2000 NHS reform plan provided equity of financing and equity of access as two main criteria against which reform proposals were to be evaluated (Secretary of State for Health, 2000, 34). The same document went on to make 'reducing inequalities in access to NHS services' an explicit goal (2000, 107).

Aside from an effort to redistribute the availability of primary care services from areas with lower need and a higher density of GPs to areas with higher relative need, though, the NHS Plan focused on updates to geographic resource allocation through the weighted capitation formula as a means of achieving equity of access. On the other hand, reductions of disparities in life expectancy and infant mortality became a performance target for the NHS, including for PCTs as commissioners. Together with Strategic Health Authorities (SHAs), PCTs received a wide range of responsibilities. These included a requirement for a public health team in each PCT headed by a board-level appointment to lead work on reducing inequalities in partnership with local authorities and other agencies (Department of Health, 2001), a requirement to target preventive services at people with the highest need (Secretary of State for Health, 2000) and conducting health equity audits, 'a mechanism to use evidence about health inequalities to inform service planning and delivery' (Department of Health, 2003, 38–39). Although another requirement was 'to improve access to high quality services for people from disadvantaged communities or where health needs are high' (Department of Health, 2003, 41), equity of access was not mentioned in these documents.

Table 12.1: Commissioning arrangements in the English NHS and selected characteristics impacting equity

Years*	Purchaser of healthcare (no. of purchasers; list size for GP-led organisations)	Level of risk pooling	Purchaser responsible for public health?	Participation in GP-led commissioning compulsory?
1948–1974	No purchaser/provider split. Allocation from the national level directly to teaching hospitals and to Regional Health Boards.			
1974–1991	No purchaser/provider split. Allocation under the RAWP formula from the national level to regions and by regions on to District Health Authorities responsible for healthcare and public health.			
1991–1996	District Health Authorities (N=192)	DHA	Yes	
1991–1999	GP fundholders (57% of GPs; 3,000–50,000 patients)	GP list	No	No
1996–2002	Health Authorities (N=100)	HA	Yes	
1994–1999	Total Purchasing Pilots (N=87; 8,000–80,000 patients)	HA**	No	No
1999–2002	Primary Care Groups (N=481)	PCG	Yes	
2002–2006	Primary Care Trusts (N=303)	PCT	Yes	
2005–2013	Practice-Based Commissioning (100% of GPs; 1,000–600,000 patients)	PCT**	No	No
2006–2013	Primary Care Trusts (N=151)	PCT	Yes	
Since 2013	Clinical Commissioning Groups (N=209, 72,000–900,000)	CCG	No[†]	Yes

Notes:

* Dates of implementation, not legislation or policy announcements; ** Budgets for Total Purchasing Pilots and Practice-Based Commissioners were indicative only.

[†] 2013 was the first time public health has not been a responsibility of the main devolved purchasing organisations in the NHS.

Source: Wenzl et al., 2015

Beyond equity of access, the reduction of avoidable health inequalities also became an explicit objective of budget allocations to commissioners. From 2002, a deprivation adjustment was made in the allocation formula to give PCTs in poorer areas larger budgets for primary, community, and hospital services (Majeed and Soljak, 2014) and, together with specific targets on outcomes such as cancer mortality, designated 'spearhead' (poorer and less healthy) areas received additional funding from 2004. SHAs were responsible for monitoring PCT performance, including achievement of targets on health inequalities (Department of Health, 2003).

Much of the empirical literature on equity of access in the NHS also focused on equity in resource allocation to commissioners (see, for example, Asthana and Gibson, 2008; Barr et al, 2014; Carr-Hill, 1989; Galbraith, 20080; Hauck et al, 2002) but not the equity implications of their purchasing decisions. Although commissioners (PCTs and PBCs) in the 1990s and 2000s were generally considered passive and weak in the face of providers with greater bargaining power, the multitude of concurrent changes in purchasing and provision of services made generating robust and longitudinal evidence on the performance of commissioners difficult (Checkland et al, 2012; Smith and Curry, 2011).

However, some studies did provide evidence of variation in access-related measures between PCTs. For instance, Appleby and Gregory (2008) analysed data on PCT spending by disease between 2004 and 2007 to assess whether spending was in line with differences in need and, thus, conducive to achievement of an equity objective. They found that spending per patient in specific disease areas, such as mental health, cancer or circulatory disease, varied by a factor of about two between PCTs after controlling for variations in need using the Department of Health's need index; reasons for such variations or their equity implications were not explored. Similarly, Delamothe (2008) cited cross-sectional data showing that spending per patient on cancer and heart disease as well as the availability of GPs varied significantly between PCTs and that the latter was positively associated with life expectancy. Coronini-Cronberg et al (2012) concluded that about half of all PCTs restricted access based on varying clinical and health economic thresholds, effectively precluding patients who may benefit from surgery from accessing services. Cooper et al (2009) provided limited but encouraging evidence on equity: their study found that, in a context of decreasing waiting times for three common types of elective surgery between 1997 and 2007, a positive correlation between an index of deprivation and the waiting time between referral and surgery also decreased; by the end of the period considered, the most deprived quintile had shorter waits than any of the other quintiles.

Smith and Curry (2011) reviewed evidence of the impact of PCT commissioning against the targets of reducing heath inequalities. They concluded that, with some exceptions such as in cardiovascular and cancer mortality, PCT commissioning had largely not been successful at mitigating health inequalities and that activity-related and financial targets prevailed over inequality concerns. They also reported that the ability of PBCs to bring about change was related to their size but that no evidence on equity of practice-based commissioning was available.

A more recent study by Cookson et al (2016) uses a range of access- and healthcare outcome-related indicators to evaluate the achievement of equity in the NHS between 2004 and 2012. Using the index of multiple deprivation to stratify the English population, they show that the NHS was successful at removing initial pro-rich inequity in the availability and quality of primary care by 2011. Initial pro-poor inequity in hospital waiting times increased through 2004, after which the trend reversed and pro-rich inequity became apparent after 2011. Inequalities in healthcare-related outcomes are shown to have been more persistent.

The paucity of longitudinal evidence and heterogeneity in methods applied by different studies, however, make it difficult to draw conclusions as to whether PCT commissioning, more specifically, had a positive impact on equity of access.

Summary of reforms under the Coalition

Following the 2010 White Paper titled, 'Equity and excellence: Liberating the NHS' (Department of Health, 2010), the NHS commissioning structure was formally changed under the 2012 Health and Social Care Act (HSCA). Among a number of other changes, Clinical Commissioning Groups (CCGs) replaced PCTs on 1 April 2013 as the main devolved commissioning organisations, albeit initially holding a smaller share of the total NHS budget than PCTs, which excluded primary care (see Chapter 8). The NHS Commissioning Board, later renamed NHS England, is responsible for the commissioning of primary care and specialised services (Figure 12.2)(see Chapter 5).

CCGs initially held some two-thirds of the NHS budget. Their share, however, can be expected to increase to eventually include primary care and most, except highly specialised, hospital services (NHS England, 2014a). From April 2015, the responsibility for

Figure 12.2: NHS Resource Allocation and Commissioning Structure as of 2013

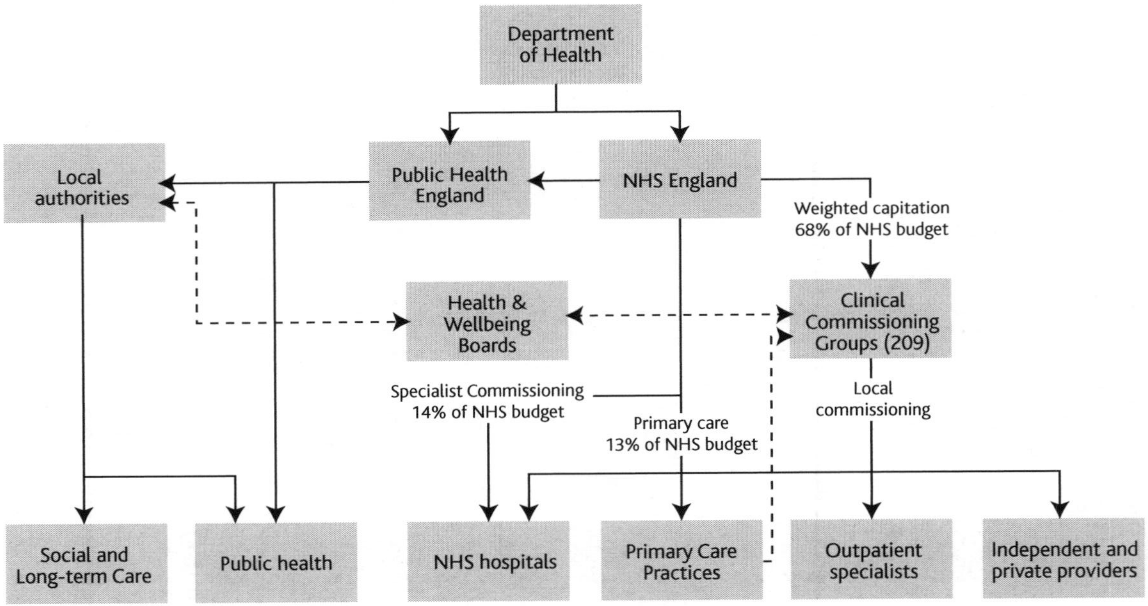

Note: Solid connecting lines denote funding flows only, not supervisory or other relationships. The dotted lines indicate that primary care practices constitute CCGs and that local Health & Wellbeing Boards (HWBs) are constituted by members of CCGs and local authorities.

Source: Authors based on National Audit Office, 2014; NHS, 2015; The King's Fund, 2015a

commissioning of primary care is gradually being delegated from NHS England to CCGs while specialised services will increasingly be commissioned jointly between CCGs and NHS England (NHS England, 2015b; 2015c; The King's Fund, 2015b).

A number of elements of the 2010 White Paper and the 2012 HSCA are notable in the context of commissioning and equity. Although the term 'equity' appeared in the title of the White Paper, the document went on to state that the NHS already achieves equity of access and to imply that *also* achieving excellence should become a focus (2010, 8). While the reduction of inequalities remained a stated goal of the NHS as whole and 'a duty to [...] tackle inequalities in access to healthcare' (2010, 5) was foreseen for NHS England, equity of access was not addressed further. Accordingly, Sections 13G and 14T of the HSCA provide a legal duty for CCGs and NHS England as commissioners to 'have regard to the need to reduce inequalities [...] with respect to [patients'] ability to access health services, and reduce inequalities between patients with respect to the outcomes achieved [...] by the provision of health services.' The duty to 'have regard' to the need of reducing inequalities is repeated a number of times in sections describing the responsibilities of commissioners but no definition is provided. With some exceptions such as immunisations, responsibilities for public health are placed with local authorities rather than NHS commissioners, including the appointment of public health directors (Section 73A). Health and Wellbeing Boards (HWBs), established by local authorities and comprising representatives of CCGs (Section 194), are to provide a structural link to coordinate activities in public health and social care with NHS healthcare and to have commissioning plans approved by local authorities (see Chapters 10 and 14). While the responsibility to deliver health services is largely delegated from the Department of Health through an annual *mandate* to NHS England, an organisation envisioned to be 'free from day-to-day political interference' (Department of Health, 2010, 30), the Secretary of State for Health has a duty to 'have regard to the need to reduce inequalities between the people of England with respect to the benefits that they can obtain from the health service' (Section 1C)(see Chapter 5).

While inequalities in health outcomes continued to receive some attention in the NHS mandates, the NHS Outcomes Framework and related policy documents issued by the Department of Health since the reform (Department of Health, 2015a; 2013a; 2013b; 2012) as well as in those issued by NHS England, equity of access remained largely absent in areas other than budget allocations to CCGs. The Five-year Forward View (NHS England, 2014a) laid out a strategic outlook for the reformed NHS, and provided a number of goals related to prevention, cooperation with local authorities, quality of care, local decision-making, patient focus and efficiency. While health inequalities were mentioned in the context of prevention, mental health and primary care, equity of access was not.

NHS England is also responsible for supervising CCGs and, in addition to allocating funds, issues a number of guidance documents, goals and operational targets. An initial document on legal duties related to inequalities (NHS England, 2014b) provided no definition of equity. Nor did it address which population groups to consider and what mechanisms and measures ought to be applied in ensuring equity of access. A revised document published in December 2015 (NHS England, 2015d), however, does give some practical guidance in two sections, which cover duties under the 2010 Equality Act and the 2012 HSCA. With reference to the duty on reducing inequalities in access and outcomes of the HSCA, it defines 'having due regard' as, 'Inequalities [being] properly and seriously taken into account when making decisions or exercising functions, including balancing that need against any countervailing factors' (NHS England 2015d, 12). In reducing inequalities in access, this requires commissioners to consider any population group experiencing inequalities (2015d, 13), assess needs across their entire population covered and not just based on registration lists of GP practices within the CCG (2015d, 16), to consider inequalities in exercising all functions (2015d, 13) and to produce evidence of the impact of actions taken in the form of an annual report (2015d, 18).

Operational goals for CCGs are based upon the NHS Outcomes Framework and defined in the NHS England Planning Guidance to CCGs. Documents issued between the reform and the end of the Coalition's term (NHS England, 2014c; 2014d; 2013; 2012b) have revolved around indicators of quality of care, usually measured in terms of averages but not in terms of needs-adjusted ranges between patients or population groups to measure equity, and financial performance. Access-related measures are limited to maximum waiting times against a target threshold, which does not account for variation between patients or for unmet need. The latest Planning Guidance (NHS England, 2015e) encourages greater integration between CCGs, NHS England and local authorities in commissioning services and provides nine *must-dos* for local commissioners (see Chapter 9). These continue to relate to improvements to quality of care, financial performance and waiting times (NHS England, 2015e, 8–9). CCG commissioning plans are required to address questions on how to assess and tackle health inequalities through better commissioning and work with local government (NHS England, 2015e, 17; 22). Equity of access, however, continues to be mentioned in relation to budget allocations only (NHS England, 2015e, 11).

Implementation and impact of the reforms

Variation between CCGs in population need, priorities in service commissioning and thus access is likely to be significant. Indeed, in making increased local autonomy a policy goal (Peckham, 2014), an increased potential for and encouragement of variation in priorities between local commissioners has perhaps been one of the clearest themes of the reform. Under efficiency pressures and in an unstable environment, historical and personal relationships between CCGs and other organisations, such as providers and local authorities, are likely to have significant bearing on CCG commissioning decisions (Warwick-Giles, 2014). For example, Docherty and Thornicroft (2015) provided anecdotal evidence of significant reductions in CCG spending on mental health services, which are unlikely to be a result of reduced need. White et al (2014) found large variation between CCG geographic areas in utilisation of inpatient psychiatric care, both in terms of crude utilisation and after standardising for variables that measure need. However, their analysis was based on data from prior to the reform (2010).

Without being able to fully control for need, it is unclear whether observed variations indicate inequity. In the context of devolved commissioning and local autonomy, a distinction between equity within and between CCGs is critical. Greater autonomy may increase the ability of a CCG to reduce inequities within the population it is responsible for. This does necessarily mean, however, that such reductions increase equity at the national level, which is a combination of equity within and between CCGs. Emerging cross-sectional evidence on CCGs indicates that variation within and between CCGs in access-related measures persist even after adjusting for need (Cookson et al, 2016). Longitudinal evidence on equity of access since the reform or, more specifically, the impact of CCG commissioning on equity, is not yet available. This limits our discussion to a review of policy documents, an assessment of the structural capabilities of CCGs and their incentives to increase equity through commissioning.

It might be argued that effective implementation of a central policy goal in a devolved system involves at least the following steps: acceptance of consistent definitions across parties involved in the implementation, conceptualisation of the policy goal and its relationship to other goals, identification of means of achieving the goal, definition of performance metrics and monitoring of performance. The latter may be of particular importance to achievement of equity in a fragmented system of resource allocation (Sheldon and Smith, 2000; Whitehead, 1994). A review of policy documents does not suggest this has taken place during the term of the Coalition government. Initial guidance and policy documents issued by the Department of Health and NHS England provided no definitions of equity of access or the practical meaning of the legal duty of CCGs laid out by the HSCA. Although complex relationships of political accountability exist with various institutions, CGGs are mainly accountable to NHS England, the relationship to which includes managerial oversight, formal goals and potential sanctions (Checkland et al, 2013; Peckham, 2014). As a result, objectives set by NHS England are significant determinants of CCG behaviour. These objectives do not cover equity of access, however. In the absence of concrete performance metrics on equity and strict *top-down* management by achievement of financial and quality metrics, the latter are likely to eclipse the former and CCGs seem unlikely to prioritise efforts to address inequities (Gridley et al, 2012; Salway et al, 2013; Turner et al, 2013)). This is supported by earlier studies of local implementation of centrally set health policy goals, which have shown that targets and oversight are key (Bindman et al, 2000; Blackman et al, 2009; Exworthy et al, 2002).

The public consultation to set the NHS mandate for 2016/17 raised concern that CCGs are not held to account sufficiently for reducing health inequalities and that there are large inequalities in access and outcomes between CCGs (Department of Health, 2015b). In response, the latest mandate (Department of Health, 2015c) provides an objective to create a new and stronger CCGs performance framework, including comparative performance reporting between CCGs and 'measurable reductions in inequalities in access to health services [...] and across a specified range of health outcomes' (2015c, 8). It is not yet clear how this objective will be implemented. The remaining targets of the mandate continue to relate to quality of care and financial balance.

Where CCGs do have an equity agenda, commissioners need to be able to measure and identify inequities to address them. This requires population-based data and technical expertise. We updated our prior review of publicly available documents of all London CCGs in Wenzl et al (2015). Since early 2015, three of 32 CCGs published updated documents containing analyses or objectives related to equity of access or health inequalities. The content of documents, usually part of the

'Equality Strategy, Policy or Information' published by all CCGs to comply with the Equality Act 2010, continues to provide little indication that equity of access is consistently considered as a basis for commissioning (see Table 12.2).

About three quarters of CCGs in London look to the Equality Delivery System 2 (EDS2), a framework produced by NHS England to help NHS organisations demonstrate compliance with the Public Sector Equality Duty of the Equality Act 2010, for guidance. Less than one-third mention their duty on inequalities in access defined in the 2012 HSCA. The nine protected characteristics of the Equality Act are used most commonly to segment populations, while other characteristics such as mental health status, deprivation or socio-economic status are used less frequently (34% and 22% respectively). The infrequent use of socio-economic measures appears particularly surprising given the continuing prominence of the socio-economic

Table 12.2: Selected details from 32 London CCGs' equity and equality publications

Characteristic	N (%) of 32 London CCGs
Publish at least one report on equality or equity	32 (100)
Use EDS2 as main source of definitions	25 (78)
Refer to their duty under the 2012 HSCA on inequalities in access to health services	9 (28)
Subgroups or characteristics mentioned	
All 9 protected characteristics in the Equality Act 2010*	26 (81)
Material deprivation	7 (22)
Mental health	11 (34)
Carers	6 (19)
Quantitative data analysis on equity or equality	
Mentioned	26 (81)
Presented	18 (56)
Characteristics analysed or identified in goals of any type	
Disability	24 (75)
Age	19 (59)
Race or ethnicity	19 (59)
Material deprivation	6 (19)
Present any measurable goals with regard to equality or equity	9 (28)

Note: * Age, disability, gender reassignment, marriage and civil partnership, pregnancy and maternity, race, religion or belief, sex, sexual orientation.

Source: Authors' analysis of published CCG reports based on Wenzl et al. (2015); updated status per January 2016

gradient in health in public debates. Data analyses are mentioned by most CCGs but only 56% also present some data in their publications. Such analyses are usually limited to testing for differences in health status between protected groups and the wider population or discrimination in service delivery. These a priori definitions of relevant population groups are unlike public health methodologies, which take the full population as a basis to identify disadvantaged sub-groups. All CCGs present a strategy or plan of some form to address inequality. The distinct concepts of health inequalities, inequities of access to care and discrimination against minorities (in provision of health services, and in CCG workforce and management structures), however, are usually approached under the single umbrella of *equality*. Related targets are mostly structural or process-related and tend not to be quantitative. Only 28% of CCGs publish operational goals in combination with an associated measure to assess progress.

Following the move of public health professionals, who are qualified to perform population-based analyses, to Local Authorities (see Chapter 10), CCGs may lack the capacity to perform such tasks. Clarke et al (2013) found that, within PCTs, managerial staff with a background in public health was more likely to use external empirical evidence as a basis for decision-making. Even in the era of PCTs, during which less financial pressure on commissioners, a relatively strong policy commitment to inequalities and integration with public health may have made for an easier environment to reallocate resources based on need, progress on inequalities was slow (Cookson et al, 2016; Turner et al, 2013). A survey of PCTs by Salway et al (2013) on commissioning for equity in a multi-ethnic population concluded that only 'isolated pockets of good practice [are found] amidst a general picture of limited organisational engagement, low priority and inadequate skills […]' (p.xv). As GP-led organisations, the professional background of CCG leadership may be better suited for responding to patient demand rather than identifying need using epidemiological methods. In addition, commissioners showed concern that CCG commitment to the equality agenda may be weaker (Turner et al, 2013).

Cooperation between local authorities and CCGs in identifying and taking action on inequities through HWBs and processes such as joint strategic needs assessments (JSNAs) is thus key. Preliminary findings from the early stages in the establishment of HWBs and CCGs by Coleman et al (2014) Coleman and Glendinning (2015), however, suggest significant barriers to effective cooperation, including a lack of statutory authority of HWBs (see also Chapter 14). The effectiveness of JSNAs has also been questioned in the past (Turner et al, 2013), although no recent evidence is available. The fact that geographic CCG boundaries are not coterminous with those of local authorities and that CCGs are funded based on registration lists of constituent GP practices rather than the population of a geographic area are likely to add to difficulties for CCGs to base needs assessments on the right population denominator (Coleman and Glendinning, 2015; Exworthy and Peckham, 1998; National Audit Office, 2014).

In contrast to increasing NHS funding throughout the 2000s (Vizard and Obolenskaya, 2015)), a largely flat real-terms budget since 2010 represents a particular challenge for CCGs at the local level (see Chapter 3), who may only have a small number of providers within their geographic area from which to commission services. Reallocating resources in an environment where increases in one area inevitably imply cuts in another is likely to encounter more resistance than when reallocation can be achieved through differentials in increases.

Discussion

Reforms under the Coalition represent a significant change to NHS policy on equity. In particular, the legal duties for commissioners in the 2012 HSCA expand equity considerations beyond the resource allocation formula and to a lower organisational level of the NHS to the process of local commissioning. Legislation also provides for a continuation of concurrent goals of reducing inequalities in outcomes and in access and perhaps strengthens this duality by virtue of making both goals statutory duties for commissioners. Limiting the reduction of health inequalities to outcomes achieved by the provision of health services may reflect the notion that healthcare only makes a marginal contribution to health. Yet, achievement of equal access for equal need, regardless of other factors such as socioeconomic status, is incompatible with a concurrent goal of reducing health inequalities (see, for example, Asthana and Gibson, 2008; Baker, 2003; Hauck et al, 2002), which might involve *positive* discrimination in favour of disadvantaged groups. A goal of reducing health inequalities also requires that commissioners are able to disentangle the effect of healthcare from determinants of health outside the realm of the health system, which may represent a significant practical challenge.

Despite a policy commitment to reducing health inequalities and other circumstances conducive to progress in reducing inequalities during the era of PCTs, prior studies suggest that local implementation of the goal was not without problems and that only limited progress was made. For the first time in the history of NHS commissioning, reforms under the Coalition have made GP-led organisations the main devolved commissioners in 2013. Given the recency of the reform and the methodological difficulty in measuring equity of access, empirical evidence on the achievement of equity goals by CCGs is largely lacking. Based on our analysis of their structural ability and contextual factors, however, it appears unlikely that CCGs will make more progress than PCTs.

The separation of public health functions from commissioning of healthcare inevitably implies a loss of expertise and commitment to inequalities in the NHS (Johnstone, 2015) (see Chapter 10). Evidence of the early work of HWBs provides little assurance that this structural link is sufficient to ensure effective cooperation between CCGs and local authorities, especially because geographic CCG boundaries are not coterminous with those of local authorities. Even if commissioners were able to identify inequities and were committed to addressing them, the stagnant NHS budget since 2010 makes for a much more difficult environment in which to reallocate resources compared to the PCT era.

In this context, the development of an equity agenda appears to be dependent on efforts by central actors such as NHS England and the Department of Health. Our review of policy documents provides little indication that there is sufficient guidance from the centre on implementation of the equity duty by commissioners. Indeed, cost containment, quality of care and efficiency appear to have been the main goals in changing the commissioning structure (Department of Health, 2015d), which is reflected by current performance metrics set for the NHS. The conclusion that equity is at best a secondary policy goal which has not been implemented effectively is supported by our updated review of CCG publications: neither equity of access as a general concept nor the duties under the 2012 HSCA receive much attention in these documents.

Conclusion

Despite the reference to equity in the title of the 2010 White Paper, equity appears to have been an afterthought in the NHS reforms under the Coalition. The consultation in the process of setting the 2016/17 NHS mandate (Department of Health, 2015b) indicates that this shortcoming is being raised almost three years after the HSCA took effect on the 1st of April 2013. The mandate only provides for a vague response, however (Department of Health, 2015c). In a context of financial pressures and other, more tangible, performance objectives, a vaguely defined concept of equity may continue to be eclipsed by other goals. Encouragingly, recent work by Cookson et al (2016) suggests a set of indicators for the NHS to start monitoring equity. It remains to be seen how these will be implemented and whether equity will become a CCG priority in the near future. Further empirical analyses will be necessary to assess NHS performance on equity once sufficient time has elapsed since the reforms and once processes in the new structure have matured.

References

Acheson, D, 1998, Independent inquiry into inequalities in health, London: The Stationery Office

Allin, S, Grignon, M, Le Grand, J, 2010, Subjective unmet need and utilization of health care services in Canada: What are the equity implications? *Social Science & Medicine* 70, 465–72

Appleby, J, Gregory, S, 2008, NHS spending: Local variations in priorities update, London: The King's Fund

Asthana, S, Gibson, 2008, Health care equity, health equity and resource allocation: Towards a normative approach to achieving the core principles of the NHS, *Radical Statistics*, 96, http://www.radstats.org.uk/no096/Cover96.pdf and http://www.radstats.org.uk/no096/

Baker, D, 2003, Primary care organization, inequalities and equity, in D Bernard, G Caroline (eds), *The New Primary Care*. Maidenhead: McGraw-Hill Education

Barr, B, Bambra, C, Whitehead, M, Duncan, WH, 2014, The impact of NHS resource allocation policy on health inequalities in England 2001–11: Longitudinal ecological study, *British Medical Journal* 348, doi:10.1136/bmj.g3231

Bindman, J, Glover, G, Goldberg, D, Chisholm, D, 2000, Expenditure on mental health care by English health authorities: a potential cause of inequity. *The British Journal of Psychiatry* 177, 3, 267–74

Black, D, 1980, *Inequalities in health: Report of a research working group*, London: Department of Health and Social Security

Black, N, Grün, R, 2005, *Understanding health services, understanding public health*, Open University Press, Berkshire, England

Blackman, T, Elliott, E, Greene, A, Harrington, B, Hunter, D, Marks, L, McKee, L, Smith, K, Williams, G, 2009, Tackling health inequalities in post-devolution Britain: Do targets matter? *Public Administration* 87, 4, 762–78

Carr-Hill, RA, 1989, Allocating resources to health care: RAWP (Resource Allocation Working Party) is dead – long live RAWP, *Health Policy* 13, 2, 135–144

Checkland, K, Harrison, S, Snow, S, McDermott, I, Coleman, A, 2012, Commissioning in the English National Health Service: What's the problem? *Journal of Social Policy* 41, 3, 533–50

Checkland, K, Allen, P, Coleman, A, Segar, J, McDermott, I, Harrison, S, Petsoulas, C, Peckham, S, 2013, Accountable to whom, for what? An exploration of the early development of Clinical Commissioning Groups in the English NHS, *British Medical Journal Open* 3. doi:10.1136/bmjopen-2013-003769

Clarke, A, Taylor-Phillips, S, Swan, J, Gkeredakis, E, Mills, P, Powell, J, Nicolini, D, Roginski, C, Scarbrough, H, Grove, A, 2013, Evidence-based commissioning in the English NHS: Who uses which sources of evidence? A survey 2010/2011, *British Medical Journal Open* 3. doi:10.1136/bmjopen-2013-002714

Coleman, A, Checkland, K, Segar, J, McDermott, I, Harrison, S, Peckham, S, 2014, Joining it up? Health and Wellbeing Boards in English local governance: Evidence from Clinical Commissioning Groups and Shadow Health and Wellbeing Boards, *Local Government Studies* 40, 560–580. doi:10.1080/03003930.2013.841578

Coleman, A, Glendinning, C, 2015, Going round in circles? Joint working between primary health and social care, *Journal of Integrated Care* 23, 2, 53–61

Cookson, R, Asaria, M, Ali, S, Ferguson, B, Fleetcroft, R, Goddard, M, Goldblatt, P, Laudicella, M, Raine, R, 2016, Health Equity Indicators for the English NHS, *CHE Research Paper* 124, Centre for Health Economics, University of York, York.

Cooper, ZN, McGuire, A, Jones, S, Grand, JL, 2009, Equity, waiting times, and NHS reforms: Retrospective study, *British Medical Journal* 339, b3264. doi:10.1136/bmj.b3264

Coronini-Cronberg, S, Lee, H, Darzi, A, Smith, P, 2012, Evaluation of clinical threshold policies for cataract surgery among English commissioners, *Journal of Health Services Research Policy* 17, 4, 241–247

Delamothe, T, 2008, Universality, equity, and quality of care. *British Medical Journal* 336, 1278–81. doi:10.1136/bmj.a169

Department of Health, 2001, *Shifting the balance of power within the NHS: Securing delivery*, London: Department of Health Publications

Department of Health, 2003, *Tackling health inequalities: A programme for action*, London: Department of Health Publications

Department of Health, 2010, *Equity and excellence: Liberating the NHS*, London: The Stationery Office

Department of Health, 2012, *The NHS outcomes framework 2012/13*, London: Department of Health

Department of Health, 2013a, *A mandate from the Government to the NHS Commissioning Board: April 2013 to March 2015*, London: Department of Health

Department of Health, 2013b, *The NHS outcomes framework 2014/15: Updated equalities analysis*, London: Department of Health

Department of Health, 2015a, *A mandate from the Government to NHS England: April 2015 to March 2016*, London: The Stationery Office, London: Department of Health

Department of Health, 2015b, *Setting the mandate to NHS England for 2016 to 2017: government response to the consultation*, London: Department of Health

Department of Health, 2015c, *The Government's mandate to NHS England for 2016/17*, London: Department of Health

Department of Health, 2015d, *2010 to 2015 government policy: NHS efficiency*, London: Department of Health

Docherty, M, Thornicroft, G, 2015, Specialist mental health services in England in 2014: Overview of funding, access and levels of care, *International Journal of Mental Health Systems* 9.

Equality Act, 2010, http://www.legislation.gov.uk/ukpga/2010/15/contents

Exworthy, M, Berney, L, Powell, M, 2002, 'How great expectations in Westminster may be dashed locally': the local implementation of national policy on health inequalities, *Policy and Politics* 30, 79–96

Exworthy, M, Peckham, S, 1998, The contribution of coterminosity to joint purchasing in health and social care, *Health and Place* 4, 233–243

Galbraith, J, 2008, The fantasy of fair funding of Primary Care Trusts, *Radical Statistics* 96, http://www.radstats.org.uk/no096/Cover96.pdf and http://www.radstats.org.uk/no096/

Goddard, M, Gravelle, H, Hole, A, Marini, G, 2010, Where did all the GPs go? Increasing supply and geographical equity in England and Scotland, *Journal of Health Services Research and Policy* 15, 1, 28–35

Goddard, M, Smith, P, 2001, Equity of access to health care services: Theory and evidence from the UK, *Social Science & Medicine* 53, 9, 1149–62

Gridley, K, Spiers, G, Aspinal, F, Bernard, S, Atkin, K, Parker, G, 2012, Can general practitioner commissioning deliver equity and excellence? Evidence from two studies of service improvement in the English NHS, *Journal of Health Services Research Policy* 17, 2, 87–93

Gulliford, M, 2003, Equity and access to health care, in M Gulliford, M Morgan (eds), *Access to Health Care*, New York City: Routledge

Gulliford, M, Figueroa-Muñoz, J, Morgan, M, 2003, Introduction: Meaning of access in health care, in M Gulliford, M Morgan (eds), *Access to Health Care*, New York City: Routledge

Hauck, K, Shaw, R, Smith, PC, 2002, Reducing avoidable inequalities in health: A new criterion for setting health care capitation payments. *Health Economics*, 11, 8, 667–77

Health and Social Care Act 2012, Chapter 7, 2012, http://www.legislation.gov.uk/ukpga/2012/7/contents

Johnstone, P, 2015, Health, equity and the north of England: A case study on a new approach. *British Medical Bulletin*, 116, 1, 29–41

Majeed A, Soljak M, 2014, Can higher NHS spending in deprived areas reduce health inequalities? *British Medical Journal* 348, doi:10.1136/bmj.g3388

Marmot, M, 2010, *Fair Society, Healthy Lives*, London: UCL Institute of Health Equity

Mooney, G, 1983, Equity in health care: Confronting the confusion, *Effective Health Care* 1, 4, 179–185

Mossialos, E, Dixon, A, 2002, Funding health care in Europe: weighing up the options, in: E Mossialos, A Dixon, J Figueras, J Kutzin (eds), *Funding Health Care: Options for Europe, European Observatory on Health Care Systems Series*, Buckingham: Open University Press

National Audit Office, 2014, Funding healthcare: Making allocations to local areas, *HC 625 Session 2014–15*, London: National Audit Office

NHS, 2015, *The structure of the NHS in England*, London: NHS, www.nhs.uk/NHSEngland/thenhs/about/Pages/nhsstructure.aspx

NHS England, 2012a, *Clinical commissioning group governing body members: Role outlines, attributes and skills*, London: NHS Commissioning Board

NHS England, 2012b, *Everyone counts: Planning for patients 2013/14*, London: NHS England

NHS England, 2013, *Everyone counts: Planning for patients 2014/15 to 2018/19*, London: NHS England

NHS England, 2014a, *NHS five year forward view*, London: NHS England

NHS England, 2014b, *Guidance for NHS commissioners on equality and health inequalities legal duties*, London: NHS England

NHS England, 2014c, *The forward view into action: Planning for 2015/16*, London: NHS England

NHS England, 2014d, *Supplementary information for commissioner planning, 2015/16*, London: NHS England

NHS England, 2015a, *The principles and values of the NHS in England*, London: NHS England, www.nhs.uk/NHSEngland/thenhs/about/Pages/nhscoreprinciples.aspx

NHS England, 2015b, *More CCGs set to take on commissioning of GP services*, London: NHS England, www.england.nhs.uk/2015/12/21/commissioning-gp-serv/

NHS England, 2015c, *CCGs approved for joint commissioning of GP services*, London: NHS England, www.england.nhs.uk/2015/03/05/joint-gp-services/

NHS England, 2015d, *Guidance for NHS commissioners on equality and health inequalities legal duties*, London: NHS England

NHS England, 2015e, *Delivering the forward view: NHS planning guidance 2016/17–2020/21*, London: NHS England

Oliver, A, Mossialos, E, 2004, Equity of access to health care: outlining the foundations for action. *Journal of Epidemiology and Community Health* 58, 8, 655–8. doi:10.1136/jech.2003.017731

Peckham, S, 2014, Accountability in the UK healthcare system: An overview, *Healthcare Policy* 10, special issue, 154–162.

Powell, M, Exworthy, M, 2003, Equal access to health care and the British National Health Service, *Policy Studies* 24, 1, 51-64

Salway, S, Turner, D, Mir, G, Bostan, B, Carter, L, Skinner, J, Gerrish, K, Ellison, GTH, 2013, Towards equitable commissioning for our multiethnic society: a mixed-methods qualitative investigation of evidence utilisation by strategic commissioners and public health managers, *Health Services and Delivery Research*

Secretary of State for Health, 2000, *The NHS Plan: A plan for investment, a plan for reform*, London: The Stationery Office

Sheldon, TA, Smith, PC, 2000, Equity in the allocation of health care resources. *Health Economics* 9, 7, 571–4

Smith, J, Curry, N, 2011, Commissioning, in A Dixon, N Mays, L Jones, L (eds), *Understanding New Labour's Market Reforms of the English NHS*, London: The King's Fund

The King's Fund, 2015a, *How is the NHS structured?* London: The King's Fund, www.kingsfund.org.uk/sites/files/kf/media/nhs-structure-2015.pdf

The King's Fund, 2015b, *An alternative guide to the new NHS in England*, London: The King's Fund, www.kingsfund.org.uk/projects/nhs-65/alternative-guide-new-nhs-england

Tudor Hart, J, 1971, The inverse care law, *The Lancet* 297, 7696, 405–12

Turner, D, Salway, S, Mir, G, Ellison, GTH, Skinner, J, Carter, L, Bostan, B, 2013, Prospects for progress on health inequalities in England in the post-primary care trust era: Professional views on challenges, risks and opportunities, *BMC Public Health* 13, 274, http://bmcpublichealth.biomedcentral.com/articles/10.1186/1471-2458-13-274

Vizard, P, Obolenskaya, P, 2015, The Coalition's record on health: Policy, spending and outcomes 2010–2015 (Working Paper 16), *Social Policy in a Cold Climate*, Centre of Analysis of Social Exclusion, London: London School of Economics

Warwick-Giles, L, 2014, *An exploration of how Clinical Commissioning Groups (CCGs) are tackling health inequalities in England*, Manchester: University of Manchester

Wenzl, M, McCuskee, S, Mossialos, E, 2015, Commissioning for equity in the NHS: rhetoric and practice, *British Medical Bulletin* 115, 1, 5–17

White, J, Gutacker, N, Jacobs, R, Mason, A, 2014, Hospital admissions for severe mental illness in England: changes in equity of utilisation at the small area level between 2006 and 2010. *Social Science and Medicine* 120, 243–51

Whitehead, M, 1994, Who cares about equity in the NHS? *British Medical Journal* 308, 6939, 1284–7

Section D:
Governance

THIRTEEN

Setting the workers free? Managers in the (once again) reformed NHS

Paula Hyde and Mark Exworthy

Introduction

Despite repeated reorganisations, the NHS continues to be under severe pressure as it faces profound challenges in terms of growing patient demand, shrinking resources and a rise in external competition. More than ever, it depends upon the effort, knowledge and expertise of its workers. Managing the healthcare workforce was a central focus for Coalition government reforms and it continues to present several challenges; not least that demand for workers often exceeds supply and workforce is often the single most expensive budget item. Thus, it attracts (political, media and public) attention during times of recession and budget constraints (Hyde and McBride, 2011).

The NHS is regularly described by the size of its workforce – often erroneously as the third largest in the world (after the Chinese army and the Indian railways). In fact, it is the fifth largest employer after the US Department of Defense (3.2m), the Chinese military (2.3m), the US supermarket chain, Walmart (2.1m) and McDonald's (1.9m) (Alexander, 2012). In 2015, the NHS workforce amounted to 1.3 million (Health Education England, nd). Together with a further 1.6 million working in social care, the health and social care workforce accounts for 1 in 10 jobs in the UK (Imison, 2015, 20).

The NHS wage bill is £45 billion (DDRB, 2016, 7), accounting for about 40% of the total NHS budget (Kings Fund, 2010) and the majority of health expenditure across all health systems. For NHS providers in England, this amounts to 'about two thirds' of their total expenditure (Lafond, 2015, 11). Moreover, the NHS is marked by the diversity of employment, with over 300 occupations and over 1,000 employing organisations (Health Education England, nd). Although managerial decision-making can go some way towards mitigating shortages and containing costs (through training and development, for example), workforce planning and establishing new ways of working are sophisticated procedures that require strategic and operational coordination if they are to improve organisational performance (Hyde and McBride, 2011). Therefore, managers matter (King's Fund, 2011).

Over the past 30 years or so, a series of health reforms have affected the NHS workforce. As a result of these and combined with the more recent austerity policies, there has been a growing impact upon pay, skill mix, morale and motivation of all staff. While not discounting the effect of reforms upon all staff (especially clinical staff), we focus, in this chapter, upon NHS managers. We do so because managers straddle the macro-, meso- and micro- levels of NHS reform and have been a central focus for recent structural reforms. Also, Powell et al (2014) show the strong link between HRM practices and organisational performance; a focus on improving staff satisfaction, wellbeing and sickness absence may act as a precursor to better services (2014, 94). Moreover, the discourse of managerialism (which managers are thought to enact) is having major ramifications across the NHS. As such, we argue that these questions and implications are emblematic of wider developments facing the NHS.

Despite the widely recognised significance of staff in the NHS, only one of the three books exploring previous NHS reforms since 1991 (Le Grand et al, 1998; Mays et al 2011; Robinson and Le Grand, 1994) includes a chapter on staffing (namely, Buchan and Seccombe, 1994). Their chapter adopted a (then) traditional focus on personnel management and industrial relations. It did not address broader considerations of the forms and consequences of staffing reforms, especially managerialism. More recent assessments of health reforms (for example, King's Fund Mid-term assessment; Gregory et al, 2012) also pay scant attention to staffing issues. The focus tends to be on technical policy instruments relating to efficiency, patient safety and so on. One exception is Appleby et al (2015), devoting 6 of its 68 pages to 'staff' but it focuses largely on staff numbers. This lack of attention on staffing is surprising considering that market-style reforms from 1991 were predicated on new forms of managerialism wrought by New Public Management (NPM) across the UK public sector (Ferlie et al, 2005) and specifically the NHS Management Inquiry report introducing NHS managers (Griffiths, 1983). Without NPM and without Griffiths managers, it would be hard to foresee how many of the subsequent NHS reforms which have been the subject of evaluation could have been effected.

By contrast, this chapter identifies recent trends in staffing across the NHS and specifically builds on a growing body of research on NHS managers and NPM. Some of this evidence has been applied to recent reforms (for example, see Hyde et al, 2016; McCann et al, 2015). We take a broad sweep from the 1980s but focus mainly on the 2010–2015 period of the Coalition government. We frame our argument in terms of the shift towards entrepreneurialism.

The remainder of this chapter is divided into two sections. The first examines the context of and background to recent reforms of NHS staffing. The second examines the state of NHS management and identifies the challenges that remain.

The changing NHS workforce during the Coalition: 'rebalancing towards clinical staffing'?

In the main section of this chapter, we explore the key dimensions of the Coalition reforms as they relate to NHS staff, specifically managers. We focus not simply on the staff as individuals but also on the discourses which the reforms espoused. These dimensions include: managerialism, hybrid managers, staff numbers, redundancy and re-employment, temporary staff, and pay

Managers and managerialism

Government reforms over the last 30 years, which have been broadly labelled as NPM (Hood, 1991), introduced powerful versions of 'managerialism' (Klikauer, 2013).[1] These reforms are not limited to health alone as they have affected housing, social care, policing, the armed forces and education. They have, however, proven particularly difficult to realise in health services (Ackroyd et al, 2007).

The Coalition reforms beginning with the White Paper 'Liberating the NHS' (2010), built on 30 years of reform that first institutionalised management in the NHS (as a result of the Griffiths Report, 1983) and then introduced a quasi-market in 1991 that positioned managers as 'business people' in preparation for market competition. Later, new business units were created in the form of Foundation Trusts (from 2004 onwards). The NHS, as a series of financially distinct entities, started to receive payments for individual patient care (through Payment by Results from 2003/04) rather than block contract. Managers were thus positioned as leaders who could both enact change and be directed by the national agenda (Bresnen et al, 2015).

During the implementation of the Coalition government reforms, NHS managers have operated in a broad sociopolitical environment which has continued the logic of NPM[2] such that managers have simultaneously been the problem and the answer (Greener, 2004). They are beset by policy reforms, system-wide restructuring, marketisation, resource shortages and increasing demand for services. A 'newspaper' view of NHS managers regards them as 'pen pushers' who represent levels of wasteful bureaucracy in large organisations. This is especially true with the rise of discourses about leadership, which often disparage management (Martin and Learmonth, 2012; Bresnen et al, 2015). Coalition government reforms to the NHS have continued the neoliberal challenge to the notion of collective provision of public health care.

As well as proposing major cuts to management costs, the passing of the Health and Social Care Act (2012) opened up the NHS further to private companies. The NHS was set to be delayered by abolishing 151 Primary Care Trusts and 10 Strategic Health Authorities. It was proposed to replace these two layers, however, with 300–500 GP Consortia overseen by an NHS Commissioning Board. (In the end, 211 CCGs were established in 2013.) 'Liberation' came to refer to the liberation of services to public or private provision in a competitive consumer market. Managers of provider services had to become increasingly entrepreneurial in a multi-commissioning, competition-driven health service. These entrepreneurial activities have been undertaken somewhat reluctantly by NHS managers to ensure year by year organisational survival (Exworthy et al, 2015) and some managers have fought for contracts outside their main area of health provision to maintain financial income year on year (Hyde et al, 2016).

Reforms brought in under the Coalition government affected middle managers specifically. Seen as being in need of reform or removal, these managers were pressed to become more effective, more efficient, more entrepreneurial (for example, Harvey et al, 2014). Senior NHS management teams had already shifted towards 'rational' cultures and away from 'clan' culture making them more likely to pursue competitive strategies (Mannion et al, 2009). Perhaps paradoxically, however, the move towards managerialism reinforced a 'utopia of rules' (Graeber, 2015) even as it rhetorically attacked management traditions of bureaucracy and control. The notion of managerial autonomy thus becomes illusory as central constraints become more powerful, though perhaps less visible (Hoque et al, 2004).

The title of this chapter ('setting the workers free') paraphrases the Coalition government's white paper 'Equity and excellence: liberating the NHS' (2010, 9) 'We will create an environment where staff and organisations enjoy greater freedom and clearer incentives to flourish'.

'Liberating the workers' can thus be understood in two ways; first, as an encouragement to staff to become more opportunistic, risk-taking and innovative, and second, by implication, staff to be less constrained by central direction or oversight. Exworthy et al (2011) distinguish between 'freedom to' (innovate) and 'freedom from' (centralisation). The 'freedoms' of Foundation Trusts did not, however, always 'liberate' staff as managers had often become inured to centralisation and adopted risk-averse behaviour in an uncertain policy climate (Exworthy et al, 2011). The innovation/centralisation distinction creates further opportunities both for disaggregation of the NHS (into discrete, autonomous organisations) and for independent sector organisations to employ (often former NHS) staff. Former public sector staff who now work in private organisations may still, however, retain strong affiliations with public sector values (Waring, 2015). Indeed, this was the justification of independent sector treatment centres (Gabbay et al, 2011).

The Coalition reforms have not always been unfavourable to all managers. By design and out of necessity, entrepreneurialism has been at the forefront of reforms. This has entailed a greater need for managers to balance their competing roles: stakeholder, entrepreneurial and political (Currie et al, 2008). As a result, Hyde et al (2016, 176) argue that '[a] new cadre of managers, working to commercial goals, are emerging, and managers in NHS departments – such as marketing, publicity, communications and human resources, where they aren't already outsourced – are coming to resemble those of other commercial corporations.' Yet managers need to also be aware of competing interests such as NHS and other organisations, local public and political institutions.

The 'new cadre' of NHS managers have been successful in delegating tasks to middle and junior managers even as their numbers decrease and their range and volume of responsibilities increase, and NHS management roles draw upon differences in professional background, career trajectory and cross-organisational mobility. Middle managers have filled gaps in service, as functional managers such as HR and Finance devolve functional responsibilities to lower levels of management (Hyde et al, 2012, 17). Moreover, managers have sought innovative ways to reconcile declining budgets with rising demand. The instruments in the Health and Social care Act (2012), for example, allowed managers in NHS Foundation Trusts to increase their organisation's income from non-NHS sources, such as car parking, retail space and medical tourists and so on (Lunt et al, 2015).

Recent research suggests that the working lives of most middle and junior managers, particularly those in clinical, hybrid and operational management roles, are considerably more pressured and insecure than they once were (Hyde et al, 2016). Moreover, the overall demotion of need for care as a determinant of resource allocation has been a widespread finding, one that was deeply troubling for NHS managers across the board (Bresnen et al, 2014; McCann et al, 2015). Managers often found themselves only being able to secure finances for services for short periods at a time before having to reapply for funding in competition with commercial providers. In this sense, falling tariffs under PbR have shifted still further the managerial landscape towards greater uncertainty. They constantly had to balance patient safety with limited available resources (consider, for example, Mid-Staffordshire NHS Trust). They carried responsibility for making cuts and for making sure there was no loss of service: an impossible demand to satisfy all the stakeholders involved. For many managers, complying with governance policies through information management was also a significant draw on their time. Aside from the actual burden of data collection, their attention was often diverted onto the short-term survival of their organisations. At a micro-level, some clinical roles such as matron were being eliminated and post-holders were moved to short-term contracts at lower grades (Hyde et al, 2016).

Middle managers continue to face intense pressure as they formed the target for cuts at the same time as being responsible for implementing change. This has had the consequential effects of increased workload, spans of control, and performance demands. The nature of NHS managerial work has changed with negative effects on careers, job tasks and responsibilities and quality of working life as a direct result of NPM and aggressive managerialism. NHS managers constantly filled the holes in a rapidly changing system and their engagement was essential to the everyday running of health services.

Hybrid managers

The turn first towards and then away from managers as a solution has also served to reduce clinical professionals' power in favour of markets and to raise questions about the balance of power (between managers and clinicians) in health care organisations. Many managers in the NHS are also clinicians of various types and are therefore exposed to tensions between professional, public service values and managerial reforms (McGivern et al, 2015). The introduction of managers to the NHS initially generated some antipathy between managers and clinicians in the NHS but their relationship is now much less clear cut than it might first appear, with both sides trying to accommodate and collaborate with various agendas (Exworthy and Halford, 1999; Noordegraaf, 2011). We therefore recognise a degree of separation between managers (as an occupational group) and managerialism (comprising the discourses and ideologies of business, leadership, commercialism and financialisation) such that managerialism may thus become enacted by various occupations (including clinicians) (Hyde et al, 2016).

This changing pattern of the (clinical) workforce is implicated in the account of new occupations and new forms of professionalism. First, reductions in staff numbers might accelerate further the configuration of and the balance of power between (clinical) occupations. For example, the medical profession has long guarded the specialty structure and hierarchy within it (between consultants and junior doctors) (Creed et al, 2010) but in recent years, the introduction of physician assistants has been prompted by demographic changes, technological changes as well as fiscal constraints (Drennan et al, 2014). Another example relates to the deregulation of nursing education and the removal of bursaries (as announced in the Comprehensive Spending Review, November 2015). Second, acknowledging the 'negotiable nature of professionalism' (Fournier, 1999, 288), the recent configuration of clinical occupations has combined with the declining deference to professionals, greater consumerism and the impact of numerous clinical scandals (such as Mid-Staffordshire hospital), to create conditions in which clinical occupations have sought to forge new forms of professionalism. These new forms comprise (for example) greater transparency of outcomes (Gabe et al, 2012) and new partnerships with patients and the public, with the aim of restoring trust in the profession (Elston, 2009).

The general direction of travel for NHS staffing has sought a rebalancing towards clinicians (Appleby et al, 2015, 9): 'the government pledged to reduce management costs by more than 45% and noted that the NHS will employ fewer staff at the end of [this] Parliament; although rebalanced towards clinical staffing and front-line support.' This figure may represent some relabelling of hybrid middle–managers, however, who are simultaneously in a hybrid clinician–management role as medical director, nurse or midwife manager, clinical team leader or paramedic area manager (Hyde et al, 2016). This is also evident in CCGs since they become member organisations, run by GPs.

While many clinical and support staff have contracts detailing hours of work and arrangements for on-call and overtime payments, the heroic expectation of managers is that they 'get the job done' and provide managerial cover outside of office hours. Managers are thus unable to limit the work (and working hours) required of them. For example, any new demands for information – to deal with a complaint, to find savings or to response to an emerging or ongoing crisis – landed at their feet, on top of an already onerous workload. They were also covering for staff shortages by 'improvising' and 'fire-fighting' to manage day-to-day patient and task demands. As financial pressures have taken greater hold over the past few years, managerial hierarchies have been delayered through reduction in headcount of managerial roles and managerial roles have been forced down the hierarchy (Hyde et al, 2016).

Staffing numbers

A hallmark of the Coalition reform programme was its reduction in managerial staffing numbers. The White Paper 'Equity and excellence' (DH, 2010) couched this in terms of financial costs and staffing numbers, stating,

> The Government will reduce NHS management costs by more than 45% over the next four years, freeing up further resources for front-line care.' (2010, 5)

> The NHS will employ fewer staff at the end of this Parliament; although rebalanced towards clinical staffing and front-line support rather than excessive administration.' (2010, 11)

Coalition policies have indeed made significant impacts upon staffing numbers across all occupational groups (see Table 13.1).

Such reductions would seem to suggest some 'success' in achieving the policy objective, a point reinforced by the reduction in administration costs from a 'baseline of £4.5 billion to £3.04 billion in 2013/14' (Appleby et al, 2015, 9), equivalent to a 36% reduction in real terms. Yet the NHS has been known for its low transaction costs (despite rising costs of managing the quasi-market); Paton (2014) cites Jennifer Dixon (currently Chief Executive of the Health Foundation) in claiming the 14% of total NHS expenditure on management costs was not high by international standards (2014, 7). The shift in staffing emphasis by the Coalition government to 'front-line' staff would also seem to have been achieved. For example, the proportion of clinical

Table 13.1: Changes in NHS staffing: 2010–2014

	May 2010	December 2014	Absolute difference	% difference
Total	1,173,248	1,187,606	+14,358	+1.22
Of which				
Hospital doctors	35,174	40,790	+5,616	+15.97
GPs	35,243	36,920	+1,677	+4.76
Nurses	310,793	317,227	+6,434	+2.07
Managers	42,267	35,594	−673	−15.79
Support staff	162,428	149,553	−12,875	−7.93

Source: Street and Grašič (2015)

and clinical support staff rose from 80.5% to 82.7% (from June 2010 to October 2014) (Appleby et al, 2015, 9), largely due to fewer managers and pressures for increased staffing following the Mid-Staffordshire scandal.

In terms of managers, abolition of PCT, SHAs and other agencies did reduce the number of managers in the NHS over the Coalition period. Notwithstanding definitional issues between administrators, bureaucrats and managers, data from the Health and Social Care Information Centre indicate that managers accounted for over one fifth of the total number of redundancies between 2011 and 2014 (Table 13.2).

The scale of the reductions is also borne out by Street and Grašič (2015) who argue that:

> The number of 'bureaucrats' has actually fallen by almost 20,000 – there being 6,700 fewer managers and 12,900 fewer support staff in December 2014 compared to May 2010. Managers now account for just 3% of the NHS

Table 13.2: Managerial redundancies, 2011–2014

	Total number of redundancies	Managers/senior managers	Managers as % of total redundancies
April 2011–March 2012	6,819	1,444	21.3
April 2012–March 2013	6,784	1,696	25
April 2013–March 2014	4,693	718	15.2
Total	18,296	3,858	21.1

Source: Health and Social Care Information Centre (2015)

workforce, a much lower proportion than the 15% in the workforce generally. (2015)

So, at first sight it may appear that the Coalition government was successful in their aim to rebalance the NHS workforce. In the first two years of the coalition government, NHS staff numbers fell by 2.6% – mainly in non-clinical parts of the workforce – while the number of managers reduced by around 8,000 to 35,555, a drop of around 18% (Gregory et al, 2012, 50). From 2004 to 2014, however, the number of hospital doctors grew by 44% and although the number of GPs per 100,000 population increased from 54 in 1995 to 62 in 2009, it has since fallen back to 59.5 (Imison, 2015). The government anticipated an overall reduction in NHS staff over the course of the Parliament but instead, total NHS staff increased by around 10,800 (between May 2010 and October 2014), a rise of just over 1% (Appleby et al, 2015, 10). Yet, in the four years to August 2013, the number of nurses fell. It might be argued that savings from any real term reductions in staffing have been counterbalanced by increases in agency costs.

Redundancy and re-employment:

The costs of managerial redundancies (linked to Coalition reforms) have caught the attention of the media and politicians. These redundancies cost £856 million, which account for about half of the £1.5 billion cost (estimated by the government) of implementing the reforms (NAO, 2013, 34). The overall implementation cost has been contested by Walshe (2014) who described this figure as 'overly optimistic' and argued that 'no allowance whatsoever [was made] for the labour costs associated with the reorganisation.' The NAO (2013) calculated that, by 2013, the average cost was £34,821 for each of the 5,600 staff who were made redundant but also that a further 12,600 staff would be made redundant in the future, each costing £51,240 (2013, 34). Reductions in NHS managerial staff appear to have been followed by the re-employment of some of these managers. Such re-employment did not counteract the loss of NHS managerial capacity which might explain why NHS spending on management consultants rose from £313 million in 2010 to £640 million in 2014 (Campbell, 2014).

Given the pressing demands of creating new organisations (such as CCGs) and managing ever more stringent efficiency programmes, such re-employment appears a rational response rather than simply a survival of a bureaucracy. During the Coalition government, some attention was paid to this re-employment issue. For example, the Health Select Committee (House of Commons Health Select Committee, 2014) inquiry into public expenditure explored the number and cost of managers being re-employed; see also NAO (2013). A committee member reported Department of Health (DH) data:

> They [DH] state that 19,126 members of staff were made redundant, 3,261 of whom have been re-hired to the NHS after redundancy, including 2,534 within one year, and, fascinatingly, 403 within 28 days of being made redundant'. (Q252; Barbara Keeley) (House of Commons' Health Select Committee, 2013)

The issue was also raised in the Parliamentary questions in April 2014:

> Mr John Spellar (Warley) (Lab): How many staff have been made redundant and subsequently re-employed by NHS organisations since May 2010. [903420]
>
> Pat Glass (North West Durham) (Lab): How many staff have been made redundant and subsequently re-employed by NHS organisations since May 2010. [903427]
>
> The Parliamentary Under-Secretary of State for Health (Dr Daniel Poulter): Since May 2010 and up to December 2013, 4,050 staff across the whole NHS have been re-employed in the NHS following redundancy. This covers all staff grades, not just managers, and is a tiny proportion of the total NHS work force of currently around 1.2 million. (House of Commons, 2014)

A particular concern (of the media and politicians) was (and remains) the redundancy of senior NHS managers. As a result, redundancy payments to senior staff (of organisations which were being abolished by the reforms) had to be approved by the NHS Chief Executive. Redundancy payments were made if there was no suitable alternative employment within the NHS. Suitability was defined in terms of location and type of job. The NAO (2013) reported that '44 of these very senior managers were made redundant under this process between August 2012 and 31 March 2013' (39). These costs amount to £12.2 million, implying an average of £277,273 per person (ranging from £33,771 to £578,470 person). (NAO, 2013, 39).

Temporary staff

Lafond (2015, 9) argues that the number of permanent NHS staff has 'remained relatively stable between 2010–11 (1.06 million) and 2013–14 (1.04 million)' (see Chapters 3 and 4). It has been the rising number of temporary staff which has caused concerns for politicians and policy makers. It also creates clinical concerns when 'whole shifts on wards [are] agency staff, making it very difficult for supervisors to know the skills and weaknesses of those they are supervising' (Powell et al, 2014, 84).

Street (2015) refers to comments by Simon Stevens (NHS Chief Executive) that 'the entire deficit of £822 million in 2014–15 could be accounted for by the "run-up in temporary staffing costs."' Other factors have also been at play, however. For example, the A&E crisis of the 2014/15 winter put the NHS's financial state in stark relief (Exworthy and Glasby, 2015). As Walshe and Smith (2015) report, the Chartered Institute of Public Finance and Accountancy predicted a £2.1bn overall deficit for the year 2015/16, two and a half times the previous year's record deficit. Even trusts that had been financially secure in the past were forecasting substantial losses.

In terms of temporary staff, however, 'between April 2012 and January 2015 the total number of hours requested by acute trusts for agency and bank staff has more than doubled to 1,917,000 hours' (Appleby et al 2015, 12). As a result, the government introduced, in November 2015, a cap on the rate that staffing agency can charge above the rate for permanent (nursing and medical) staff. The shift towards a 'flexible workforce' reflects, according to Hyde et al (2016), the way in which clinicians with previously long-term contracts are being moved onto short-term contracts as funding becomes increasingly short term. This shift is contrary to clinician's own wishes, not least because it adversely affects redundancy pay if/when their new short-term contract is not renewed. By contrast, Street (2015) argues that some staff are looking for flexibility in their working life, and that numbers of clinically trained staff are falling (partly filled by the migration of clinical staff to the UK).

Pay

The fiscal crisis during the Coalition government prompted the government to curtail public sector pay through a freeze in pay increases of those earning over £21,000 per annum (up to April 2013). Furthermore, in March 2014, the Government announced that, in England, only staff that are at the top of their pay band would receive a 'non-consolidated' 1% pay uplift for 2014/15 and staff who are receiving increments would not get the 1% pay uplift and would only receive their increment. In the summer budget of 2015, it was announced that public sector workforces would get pay awards of 1% for four years from 2016/2017 onwards (DDRB, 2016, 15).

NHS Employers (2010) suggested that 'A 2-year incremental freeze would generate savings of £1.9bn' and represent 2.1% of the pay bill. Gregory et al (2012, 49), however, argue that the government has achieved significant reductions in the cost of employing staff, although the NHS pay bill has continued to rise due to wage increments. The government is therefore keen to remove such increments. For clinical staff, this is a significant issue because, '[in] the NHS, a typical nurse currently receives seven years of pay progression, employed doctors in training currently receive automatic incremental pay for time served and consultants have a 19 year pay progression system' (DDRB, 2016, 11).

The effects of reforms on NHS staffing have involved a change not only in the type and numbers of managerial staff but also in the pay hierarchy (see Chapter 3). While we acknowledge that managers cannot easily be separated from the NHS workforce generally, Allied Health Professionals, including nurses, appear to be falling down the pay scale while a new cadre of managers (HR and others) work under extreme pressure but on higher rates of pay (Hyde et al, 2016). The increased use of temporary and short term contracts are linked to insecure organisational income and for many this means work intensification, truncated careers, reduced autonomy and increased responsibility. The overall effect is the relegation of clinical expertise in favour of performance management (Hyde et al, 2012, 2016; McCann et al, 2015). As a result, most health professionals have experienced loss of real terms income both in terms of delegating tasks to lower pay grades and in the form of pay freezes.

By and large, doctors' pay appear to be less threatened than other clinical occupations, so there may be a separating out of NHS professions in terms of pay and job security. Prior to the Coalition, in 2004, primary care and hospital doctors negotiated a new employment contract with the government, which led to significant 'basic' pay increases (of 24 per cent for lower grades, rising to 28 per cent for higher grades)(NAO, 2013). (Such pay increases did not, however, translate into commensurate productivity gains; see NAO, 2010). In addition, consultants have retained significant incentive payments in the form of Clinical Excellence Awards (Exworthy et al, 2016).

It is therefore significant that the renegotiation of the doctors' contract in 2015 and 2016 has generated much attention. While the consultants' contract negotiations appear to have been smooth, the case of the junior doctors has been protracted. Linked to efforts to introduce 'seven day working', the new contract has been rejected by the junior doctors. This denotes a wider readjustment of relations between the state and medical profession (Exworthy, 2015).

Where are NHS managers heading and what does this tell us about the NHS?

Despite the continual reforms over the past 25 years, the vast majority of patients get the appropriate treatment at right time and at a good quality. While the NHS has survived financial problems before, though, Walshe and Smith (2015, 4670) argue that 'much of the NHS organisational architecture and *management capacity* that used to deal with these pressures and broker local solutions was foolishly stripped out of the NHS in the Lansley reforms of 2012' (emphasis added). NHS managers, particularly hybrid clinical managers and operational managers, have traditionally plugged gaps in the system but managers are increasingly being stretched to breaking point. The situation leads, we argue, to three main conclusions about the direction of NHS management.

First, the managerial discourse that was embodied by the Coalition reforms marked a continuation and even an extension of the previous NPM reforms. In particular, the reforms highlighted a marked distinction between managers (as an occupational group) subject to staff reductions and reform, and the rise of managerialism which continues to test out private sector approaches (such as lean management) and private sector provision. The transition of NHS administrators into managers and subsequently into entrepreneurs continued apace, accelerated by fiscal constraints (Macfarlane et al, 2011). Moreover, reforms of the Coalition government seemed to precipitate NHS managers moving beyond 'leaderism' (Bresnen et al, 2015) towards a form of short-term, reluctant entrepreneurialism aimed at keeping NHS organisations financially secure through widespread temporary contracting for services.

The reduction of (often experienced) managers at a time when the management of reorganisation was such a high priority seemed nonsensical (Walshe, 2010; 2014). If the reorganisation was so significant, the implication was that managers were not trusted to deliver such change. (Some managers who were made redundant had, however, been running so-called 'failing Trusts'). The emphasis on 'front-line' clinical staff is to be welcomed but it does not remove the managerial challenge of delivering organisational change on such a scale. Furthermore, while managers were initially framed as the problem, their (partial) re-employment to deliver the policy goals and the subsequent reinvention of local and regional structures (often associated with devolution – see Smith, 2015 – and integration) underline the need for managerial capability and capacity.

Second, consistent with the tenets of NPM, the policies the Coalition government saw active encouragement of the private sector in providing health services and delivering support to commissioning organisations. This is despite the mixed performance of private sector provision during recent years (for example, Perotin et al, 2013); some private providers had struggled to run hospitals as viable organisations (for example, Circle). Furthermore, the new commissioning structures (and consequent increase in costs for commissioners and providers) place local health systems under further strain.

The emphasis on markets was waning in the latter years of the Coalition government, however, in favour of solutions which sought to restore the fragmented system that marketisation and failed inter-sectoral collaboration had wrought (see Chapter 9). While commissioning remains in name and action, it is debatable whether it will retain anything like the salience of previous reforms; NHS England's strategy *Five year forward view* (NHS England, 2014) offers a tacit acknowledgement of this (Chapter 5). Clearly, this has implications for the management skills that health organisations will require in the future as managers navigate the transition to yet another paradigm (Macfarlane et al, 2011).

Third, the effects of the acceleration in NPM, an aggressive form of managerialism, have revealed an emergent trend that seems to divide NHS staff between doctors and other NHS professional groups including managers. To date, doctors have not suffered pay restraint to the same extent as other NHS staff (not least since consultants' clinical excellence awards have hardly been affected by recent reforms; Exworthy et al, 2016). This is happening alongside fewer, overworked middle managers and an emergent cadre of managers with predominantly business concerns. The shift towards greater reliance on temporary and agency staffing has further underlined the increasingly fragmented nature of NHS staffing. While some of this shift reflects staff preferences and choice, it equally shows the way in which traditional structures of staffing continue to be dismantled. Pay perhaps best illustrates this. The cost of staffing the NHS remains a central problem for government in the longer term as Gregory et al (2012) argue that the main policy instrument during the Coalition government (a real reduction in NHS staff pay) cannot be repeated indefinitely if the NHS is to attract and retain staff (54).

So, in summary, NHS staffing (and especially managers) remains crucial to the 'success' of policy reforms. The accumulated effect of previous reforms, and most recently the Coalition reforms, however, has created a perpetual crisis in 'managing' the NHS; crisis has become part of the lexicon of how the NHS is run. In turn, this is aggravating the tension between managerialism and NHS core values. Economic imperatives under the reformed system have come to overshadow ethics of care with profound effects for patients (for example, more limited eligibility criteria for services). Therefore, the 'success' in reducing management costs is, we argue, a heavy price to pay for unintended consequences relating to work intensification, redundancy, re-employment, agency costs and gaps in service provision.

The longer term effects of these reforms are harder to predict but rapid staff turnover at all levels will have several significant effects; work intensification for those who remain, a loss of organisational memory, reform fatigue and short life organisations (Pollitt, 2009; Morris and Farrell, 2007; Salaman, 2005). Hence, '...almost a third of hospital Trusts had at least one board level position that was not permanently filled' (Imison, 2015, 20) and the average tenure of an NHS Chief Executive is 2 years and 4 months (Exworthy et al, 2015). Furthermore, a more engaged workforce, not under intense pressure, is likely to improve the satisfaction of patients they care for (Powell et al, 2014, 95).

The need will thus become ever more pressing for NHS managers to balance a series of dualities; namely, 'empowering frontline leaders while also providing leadership in organisational and local and national systems' (Gregory et al, 2012, 65). In short, reforms of NHS management may say as much about liberating staff as redefining the organisation which they are managing.

Notes

[1] The distinction between managers and 'managerialism' is important to note because reforms have played out through managers as an imposed form of managerialism.

[2] Several authors argue that NPM has been superseded by New Public Governance (NPG); that is, 'the machinery of self-organising inter-organisational networks that function both with and without government to

provide public services' (Osborne, 2006, 381). NPG has not replaced NPM in practice, which continues to dominate through preference for private sector management techniques, hands-on management, focus on entrepreneurial leadership, emphasis on input and output control, disaggregating public services and focusing on cost management, and the growth of markets, competition and contracts for resource allocation (Osborne, 2006, 379).

References

Ackroyd, S, Kirkpatrick, I, Walker, RM, 2007, Public management reform in the UK and its consequences for professional organisation: A comparative analysis, *Public Administration* 85, 1, 9–26

Alexander, R, 2012, *Which is the world's biggest employer?* BBC, www.bbc.co.uk/news/magazine-17429786

Appleby, J, Baird, B, Thompson, J and Jabbal, J, 2015, *The NHS under the coalition government, Part two: NHS performance,* London: King's Fund

Bresnen, M, Hodgson, D, Bailey, S, Hyde, P, Hassard, J, 2014, Being a manager, becoming a professional? A case study and interview based exploration of the use of management knowledge across communities of practice in healthcare organisations, *Health Services and Delivery Research,* 2, 14, 1–166, http://www.journalslibrary.nihr.ac.uk/__data/assets/pdf_file/0019/118252/FullReport-hsdr02140.pdf

Bresnen, M, Hyde, P, Hodgson, D, Bailey, S, Hassard, J, 2015, Leadership talk: From managerialism to leaderism in healthcare after the crash, *Leadership,* 11, 4, 451–70

Buchan, J, Seccombe, I, 1994, The changing role of the NHS personnel function, in R Robinson, J Le Grand (eds) *Evaluating the NHS reforms,* London: King's Fund Institute

Campbell, D, 2014, NHS bill for management advisers doubles to £640m, *The Guardian,* 9 December 2014, www.theguardian.com/society/2014/dec/09/nhs-management-consultants-bill-doubles-640m

Creed, PE, Searle, J, Rogers, ME, 2010, Medical specialty prestige and lifestyle preferences for medical students, *Social Science and Medicine,* 71, 1084–8.

Currie, G, Humphreys, M, Ucbasaran, D, McManus, S, 2008, Entrepreneurial leadership in the English public sector: Paradox or possibility?' *Public Administration,* 86, 4, 987–1008

DDRB (Review Body on Doctors' and Dentists' Remuneration) Review, 2016, *Written Evidence from the Health Department for England 2016,* London: Department of Health

Department of Health, 2010, *Equity and excellence: Liberating the NHS*, London: DH

Drennan, V, Halter, M, Brearley, S, Carneiro, W, Gabe, J, Gage, H, Grant, R, Joly, L, de Lusignan, S, 2014, Investigating the contribution of physician assistants to primary care in England: a mixed-methods study, *Health Services and Delivery Research* 2, 16, www.journalslibrary.nihr.ac.uk/hsdr/volume-2/issue-16#abstract

Elston, M-A, 2009, Re-making a trustworthy medical profession in twenty-first century Britain, in Gabe, M Calnan (eds), *The new sociology of the health service*, London: Routledge

Exworthy, M, 2015, #iminworkjeremy: Why doctors are rejecting Jeremy Hunt seven-day roster, *The Conversation*, 23 July 2015 https://theconversation.com/iminworkjeremy-why-doctors-are-rejecting-jeremy-hunt-seven-day-roster-45117

Exworthy, M, Glasby, J, 2015, Five key moments that shaped the NHS under the coalition, *The Conversation*, 16 March 2015, https://theconversation.com/five-key-moments-that-shaped-the-nhs-under-the-coalition-38677

Exworthy, M, Halford, S, 1999, Assessment and Conclusions, in M Exworthy, S Halford (eds), *Professionals and the New Managerialism in the Public Sector*, Buckingham: Open University Press

Exworthy, M, Frosini, F, Jones, L, 2011, NHS Foundation Trusts: 'you can take a horse to water...' *Journal of Health Services Research and Policy* 16, 4, 232–7

Exworthy, M, Macfarlane, F, Willmott, M, 2015, NHS managers: from administrators to entrepreneurs? in SB Waldorff, AR Pedersen, L Fitzgerald, E Ferlie (eds), *Managing change: From health policy to practice.* Basingstoke: Palgrave Macmillan

Exworthy, M, Hyde, P, McDonald-Kuhne, P, 2016, Knights and knaves in the English medical profession: The case of Clinical Excellence Awards, *Journal of Social Policy* 45, 1, 83–99

Ferlie, E, Lynn, LE, Pollitt, C (eds), 2005, *Oxford handbook of public management*, Oxford: Oxford University Press

Fournier, V, 1999, The appeal to 'professionalism' as a disciplinary mechanism, *The Sociological Review* 47, 2, 280-307

Gabbay, J, LeMay, A, Pope, C, Robert, G, Bate, P, Elston, M-A, 2011, *Organisational innovation in health services: lessons from the NHS Treatment Centres*, Bristol: Policy Press

Graeber, D, 2015, *The Utopia of Rules: On technology, stupidity, and the secret joys of bureaucracy*, New York: Melville House

Greener, I, 2004, Talking to health managers about change: Heroes, villains and simplification, *Journal of Health Organization and Management* 18, 5, 321–35

Gregory, S, Dixon, A, Ham, C, 2012, *Health policy under the coalition government: A mid-term assessment,* London: King's Fund

Griffiths, R, 1983, *NHS Management Inquiry Report,* London: DHSS

Harvey, J, Annandale, E, Loan-Clarke, J, Suhomlinova, O, Teasdale, N, 2014, Mobilising identities: The shape and reality of middle and junior managers working lives: A qualitative study, *Health Services and Delivery Research* 2, 11 http://www.journalslibrary.nihr.ac.uk/hsdr/volume-2/issue-11#abstract

Health and Social Care Information Centre, 2015, Timeseries of Redundancies (Headcount) for main staff groups by Agenda for Change payband, www.hscic.gov.uk/media/16502/Redundancies-for-main-staff-groups-by-Agendafor-Change-payband/xls/Redundancies_for_main_staff_groups_by_Agenda_for_Change_payband.xlsx

Health Education England, *Workforce planning*, London: NHS Health Education, https://hee.nhs.uk/our-work/planning-commissioning/workforce-planning

Hood, C, 1991, A public management for all seasons, *Public Administration* 69, 1, 3–19

Hoque, K, Davis, S, Humphreys, M, 2004, Freedom to do what you are told: Senior management team autonomy in an NHS Acute Trust, Public Administration 82, 355–75

House of Commons, 2014, *Hansard: oral answers to questions.* 1 April 2014. Col.703. London: House of Commons, http://www.publications.parliament.uk/pa/cm201314/cmhansrd/cm140401/debtext/140401-0001.htm#140401-0001.htm_wqn4

House of Commons' Health Select Committee, 2013, *Oral evidence: public expenditure on health and social care.* HC793. Tuesday 17 December 2013. London; House of Commons. http://www.parliament.uk/business/committees/committees-a-z/commons-select/health-committee/inquiries/parliament-2010/pex-2013/

House of Commons Health Select Committee, 2014, *Public expenditure on health and social care.* Seventh report of session 2013-2014. HC793. London: The Stationery Office

Hyde, P, McBride, A, 2011, The healthcare workforce, in K Walshe, J Smith (eds), *Healthcare Management* (2nd edition), Buckingham: Open University Press

Hyde, P, Granter,E., McCann, L, Hassard, J, 2012, The lost health service tribe: In search of middle managers, in H Dickinson, R Mannion, *The Reform of Health Care: Shaping, Adapting and Resisting Policy Developments*, Basingstoke: Palgrave Macmillan

Hyde, P, Granter, E, Hassard, J, McCann, L, 2016, *Deconstructing the welfare state: Managing healthcare in the age of reform*, London: Routledge

Imison, C, 2015, Equipping the NHS with the staff it needs, in All Party Parliamentary Health Group, *Health policy priorities for a new Parliament*, London: King's Fund

King's Fund, 2010, *General election 2010*, www.kingsfund.org.uk/ projects/general-election-2010/faqs

King's Fund, 2011, *The future of leadership and management in the NHS: No more heroes*, London: King's Fund

Klikauer, T, 2013, *Managerialism: A critique of an ideology* Basingstoke: Palgrave

Lafond, S, 2015, *Current NHS spending in England*, London: Health Foundation

Le Grand, J, Mays, N, Mulligan, J-A (eds), 1998, *Learning from the NHS internal market: A review of the evidence*, London: King's Fund

Lunt, N, Exworthy, M, Hanefeld, J, Smith, RD, 2015, International patients within the NHS: A case of public sector entrepreneurialism, *Social Science and Medicine* 124, 338–45

Macfarlane, F, Exworthy, M, Greenhalgh, T, Willmott, M, 2011, Plus ça change, plus c'est la même chose: senior NHS managers' narratives of restructuring, *Sociology of Health and Illness* 33, 6, 914–29

Martin, G, Learmonth, M, 2012, A critical account of the rise and spread of 'leadership': The case of UK health care, *Social Science and Medicine* 74, 3, 281–8

Mannion, R, Harrison, S, Jacobs, R, Konteh, F, Walshe, K, Davies, HTO, 2009, From cultural cohesion to rules and competition: The trajectory of senior management culture in English NHS hospitals, 2001–2008, *Journal of the Royal Society of Medicine* 102, 8, 332–6

Mays, N, Dixon, A, Jones, L (eds), 2011, *Understanding New Labour's market reforms of the NHS*, London: King's Fund

McCann, L, Granter, E, Hassard, J, Hyde, P, 2015, 'You can't do both: something will give': Limitations of the targets culture in managing UK health care workforces, *Human Resource Management* 54, 5, 773–91

McGivern, G, Currie, G, Ferlie, E, Fitzgerald, L, Waring, J, 2015, Hybrid manager-professionals' identity work: The maintenance and hybridization of professionalism in managerial contexts, *Public Administration* 93, 2, 412–32

Morris, J, Farrell, C, 2007, The 'post-bureaucratic' public sector organization: New organizational forms and HRM in ten UK public sector organizations, *International Journal of Human Resource Management* 18, 9, 1575–88

NAO (National Audit Office), 2010, *Management of NHS hospital productivity*, HC491, London: NAO.

NAO (National Audit Office), 2013, *Managing the transition to the reformed health service*. HC537. London; The stationery Office

NHS Employers, 2010, *Summary of proposal on freezing pay increments.* London: NHS Employers

NHS England (2014) *Five year forward view*. https://www.england.nhs.uk/wp-content/uploads/2014/10/5yfv-web.pdf

Noordegraaf, M, 2011, Risky business: How professionals and professional fields (must) deal with organizational issues, *Organization Studies* 32, 10, 1349–71.

Osborne, S, 2006, The new public governance, *Public Management Review*, 8, 3, 377–87

Paton, C, 2014, *At what cost? Paying the price for the market in the English NHS*, Centre for Health and Public Interest, http://chpi.org.uk/wp-content/uploads/2014/02/At-what-cost-paying-the-price-for-the-market-in-the-English-NHS-by-Calum-Paton.pdf

Perotin, V, Zamora, B, Reeves, R, Bartlett, W, Allen, P, 2013, Does hospital ownership affect patient experience? An investigation into public–private sector differences in England, *Journal of Health Economics* 32, 3, 633–46

Pollitt, C, 2009, Bureaucracies remember, post-bureaucratic organizations forget? *Public Administration* 87, 2, 198–218

Powell, M, Dawson, J, Topakas, A, Durose, J, Fewtrell, C, 2014, Staff satisfaction and organisational performance: Evidence from a longitudinal secondary analysis of the NHS staff survey and outcome data, *Health Services and Delivery Research* 2, 50, www.journalslibrary.nihr.ac.uk/hsdr/volume-2/issue-50#hometab0

Robinson, R, Le Grand, J (eds), 1994, *Evaluating the NHS reforms*, London: King's Fund Institute

Salaman, G, 2005, Bureaucracy and beyond: Managers and leaders in the post-bureaucratic organizations, in P Du Gay, (ed) *The values of bureaucracy*. Oxford: Oxford University Press

Smith, J, 2015, On devolving health and social care: Don't let devolution become yet another fad, *Health Service Journal*, 5–12 August, 125, 6455, 16–7

Street, A, 2015, Are agency staff to blame for hospital deficits? *The Conversation*, 3 December. https://theconversation.com/are-agency-staff-to-blame-for-hospital-deficits-51605

Street, A. and Grašič, K, 2015, Fact Check: Are there more NHS doctors and nurses than before the coalition? *The Conversation*, 2 April, https://theconversation.com/fact-check-are-there-more-nhs-doctors-and-nurses-than-before-the-coalition-39607

Walshe, K, 2010, Reorganisation of the NHS in England, *British Medical Journal*, 341, c3843

Walshe, K, Smith, J, 2015, Tackling the NHS's unprecedented deficit and securing reform, *British Medical Journal*, 351, h4670

Waring, J, 2015, Mapping the public sector diaspora: Towards a model of inter-sectoral cultural hybridity using evidence from the English healthcare reforms, *Public Administration*, 93, 2, 345–62

FOURTEEN

Health and Wellbeing Boards: The new system stewards?

Anna Coleman, Surindar Dhesi and Stephen Peckham

Introduction

Health and Wellbeing Boards (HWBs) emerged from debates about the Health and Social Care Bill (2011) as a key coordinating mechanism or steward for local health and social care systems (House of Commons Communities and Local Government Committee, 2013, 14). For many this is yet a further attempt to improve coordination between health and social care services which historically has been a mixed experience (Lewis, 2001; Glendinning and Means, 2004; see chapter 9). The rationale for HWBs, however, includes a broader coordinating function across local authority (LA) services with a role in addressing the wider social determinants of health such as housing, education and planning, as well as social care (see Chapter 10). This wider context of joint-working is generally unexplored despite the emergence in some areas of joint public health directors pre-dating the formal shift of Primary Care Trust public health responsibilities to local government in 2013 (Marks et al, 2011).

While partnerships are seen to be a prerequisite for tackling 'wicked issues' (issues so complex that their solution lies with a multi-agency response), historically they seem unable to break free from the 'silo-based' structures which govern how many UK public services are organised and delivered (Coleman, 2014). Past initiatives to achieve joined up, well coordinated and jointly planned services have previously had limited success.

Various approaches to local authority and NHS partnerships have been introduced since the 1970s with varied success (Hunter and Perkins, 2014). Funding structures remained a key barrier partially addressed by the 1999 Health Act which introduced new 'flexibilities' allowing health bodies and LAs to

- set up pooled budgets

- delegate function, by nominating a lead commissioner or integrating provision, and
- transfer funds between bodies.

The aim was that services should become far more coordinated, designed around users and potentially a cost saving. For example, keeping an elderly person in hospital can be more expensive than the more appropriate package of social care needed to allow the patient to be discharged. With pooled budgets, funds would no longer be tagged as belonging to health or social services, and managers would be able to take more sensible, holistic decisions; however, issues remained, such as non-compatibility of budgetary cycles, audit and governance arrangements and non-coterminous boundaries.[1]

In addition, a reduction of health inequalities and desire to integrate health and social care were prominent objectives in many Local Area Agreements, also reflected in the 2007 Local Government and Public Involvement Act. Health inequalities were also identified as an issue for HWBs to tackle locally.

Faced with complex organisational change under the Health and Social Care Act 2012 (HSCA), unprecedented financial constraints (austerity and cuts) and increasing demand for services, we look at whether HWBs can do any better than previous initiatives. This chapter examines the development of HWBs and draws on the findings of studies conducted by the authors (Coleman et al, 2014, Dhesi, 2014, Jenkins et al, 2015, Peckham et al, 2015) and considers whether or not HWBs are emerging as system stewards. By this we mean HWBs acting at a strategic level to coordinate and set the direction of health and social care developments at the local level, as well as encouraging integrated working (Department of Health, 2013)

Health and Wellbeing Boards

Addressing 'wicked issues' such as increasing costs of health and social care, poorer health outcomes for some groups and the persistence of health inequalities requires a multi-agency approach (Murphy, 2013). The Coalition Government introduced many new organisations and structures resulting in whole system change across health, public health and social care settings which led to greater fragmentation. This in turn led to an increased interest in the wider strategic and coordination role of HWBs and initiatives encouraging increased integration around common objectives articulated in common strategies and plans, often based on community or population outcomes, which have been used as the foundations for their development.

The concept of HWBs was initially proposed in the 'Healthy Lives, Healthy People: Our Strategy for Public Health' White Paper (Department of Health, 2010a) and the White Paper 'Equity and Excellence' (Department of Health, 2010b). Moves were made to create and develop HWBs locally as the Health and Social Care Bill was published in 2011. The passage of the bill was troubled (Timmins, 2012; Chapters 2 and 18) and the HSCA was not passed until March 2012, with HWBs expected to be set up in shadow form from April 2012. All unitary/upper-tier LAs were expected to have HWBs fully operational 12 months after this (April 2013) under section 194 of the Act.

HWBs are tasked with creating a forum of relevant professional groups, local elected members and others, and carrying out a joint strategic needs assessment (JSNA) for the local population – described as 'the means by which local leaders work together to understand and agree the needs of all local people, with the joint health and wellbeing strategy setting the priorities for collective action' (Department of Health, 2011, 7). They are also responsible for developing a joint health and wellbeing strategy (JHWS) for their area with a 'core purpose …to improve local health and social care and to reduce health inequalities' (Local Government Improvement and Development, 2011, 7). The JHWBS is the overarching framework within which commissioning plans are developed for health services, social care, public health and other services which the board agrees are relevant.

HWBs are also expected to promote greater integration and partnership, including joint commissioning, integrated provision, and pooled budgets where appropriate and are described as 'sitting at the heart of local commissioning decisions, underpinning improved health, social care and public health outcomes for the whole community' (Department of Health, 2011, 7). These will be the pillars of local decision-making, focussing leaders on priorities for action and providing the evidence base for decisions about local services. There was thus a clear emphasis on joint working and integrated care with HWBs being given responsibility for oversight of their local area's Better Care Fund (BCF),[2] set up with the intention to increase the scale and pace of integrated working with a particular focus on reducing hospital admissions and length of hospital stay (Chapter 3).

Although the passage of the HSCA was somewhat fraught, the idea and introduction of HWBs was generally welcomed by public health professionals and LAs and was seen as the least controversial part of the reforms, with over 90% of LAs volunteering to become early implementers (Chapter 10). Nevertheless, some critics dismissed claims that HWBs would improve the democratic legitimacy of the NHS (Fitzpatrick, 2011) and others felt that they 'will not be sufficient to ensure a partnership approach to improving health and wellbeing' (Kingsnorth, 2013, 73). Their mandated membership (see below) necessitates that a diverse mix of stakeholders are consulted in the strategic and policy tasks of key commissioners in the HWBs (Coleman et al, 2014).

Established as sub-committees[3] of upper tier/unitary LAs, the exact membership of HWBs was not mandated, but was subject to a minimum core membership, and HWBs could choose how they wished to work. However, the Department of Health emphasised the role of local elected members to provide greater local democratic legitimacy of commissioning decisions (Department of Health, 2011). The core membership should consist of:

- at least one nominated councillor of the LA
- the director of adult social services for the LA
- the director of children's services for the LA
- the director of public health for the LA
- a representative of the local HealthWatch organisation
- a representative of each relevant commissioning group
- such other persons, or representatives of such other persons, as the LA deems appropriate.

All members have equal voting rights on HWBs – unusual for an LA (sub)committee including non-elected members. Dhesi (2014) and Coleman et al (2014) found that LAs were conscious of the need for balance in the number of LA and CCG members, where the view was either that the democratic voice of the LA should have the greatest weight or that health and LA representatives should be evenly balanced.

Upper-tier/unitary LAs are the authorities responsible for HWBs and, unlike in previous joint health and social care initiatives, there is no duty or requirement for district and borough councils to have a seat at the board, to be consulted or to be otherwise involved, (with the exception of the drafting of the JSNA, see Chartered Institute of Environmental Health, 2010), an omission for which the government was criticised by the Health Select Committee (Williams, 2012). LAs are free to determine the number of elected members on HWBs, though this has promoted concerns about the politicisation of decision-making and the need to ensure that the most suitable members are present (Ford and Calkin, 2011). There is also the option for HWBs of using co-option to increase variety and suitability of membership.

Given the variety of potential representatives on HWBs, this gives opportunities for cross-organisational work at a strategic level, and being able to co-opt enables variation suited to local needs/context to be developed. Other potential representatives, include the fire service, police, voluntary organisations and housing associations, all of whom can influence the wider determinants of health. It is important that representatives are senior enough to make decisions on behalf of their organisations, and to attend meetings regularly in order to maintain the position of the HWB as a respected forum (Coleman et al, 2014; Dhesi, 2014).

Humphries (2013) suggested several features of HWBs which could set them apart from previous partnership initiatives. These included: involvement and engagement of GPs; better governance and accountability (due to being sub-committee of the LA); encouragement of wider relations between the NHS and broader LA (not just Social Services); and opportunities afforded by the move of Public Health functions to local government (Coleman and Glendinning, 2015). However, as we have noted, similar initiatives had historically fallen short of expectations.

Following publication of the White Paper (Department of Health, 2010a), the idea of HWBs developed – including potentially having a lead commissioning role (Behan, 2011). HWBs have no direct commissioning responsibilities, however, and instead are expected to influence the commissioning decisions of LAs and CCGs by providing local strategic oversight (stewardship). They are the single element in a fragmented system with a specific mandate to promote integration between local services. CCGs and LAs, together with other key stakeholders, are members of these pivotal joint local fora (Coleman and Glendinning, 2015).

A recent publication (LGA, NHSCC, 2015:2) suggests that 'HWBs provide a genuine opportunity to develop a place-based, preventive approach to the commissioning of health and care services, improving health and tackling health inequalities and the wider determinants of health'. Since HWBs have no formal powers, however, their ability to influence others will depend upon their success in building relationships (Coleman, 2014).

In the following section we use empirical evidence from research, with which we have been involved looking at changes in the system following the implementation of the HSCA (Coleman et al, 2014;

Dhesi, 2014; Jenkins et al, 2015; Peckham et al, 2015), to illustrate some of the issues faced by HWBs as they developed.

Implementation and impact of reform 2010–2015: Membership, structures and relationships

Dhesi (2014) found that the matter of HWB membership was a thorny issue for many, with Chairs and support officers attempting to achieve a balance between inclusion of all relevant parties and creating an unwieldy board with too many members for effective decision-making. HWB membership numbers varied considerably, ranging from little more than the statutory minimum (6), to around 40 members at one authority in a largely rural two-tier system.

Many HWBs faced challenges when deciding which, if any, non-statutory members should be included. The following comment gives a HWB member's opinion on the lack of representation of district council based services in a two-tier area:

> *my specific suggestion was that the seats, however many, given to the District Council should go to the key roles, because, I think, it's really damaging not to have Environmental Health and not to have Housing represented around the table, that, I think, is a real disadvantage for us.* (HWB member; Dhesi, 2014)

Our studies suggest that in some two-tier areas, due to the large number of district councils, not all were directly represented on the county level HWB. However, there were representative district councils on these HWBs, and in several areas there were also local versions of HWBs operating. To illustrate, in one area (Peckham et al, 2015, 17) the local HWB matched CCG boundaries, so all district councils sit on at least one local HWB, and in another site, there was one local HWB for each district council. In another site, each local HWB had an integrated commissioning board, which was attended by a member of the public health team (such as a business manager or commissioning manager). This was to ensure commissioning was aligned and integrated where possible. The District Council's Network highlighted the issue of adequate district council representation 'it seems contradictory... given the prominence of the prevention agenda – that while CCGs have a statutory role, there is no obligation to involve districts beyond the production of JSNAs' and the committee recognised the issue as a concern (House of Commons Select Committee on Health, 2013, 32).

The existence of sub-structures did not appear to be related to the size of the HWB, and sub-structures changed over time during the developmental stages. In many areas the HWB and sub-structures had been developed from existing groups (Dhesi, 2014, Coleman et al, 2014). Others have also observed that in some areas there was an existing system of close collaboration (Tudor Jones, 2013). An environmental health manager noted this trend and described the need to change the people and not just recycle the previous arrangements:

> *I'll look back in a year's time and think, well, it's just the same old, same old, nothing has really changed, because I've been involved with the NHS for a couple of decades now and I've seen restructures, I've seen different GP structures, to the PCT's, they come and go with just the different names, and it's the same people pop up in different structures... You need to change the people sometimes, not just the structure and I'm seeing it happen now'.*
> (EH manager, Dhesi, 2014)

In other areas of the country, an administrative layer has been created above the statutory HWB (often where there was a history of joint working at this scale). This shows that the imposition of LA–wide HWBs does not always sit comfortably with existing partnerships and that different areas have created local arrangements to accommodate this.

Despite concerns expressed that HWBs might be mere 'talking shops' as they did not have statutory powers (HCLGC, 2012; Humphries and Gelea, 2013) public health staff, LA staff and councillors interviewed by Peckham et al (2015, 18) were generally positive about the future role of HWBs and who was involved, despite some feelings that HWBs were still developing their roles.

It is clear both from policy documents and from our research data that HWBs have an important role to play in cross–system coordination. When interviewees in Peckham et al's (2015) study talked about HWBs, it was usually with a sense of optimism. HWBs were seen to play a key part in (potentially) pushing ahead system change, particularly around the integration agenda. Their position in the council, and their membership – often chaired by a senior councillor, was seen to give the HWB the opportunity to progress on the whole redesign of the system, taking the public with them as they do. In a survey of Directors of Public Health (DsPH) (Jenkins et al, 2015) respondents reported that the main benefit of the HWB was that it was 'definitely' instrumental in identifying main health and wellbeing priorities (61%), although as many as 63% of DsPH felt that the HWB was 'not really' making difficult decisions. One senior manager described it as 'the place to come to', given its high profile and membership. As Figure 14.1 shows, the responses for elected members were slightly more positive, with more saying that membership of the HWB allowed them to influence decision-making in the authority (73%) and to engage with the development of the BCF (73%).

Peckham et al (2015, 27–28), highlighted the HWB role in forging new or better relationships between different actors within the system – in particular between elected members and clinicians, which in turn offers opportunities for change and improvement:

> *we insisted…that the one relationship we had to get right was between elected members and clinicians, because they were the only two new entrants into the health and wellbeing board as far as we were concerned, everybody else had been there before.* (Senior strategy manager, Peckham et al, 2015, 27–8)

In addition, HWBs have a role in encouraging new ways of working for health improvement, perhaps by focusing on a particular health

Figure 14.1: Role on Health and Wellbeing Board

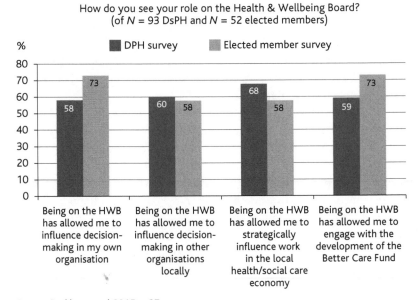

How do you see your role on the Health & Wellbeing Board?
(of *N* = 93 DsPH and *N* = 52 elected members)

Source: Peckham et al 2015, p 27

issue and tasking others across the system with looking at how they might be able to assist, or by 'shaking things up' and putting pressure on system actors, or by system actors putting pressure on each other, asking what more they can do, or what they can do differently. This role of applying pressure has a performance management/scrutiny aspect to it, which one senior manager described as 'hold[ing] public health activity to account' (Peckham et al, 2015).

Priority Setting

The influence of the Marmot review (2010), where two policy objectives relate specifically to children and young people, can be seen in the prioritisation of children in many locally developed JHWBS. A commitment to addressing the social determinants of health was notable during shadow stage interviews with HWB members and support officers, although observations at all case study sites noted a focus on healthcare and social care during many HWB meetings, particularly at the CCG authorisation stage reflecting both internal and external policy pressures (Dhesi, 2014). Dhesi's research (2014) found that many early agendas had the authorisation of CCGs[4] as standing items for some time and integrated care was also a regular feature on the agenda at meetings across the case study sites. There were two approaches to issue-based prioritisation: focussing on specific population groups, such as children or vulnerable people; and focussing on health issues, such as smoking, drugs and alcohol, dementia or obesity. Sites (Dhesi, 2014) generally adopted a mixture of both issue-based approaches and there was little real support seen for geographical prioritisation other than in primary care, where the provision and quality of care were sometimes referred to as issues.

However, Dhesi (2014) highlighted differences in opinion about priorities, and in some cases uncertainty about the best course of action to take. This is illustrated by the views of an elected member of a HWB when asked how best to tackle health inequalities locally:

> What more can [LA] do to help [DPH] and CCGs in driving down health inequalities? I mean we all know what they are, you know, we live 10 years shorter in [area] than we do in [area] and you know, teenage pregnancies, obesity, it's all worse in the North than it is in the South… think we've got to see what we can do about [it], I'm not sure we actually know.' (HWB member; Dhesi, 2014)

Several interviewees noted the impact of wider policy initiatives, and the limited scope of the HWB in tackling an issue with structural causes. Concerns were raised around central government welfare policy exacerbating health inequalities, while others emphasised the impacts of other policy areas, 'so it's really to do with economics, war, housing, education, all these big things…' (EH practitioner; Dhesi, 2014). Another interviewee considered that expectations on what was possible in tackling health inequalities locally needed to be managed, but felt that improvements in certain specific areas were possible.

In contrast to the majority of other sites in Dhesi' study (2014) an EH manager explained that the existing strategies did not include priorities relating to the social determinants of health, but that this was based on previous initiatives and likely to change as they were reviewed:

> when you go back to the JSNA, those wider determinants aren't really in there, it's very much around the legacy of what was the local area agreement and the [area] Strategic Partnership and the priorities that were there got carried over and the strategy, you know, everybody will admit, was put together in a hurry really, so that the board had something to work to and could launch and that was it, but they've also recognised that in the next 12 months, we do need to refresh that. (EH manager; Dhesi, 2014)

In some areas there were reports of health inequalities being seen as low priority or as in one case being unacknowledged. There were some indications that a commitment to prevention and focus on the social determinants of health were starting to result in changes in local arrangements. An elected member described what they viewed as a change under the new system:

> It can't be just about treating ill people. But it never had the chance, I don't think, under the old regime, to have a proper prevention agenda.' (HWB member; Dhesi, 2014)

However, others raised concerns about the level of funding available for preventative services, and also the need for priorities to work in practice, within the sphere of HWB influence, if they were to have some meaning and impact.

Looking at perceptions of the role of HWBs, a survey found that while DsPH and elected members were very similar in the way they ranked the benefits of being on the HWB (Jenkins et al, 2015;

Peckham et al, 2015, 27–28), Councillors were more positive about the powers of the HWB on every aspect. For example, they rated identifying the main health and wellbeing priorities most highly (86% said 'definitely' compared to 61% of DsPH). At the other end of the rankings, 35% of Councillors compared to only 6% of DsPH felt that the HWB was 'definitely' making difficult decisions (see Table 14.1; Peckham et al, 2015, 28).

Operational Matters

The tone of HWB meetings and decision-making processes varied considerably, with some chairs permitting much debate, while others felt that discussion and any disagreement should take place outside HWB meetings. Research (Dhesi, 2014; Coleman et al, 2014) indicated that there was variation in how decisions were made at HWBs, but there was a significant level of work which was, or was planned to be, carried out outside the HWB. This is interesting due to the requirement of HWBs to meet in public from April, 2013. However observations have revealed that the content and level of debate heard in public at some sites was minimal, with a clear intention

Table 14.1: In your opinion is the Health and Wellbeing Board... (% of replies in DPH and elected member surveys)

		Definitely	To some extent	Not really	No
Instrumental in identifying the main health and wellbeing priorities?	DPH	60.5	33.3	6.2	81
	EM	86.0	14.0	0.0	43
Strengthening relationships between commissioning organisations?	DPH	39.5	51.9	8.6	81
	EM	77.3	18.2	4.5	44
Beginning to address the wider determinants of health?	DPH	23.5	49.4	27.2	81
	EM	59.1	36.4	4.5	44
Influencing cross-sector decisions and services to have positive impacts on health and wellbeing	DPH	14.8	64.2	21.0	81
	EM	50.0	43.2	6.8	44
Facilitating the greater use of collective budgets?	DPH	12.3	55.6	32.1	81
	EM	43.2	50.0	6.8	44
Helping to foster a collective responsibility for the use of budgets?	DPH	9.9	63.0	27.2	81
	EM	40.9	45.5	13.6	44
Making difficult decisions?	DPH	6.2	30.9	63.0	81
	EM	34.9	51.2	14.0	43

Note: EM = (Elected) Member

at some sites that disagreements will be debated privately. One site (Dhesi, 2014) in particular held very little debate during meetings and this approach was explained by the chair:

> *I'm determined that we will never have a vote on the board. We'll do it all by consensus. And if there is a danger of falling out over something we'll take it away and sort it, but not in public at the board.* (HWB member, Dhesi, 2014)

Public access to the work of sub-structures appeared to be an area of development. In addition, it was clear that at many sites, officers rather than elected HWB members (with the exception of some chairs) were driving the agendas of HWBs, although HWB members did feel able to add agenda items if they wished.

Both Dhesi (2014) and Coleman et al (2014) showed clearly that there were differing views about the role of party politics, with some members feeling that there was no role for it in HWBs. Officers involved in HWBs often expressed the need to gain cross-party support, although it was evident that people with different political persuasions could take different views on health decisions for their local areas. As sub-committees of the council, HWBs operate with equal voting rights for all Board members, including the LA officers – which is different to any other LA committee where officers advise and councillor's vote.

Humphries (2013) identified key factors for HWB success. These were the role of local government, the role of national government, strategy vision and purpose, promoting integration, beyond the meetings and establishing relationships. Early evidence from work by Peckham et al (2015) suggests that public health is an integral part of HWBs and with PH now being located in LAs rather than health (PCTs) there are many more opportunities for better work across traditional professional boundaries. Despite some tensions identified in case study work (Peckham et al, 2015), Jenkins et al's (2015) survey of DsPH indicated that the overwhelming majority (82%) of respondents felt more able to influence the work of the LA as a whole than they could prior to the reforms.

HWBs were seen as important for public health despite their broader function and current strong focus on integrated care. The DPH is a statutory member of the HWB but there were different expectations about how engaged HWBs actually were, or should be, with the wider public health agenda:

We have a very strong focus on integration, Better Care Fund – all that side of things. I'm conscious sometimes of an element of criticism. Well I mean when I say criticism it's probably a bit strong; there's always a challenge to say, 'Are you actually thinking enough about long term determinants and all the sort of public health agenda?' (Councillor; Peckham et al, 2015 17)

Evidence from a Regional Voices (2015) survey asked representatives about their engagement with HWBs and their success in influencing it. The results suggested that over a three-year period the voluntary and community sector found it easier to influence the JSNA than the JHWS and consequently commissioning. Two further findings were that organisations working with equality groups highlighted how difficult and resource intensive it can be to engage with HWBs resulting in issues considered to be important being omitted from strategic agendas. Where voluntary bodies span geographical boundaries and end up working with multiple HWBs, they particularly struggle to engage and influence adequately.

Health and Wellbeing Boards: developing their roles

Findings from our research projects (Coleman et al, 2014; Dhesi, 2014; Peckham et al, 2015) and the work of others (LGA, NHSCC, 2015; Humphries et al, 2012) suggests that the system within which HWBs are operating is still under development and given the scale of change (for organisations and individuals within these), this is not altogether surprising.

It has been noted that 'In such a fragmented system, the HWB is crucial in ensuring local governance and stewardship. However, while the HWB was seen as having a role in "holding public health activity to account", it did not have any inherent power to fulfil this role, and it was unclear how this might work' (Peckham et al, 2015, 38). In addition the dual roles held by HWBs – building partnerships across the local area and applying pressure and scrutiny – may prove uneasy bedfellows. Given the broad remit of HWBs and that they were still very much in development 'the dominant priorities were integrated care and the Better Care Fund' (LGA, 2014) often at the expense of other roles/functions. Peckham et al (2015) found that councillors were more optimistic about the roles of HWBs than DsPH, which may reflect the institutional positions they hold. Also, HWBs have not developed an executive decision making role but remain information exchangers and focused on a coordination role – supporting the findings of other research (Humphries and Galea, 2013).

HWBs are struggling in many cases to carry out all their roles and have focussed on selected areas such as integrated care or very locally specific issues. In addition other imposed national change such planning the use of the BCF need to be coordinated and overseen by the HWB. The BCF involves NHS funding being pooled with money from other funding streams and spent jointly by the NHS and LAs on promoting integrated care. The compulsory pooling of significant amounts of funding when budgets are already under huge strain will add to pressures facing NHS providers; furthermore, changes to the operation of the BCF have undermined support for it within local government (Kings Fund, 2015). There is some current disquiet about the BCF and delays in announcing a way forward for it in 2016/17, and planning time is being diminished (Peters, 2015). Under the changes announced in July 2014 (Johnstone, 2015), HWBs were to set a local target for reducing the number of unplanned hospital admissions by at least 3.5%, or 185,500 nationwide. All these changes have led, in many areas, to a lack of strategic oversight by HWBs and many questioning their role.

New arrangements are bedding in at a time of unprecedented austerity and budgetary pressures on both the NHS and LAs. Adult social care services have inevitably been adversely affected by cuts to LA budgets, both in the range of services they can fund and the organisational structures within which they operate. Funding constraints such as these do not provide an encouraging environment for new, robust collaborative relationships to develop (Coleman and Glendinning, 2015). The announcement of a £200 million cut in public health funding, constitutes a 7.4% reduction in the public health budget (Barr and Robinson, 2015) potentially costing the Treasury much more than £200 million in the long term (Owen et al, 2012).

There are also more fundamental changes happening at a local and national level at different speeds around England. These include the devolution of health and care budgets; developing Sustainability and Transformation Plans (NHSE 2016) and new models of commissioning and care provision as set out in the Five Year Forward View (NHSE, 2014). In addition the Care Act 2014 places new responsibilities on LAs responsible for adult social care with a particular emphasis on prevention and the need to develop greater health and social care integration (Department of Health, 2012).

In 'Making it better together', the LGA and NHSCC (2015) call for action and set out proposals for strengthening the impact of HWBs.

They stress the importance of developing a place-based preventative approach to commissioning health and care services and tackling health inequalities and the wider determinants of health. In a time of developing new models of care they believe HWBs could play a bigger role as local system leaders, building on the good work they are already undertaking (2015, 2). This they suggest can be facilitated, not by significant legislative change, but through the bold use of existing powers (2015, 4). The report states that 'in some areas members [of HWBs] have begun to make use of the powers and freedoms HWBs have to make a significant impact.... while others were more sceptical about the boards' capacity and have made only tentative steps so far' (2015, 9). A plea is made for a balance between national accountability and local flexibility, the removal of barriers to integration and increased place-based leadership, enabling HWBs to look at both immediate priorities for integration and action for upstream prevention. They set out what a 'good' HWB would look like and include:

- shared leadership – equal partnership between local commissioners enabling a shared understanding to facilitate services which address the wider determinants of health;
- a strategic approach – shared ownership of problems and solutions, focussing on manageable local priorities and making change at a sensible local pace;
- engaging with communities – working with and accountable to local communities together;
- collaborative working – pooling and sharing risks, budgets, data and intelligence
- and developing good working relations throughout the local health economy (including providers).

This latter point is supported by the findings of Peckham et al where it was found that:

> In influencing the system, participants often talked about using specific relationships as levers; key relationships would be used to help to smooth the process, understand what is required to get papers through the local authority and also to get political priorities agreed. (Peckham, 2015, 26)

Calls have long been made for aligning finance and budgets between the NHS and local government (for example Hudson, 1998; Ling, 2002) and this is now repeated (LGA, NHSCC, 2015). Aligning finances and budgetary timetables would simplify integration and the creation of joint incentives could facilitate prevention and early intervention. To allow strategic planning and monitoring of outcomes facilitating an easier flow of information across health and local government would seem key, as would aligned accountability frameworks across local health systems. Coordinated workforce planning to include recruitment and training would also encourage better cross-professional working.

Conclusions

We demonstrate that HWBs display similarities and differences with previous partnership approaches. Distinct differences include equal membership rights of LA officers and external members on a local government committee, new governance forms in local government, problems regarding structures and patterning – especially in two-tier areas but also in areas where new structures (at regional level, for example) are also present. The system surrounding HWBs and the Boards themselves are still developing, with national imposition of new responsibilities, local variations and establishing working relationships and appropriate agendas being challenging. There is an ongoing struggle between local agendas (for example, tackling inequalities) and a central Government push (for example, integration) where HWBs can only be a part of the solution suggesting they may be best focusing on their local system oversight and coordination role. The context of financial austerity in local government and recent additional public health cuts, does not facilitate joint working and can lead to suspicion locally between organisations about potential budget raids although, conversely it may force different approaches to be examined – such as through devolution.

Given these challenging contexts it is perhaps not surprising that the role of HWBs remains unclear in practice. The HWB sits at the intersection of three broad movements. The first is that of developing local collaboration and coordination. To date this has been dominated by the integrated health and social care agenda to the detriment of broader health and wellbeing goals – particularly in the context of public health budget cuts. The mixed reception to devolved autonomy also suggests that this will continue to be an area of concern and complexity. Second, this is likely to be exacerbated by the need to address more substantial budget restrictions and reductions across both LAs and healthcare. While integration is seen as a response to this, structural constraints in terms of organisational, professional and accountability differences continue to create a complex arena within which the HWB has to operate. Given the complexity of 'wicked issues' and the need for action not only across local organisations but also between local and national government does raise the question of whether the HWB can ever provide adequate strategic leadership and coordination. Finally, the key issue relating to internal governance and accountability, membership of HWBs is based on equality of membership with LA officers and non-LA representatives having voting rights with elected members. This makes HWBs unusual governance structures within local government. Achieving the potential of HWBs to deliver democratic accountability and 'joined-up' solutions depends on how well local organisations can, not just manage these, but also shape the environment within which the HWB operates locally.

There is unlikely to be a single response given the extent of local variations in LA and health and social care systems, and the wider context of developments following the Five Year Forward View (NHSE, 2014) and local progress on devolution. Pushing more and more onto HWBs is unlikely to help them develop their key strategic roles and enable them to take on a clear leadership and coordination role in the local health and social care system. There is likely to remain a tension between local determination and national policy – notwithstanding new approaches to devolution. In addition many of the social determinants of health rely on national policy initiatives rather than being solely amenable to local policy solutions.

Notes

[1] Section 31 of the Health Act 1999 has now been repealed and replaced, for England, by section 75 of the National Health Service Act 2006, which consolidated NHS legislation.

[2] The August 2013 Spending Review established the £3.8 billion BCF 'to deliver better outcomes and greater efficiencies through more integrated services for older and disabled people.' The total pooled budget is now £5.3 billion and is to be used to integrate health and social care.

[3] Most LA committees allow only elected members to vote, having taken guidance from officers. However, on HWBs elected members, officers and others who are full members all have an equal entitlement to vote on decisions taken.

[4] In order to become a statutory body each CCG had to go through an authorisation process. This was a set of checks and balances set against 6 domains set out by the NHS Commissioning Board (later known as NHSE).

Within each domain, aspirant CCGs would be expected to produce a range of evidence, including documents such as plans and proposals, examples of work undertaken and feedback from local stakeholders. http://www.dh.gov.uk/en/Publicationsandstatistics/Publications/PublicationsPolicyAndGuidance/DH_130293

References

Barr, B, Robinson, D, 2015, Cutting public health funds: Implications for health inequalities, http://betterhealthforall.org/2015/06/16/cutting-public-health-funds-implications-for-health-inequalities/

Behan, D, 2011, *Letter from Director General for Social Care, Local Government and Care Partnerships to all leaders and chief executives of Local authorities*, London: Department of Health

Ford, S, Calkin, S, 2011, Beefed up health and wellbeing boards extend council powers, *Health Services Journal*, 14 June 2011, http://www.hsj.co.uk/topics/policy/beefed-up-health-and-wellbeing-boards-extend-council-powers/5031167.article

Chartered Institute of Environmental Health, 2010, *Equity and excellence: Liberating the NHS: Response to the Department of Health's consultation*, London: Chartered Institute of Environmental Health

Coleman, A, January 2014, Health and Wellbeing Boards: A new type of partnership, Birmingham University: INLOGOV, http://inlogov.wordpress.com/2014/01/28/health-and-wellbeing-boards/.

Coleman, A, Checkland, K, Segar, J, McDermott, I, Harrison, S, Peckham, S, 2014, Joining it up? Health and Wellbeing in the new English National Health Service organisation: Early evidence from Clinical Commissioning Groups and shadow Health and Wellbeing Boards, *Local Government Studies* 40, 4, 560–580

Coleman, A, Glendinning, C, 2015, Going round in circles? Joint working between primary health and social care. Journal of Integrated Care 23, 2, 53–61

Department of Health, 2010a, *Healthy Lives, Healthy People: Our strategy for Public Health in England*, London: The Stationery Office

Department of Health, 2010b, *Equity and excellence: Liberating the NHS*, London: The Stationery Office

Department of Health, 2011, *Joint Strategic Needs Assessment and joint Health and Wellbeing strategies explained: Commissioning for populations*, Gateway Ref 16731

Department of Health, 2012, *Caring for our future: Reforming care and support*, Cm8378, London: The Stationery Office

Department of Health, 2013, Summary table of the duties and powers introduced by the Health and Social Care Act 2012 relevant to JSNAs and JHWSs, London: The Stationery Office, www.gov.uk/government/uploads/system/uploads/attachment_data/file/223845/Summary-table-of-the-duties-and-powers-introduced-by-the-Health-and-Social-Care-Act-2012-relevant-to-JSNAs-and-JHWSs-March.pdf

Dhesi, S, 2014, *Exploring how Health and Wellbeing Boards are tackling health inequalities with particular reference to the role of environmental health*, PhD Thesis, Manchester University

Fitzpatrick, M, 2011, Health and Wellbeing Boards. *The British Journal of General Practice* 61, 587, 406

Glendinning, C, Means, R, 2004, Rearranging the deckchairs on the Titanic of long-term care? *Critical Social Policy*, 24, 4, 435–57.

Health and Social Care Bill (2011) London: Department of Health

House of Commons Communities and Local Government Committee, 2013, *The role of local authorities in health issues*, www.publications.parliament.uk/pa/cm201213/cmselect/cmcomloc/694/694.pdf

House of Commons Select Committee on Health, Communities and Local Government Committee, 2013, The role of local authorities in health issues. *Eighth Report of Session 2012–13*, London: The Stationery Office

Hudson, B, 1998, Circumstances change cases: Local Government and NHS. Social policy and Administration, 32, 1, 71–86

Humphries, R, 2013, Health and wellbeing boards: Policy and prospects, *Journal of Integrated Care* 21, 1, 6–12

Humphries, R, Galea, A, 2013, *Health and Wellbeing Boards: on year on*. London: The King's Fund

Humphries, R, Galea, A, Sonola, L, Mundle, C, 2012, *Health and Wellbeing Boards: System leaders or talking shops?* London: The Kings Fund

Hunter, DJ, Perkins, N, 2014, *Partnership working in Public health*, Bristol: Policy Press.

Jenkins, L, Bramwell, D, Coleman, A, Gadsby, E, Ogilvie, J, Peckham, S, Perkins, N, Segar, J, Rutter, H, 2015, Public Health and Obesity in England: The new infrastructure examined, *First survey report: Findings from a survey of Directors of Public Health and Elected Members*, Kent: PRUComm

Johnstone, R, 2015, Health Ministers defend Better Care Fund changes, *Public Finance*, 10 July, www.publicfinance.co.uk/news/2014/07/health-minister-defends-better-care-fund-changes/

Kings Fund, 2015, *The Budget: Health and Social Care Funding Briefing*. London: Kings Fund, www.kingsfund.org.uk/sites/files/kf/field/field_publication_file/Budget%20briefing%20July%202015%20final_0.pdf

Kingsnorth, R, 2013, Partnerships for health and wellbeing: Transferring public health responsibilities to local authorities. *Journal of Integrated Care* 21, 2, 64–76

Lewis, J, 2001, Older people and the health–social care boundary in the UK: Half a century of hidden policy conflict, *Social Policy and Administration*, 35, 4, 343–59

LGA, NHSCC (Local Government Association and NHS Clinical Commissioners), 2015, Making it better together: A call to action on the future of health and wellbeing boards, www.nhscc.org/wp-content/uploads/2015/06/Making-It-Better-Together-30June2015.pdf

Ling, T, 2002, Delivering joined-up government in the UK: dimensions, issues and problems. *Public Administration* 80, 4, 615-642

Local Government Improvement and Development, 2011, *Joint Strategic Needs Assessment: A springboard to action*, London: Local Government and Improvement

Marks, L, Cave, S, Hunter, DJ, Mason, J, Peckham, S, Wallace, A, 2011, Governance for health and wellbeing in the English NHS. *Journal of health services research and policy* 16, (Suppl 1), 14–21

Marmot, M, 2010, *Fair Society, Healthy Lives: Strategic Review of Health Inequalities in England post 2010*, London: UCL

Murphy, P, 2013, Public health and health and wellbeing boards: Antecedents, theory and development, *Perspectives in Public Health* 133, 5, 248–53

NHS England, 2014, *Five Year Forward View*, London: NHS England

NHS England, 2016, *Sustainability and Transformation Plans*, https://www.england.nhs.uk/ourwork/futurenhs/deliver-forward-view/stp/

Owen, L, Morgan, A, Fischer, A, Ellis, S, Hoy, A, Kelly, MP, 2012, The cost-effectiveness of public health interventions, *Journal of Public Health* 34, 1, 37–45

Peckham, S, Gadsby, E, Coleman, A, Jenkins, L, Perkins, N, Rutter, H, Segar, J, Bramwell, D, 2015, PHOENIX: Public Health and Obesity in England – the New Infrastructure Examined *Second interim report*, London: PRUComm

Peters, D, 2015, Areas still receiving support with Better Care Fund plans. *Municipal Journal*, 29 July, http://www.themj.co.uk/Areas-still-receiving-support-with-Better-Care-Fund-plans/201378

Regional Voices, 2015, Survey of engagement with Health and Wellbeing Boards, www.regionalvoices.org/hwb-reps/survey

Timmins, N, 2012, *Never again: Or, the story of the Health and Social Care Act 2012*, London: Institute for Government and The King's Fund

Tudor Jones, G, 2013, Assessing the transition to a more localist health system: The first step towards a marriage between the NHS and local government, *Localis*, http://www.localis.org.uk/article/1485/In-Sickness-and-in-Health.htm

Williams, C, 2012, Districts fail to get guarantee. *EHN online*, 9 February

FIFTEEN

Blowin' in the wind:
The involvement of people who use services, carers and the public in health and social care

Karen Newbigging

Introduction

The origins of service user (or patient), carer and public (and community) involvement in health and social care, commonly known as patient and public involvement (PPI), can be traced well back before the inception of the NHS (Gorsky, 2008), influenced by the emergence of health-related social movements and to the civil rights movements of the 1960s. The consequent evolution of a wide range of deliberative processes has spawned a varied and contested terminology, masking different purposes and intentions resulting in different understandings (Baggott, 2005; Stewart, 2013). The purpose of PPI is typically conceived of as shifting the balance of power within the health system so that service users, carers and the public have a greater say in the organisation and delivery of care at the macro-, meso- and micro-levels, in terms of decisions about individual and collective health and social care. PPI is often framed in terms of addressing the democratic deficit in the NHS (Baggott, 2005) but in England, since 2000, it has become increasingly aligned with the reform of the NHS to become patient centred by enabling people to exercise choice as a right and responsibility across all aspects of health care. Since then, there has been a rapid diversification of approaches to and methods for PPI, which experienced organisational turbulence under the Labour administration. The complexity and ambiguity of purpose of Labour's PPI reforms were widely criticised for privileging choice over voice, indicative of a changing relationship between the individual and the state with increased marketisation of the health and social care sector and devolution, in tandem with globalisation

(Tritter, 2009). PPI was, therefore, far from a tabula rasa, when the Conservative–Liberal Coalition government came into office in 2010.

Conceptualising PPI

Viewed as intrinsically good (Florin and Dixon, 2004), the purpose of PPI is variously framed in terms of self-determination and challenging professional paternalism (Williamson, 2014); promoting social justice though recognising the different epistemologies of health and illness of service users, carers, the wider public and health professionals (Beresford, 2005; Carel and Kidd, 2014); increasing the accountability of the health sector and defending social citizenship (Martin, 2008; Warsh, 2014); generating public value and legitimacy, including more effective use of public resources (Tritter and Koivusalo, 2013); promoting rights, and increasingly, responsibilities (Department of Health, 2009), and potentially leading to better health outcomes and reducing health inequalities (Popay, 2006). Alford's typology (1975) of actors with a structural interest in health reform identifies those reflecting diverse community interests, as bonded by a concern to maximise the responsiveness of the health system to their needs and to secure access to high quality health care that responds to these. Thus PPI is seen as offering real possibilities to democratise the health sector, improve the quality and outcomes of health and social care and generate radical and innovative solutions to care issues (Parliament, House of Commons Health Select Committee, 2007) including new forms of expertise and models of good practice for quality and safety (Francis, 2013) and access to wider networks and resources (Parkinson, 2004).

These different, intersecting and potentially conflicting discourses indicate the multi-faceted and pluralistic nature of PPI (Conklin et al, 2010; Gibson et al, 2012). Various frameworks have been offered as a guide to navigate this and evaluate approaches to PPI. Arnstein's (1969) ladder of participation, frequently cited as a touchstone for such purposes, raises fundamental questions about the role of power and authenticity of involvement in terms of the degree of control that service users and the public have in agenda-setting and leadership of PPI initiatives. Consequently, various tensions between different PPI approaches have been identified and their enactment interpreted as a reflection of political ideology. Beresford (2002), for example, contrasts consumerist approaches to PPI –associated with the political right and concerned with marketisation in terms of profitability and effectiveness – with democratic approaches, associated with disabled peoples' movements, concerned with people having more say and control over their lives. The latter framing of PPI is concerned with its emancipatory potential through the empowerment of patients and service users to fully participate both in individual level decisions and wider democratic processes. Thus, consumerist approaches to PPI are often viewed as essentially instrumental with PPI, not an end in itself but a means to achieve the efficiency and quality of health and social care. The plurality of approaches to PPI at micro-, meso- and macro-levels means that in practice both approaches may be evident, creating tensions and raising questions about the goals of specific PPI initiatives.

The evolution of PPI in England before 2010

Widely promoted in an international context (World Health Organization, 1978; Council of Europe, 2000), the formal structures for PPI, Community Health Councils (CHCs) were introduced in 1974. They were initially seen as a way of providing a voice for people from deprived communities and neglected in long-term care and were set up as one strand of NHS reform to represent the interests of local people to managers (Hogg, 2009). The pace of development of PPI in the UK is attributed to the advent of neoliberalist welfare policies and in particular, Thatcher's introduction of the internal market into healthcare: positioning service users and members of the public as consumers (Mold, 2010). From 1997, New Labour, embarked on further shifting the relationship between the state and its citizens: 'transforming citizens from passive recipients of state assistance into self-sustaining individuals' (Clarke, 2005, p.447). While this was evidently a drive towards responsibilisation of citizens for their own health (Clarke, 2005), it also reflected the diminution of the legitimacy of professions as the sole arbiters of knowledge (Carel and Kidd, 2014) and the need for greater openness and transparency within health and social care, in the context of the inquiries into the Bristol heart scandal, Alder Hey and Shipman (Elston, 2009). Under the leitmotif of modernisation, Labour's widespread reforms included proposals to 'modernise, deepen and broaden the ways that patient views are represented in the NHS' (Department of Health, 2000, 95) and the associated PPI reforms included mechanisms and structures for PPI at both micro-, meso- and macro-levels with the functions of voice, choice, redress, representation and scrutiny (as outlined in Table 15.1).

Whilst there had been concerns about the variability of CHCs' working practices and poor representation of the diversity of local communities (Tritter and McCallum, 2006), the justification for their abolition was unclear and the decision highly controversial.[1] In 2003,

Table 15.1: Key PPI reforms under New Labour

New Labour legislation and policy reforms	PPI focus
NHS Plan 2000	• Abolition of CHCs proposed and funding to be redirected to Independent Complaints Advocacy (ICAS), PALS, Patient and Public Involvement Forums (PPIFs). in every NHS Trust and PCT supported by Commission for Patient and Public Involvement in Health (CPPIH) • Transfer of power to refer to the Secretary of State regarding the right to be consulted on major changes from CHCs to Local Authority (LA) Overview and Scrutiny Committees (OSCs), established by the Local Government Act 2000, to review health and social care • Commission for Health Improvement (CHI) to include citizen and lay inspectors on all review teams • An expert patient programme • Patient choice of GP and hospital treatment
Health and Social Care Act 2001	• Section 11 placed duty on the NHS to consult and involve patients and the public in the planning, development and operation of services • Set out the function of OSCs in respect of local health services, both PCTS and NHS Trusts
National Health Service Reform and Health Professions Act 2002	Abolition of CHCs in England and replacement by PPI Forums, managed by CPPIH, for every PCT and NHS Trust in England.
Health and Social Care (Community Health and Standards) Act 2003	Establishment of Foundation Trusts (FTs), placing them under a duty to engage with local communities and encourage local people to become members of their organisations.
Our health, our care, our say 2006	White Paper with a focus on giving patients greater choice and strengthening PPI in commissioning.
Local Government and Public Involvement in Health Act 2007	• Abolished CCPIH and replacement of PPIFs by Local Involvement Networks (LINKs), with a statutory duty on LAs to provide them • Power to inspect replaced by 'enter and view'. • Strengthened Section 11 of the Health and Social Care Act for consultation and involvement of the public and patients in service planning and provision.
Health and Social Care Act 2008	Established the Care Quality Commission (CQC),[1] strengthening the regulatory framework, including responsibility for the regulation of involvement, supported by enforcement powers
NHS Constitution for England 2009	Replaced and enhanced the Patients Charter, introduced in 1991, outlining the rights and responsibilities for NHS patients: including the right to be involved in your own health care, the right to have choices and the right to redress.

Note: [1] Merging the Healthcare Commission, the Mental Health Act Commission and the Commission of Social Care Inspection.

185 CHCs were replaced at a local level by 572 PPIFs coordinated by an independent national organisation, the Commission for Patient and Public Involvement in Health (CPPIH) (Hogg, 2009). Unlike their predecessors, Patient and Public Involvement Forums (PPIFs) were organised around NHS organisations as opposed to local geography (Baggott, 2005). Framed in more individualistic terms, (O'Hara, 2013), their role was to ensure the voice of local people in service improvements and they had more limited powers than CHCs, with the right to refer matters of concern to the Secretary of State now lying with the newly formed local authority (LA) Overview and Scrutiny Committees (OSCs). Baggott's (2005) analysis highlights the complexity, fragmentation and under-resourcing of this new PPI system, which proved to be short-lived. The decision to abolish CPPIH came in 2004, just a few months after the organisation recruited thousands of volunteers to serve on the PPIFs, as a consequence of the review of arms-length bodies. In 2008, PPI Forums were replaced by 152 LINks with their remit formally and importantly extended to cover social care, and a national association of LINk members. The failure of PPIFs and CPPIH was interpreted as 'a confusion of consumerist and democratic' goals (Hogg, 2009, 5) and reflected a lack of conviction concerning their impact and value for money within a changing context of an increasing emphasis on primary care and the integration of health and social care (House of Commons Health Select Committee 2007). With LINks, 'a network of networks', the emphasis shifted from institution to place, reflecting the 'new localism' permeating public services (Hogg, 2007). On the face of it, LINks provided greater opportunities for local democracy, representing a more pluralistic model with stronger grassroots connections (Hogg, 2007). The model was widely criticised before its implementation, however, for the lack of clarity about the role and structure of LINks; potential duplication with the other PPI networks; the inadequate level of resourcing, and the likely failure to hold the government to account (Parliament, House of Commons Health Select Committee, 2007).

New Labour's reforms demonstrate how vulnerable PPI is to the changing winds of government with the learning from earlier models overlooked. By 2010, the PPI topography had changed with the abolition of CHCs and the fragmentation of their key functions: supporting individuals and complainants (redress); monitoring local hospitals and community services (scrutiny), and representing public views on the NHS (voice and representation). PPI duties had however been extended to cover commissioning and social care, with the latter being more closely allied to local democratic structures and less under the dominance of health managers and professionals. For some commentators, however, Labour's claims for greater local public accountability in a context of a centralised model driving the NHS rang hollow (Peckham et al, 2005). Foundation Trust (FT) membership and LINks were widely viewed as enactment of the increasing marketisation of the health and social care sector with choice, individual rather than collective, overshadowing voice in the changing arrangements for PPI, further positioning service users as consumers and diminishing the scope for public participation (Baggott, 2005; Vincent-Jones et al, 2009).

The Francis inquiry (2013) into the system-wide failures in the quality of care at Mid Staffordshire NHS Foundation Trust (Chapter 16), while illustrating the fundamental importance of the voice of service users and carers in ensuring safety and high quality care, provides a damning indictment of Labour's PPI reforms. Francis identifies the preoccupation with organisational form and processes at the expense of the public voice, monitoring and scrutiny of services, organisation of advocacy and handling of complaints as particularly problematic. Empirical data to further understand the impact of New Labour's PPI reforms is dogged by conceptual vagueness and methodological weaknesses. Nonetheless, a systematic review of PPI in healthcare from 1997 to 2009 identified some modest achievements in service design, evaluation and reconfiguration (Mockford et al, 2012). This review and other studies of PALs (South, 2007; Booker et al, 2008) and FT membership (Allen et al, 2012) reiterated the importance of clarity of purpose and contextual factors, including senior leadership, organisational commitment and adequate and dedicated resources as influencing the impact of PPI.

The Coalition's reforms of PPI

In a context of austerity, and another round of high profile failures in safety and the quality of health and social care, the Coalition government embarked on its highly contested programme of reform. The White Paper, 'Equity and Excellence' (Department of Health, 2010) aimed to provide a more responsive and patient-centred NHS: 'placing patients at the heart of everything we do' (Department of Health, 2010: 1) and positioning patient experience as a method for driving quality improvement. Proposals were made to strengthen the voice of service users through emphasising shared decision-making; access to information and Patient Reported Outcome Measures (PROMs); and to promote greater choice and control through the expansion of personal budgets and control over care records. The collective voice of service users and the public was to be via local Healthwatch organisations (LHWs), to replace LINks. In addition, the proposed new NHS Commissioning Board[2] was tasked with promoting patient and carer involvement, so that it championed their interests rather than providers. The proposed GP consortia (that is, CCGs) were also placed under a duty to promote individual choice and to involve current and potential service users in the commissioning process.

The Health and Social Care Act 2012 extended PPI duties to Monitor, Health and Wellbeing Boards, CCG governance arrangements, and promoted greater transparency with CCG and FT Boards required to meet publicly. Part 5 of the 2012 Act, dedicated to public involvement and local government amended Labour's 2007 Act to make provisions for the introduction of LHWs. LAs were, controversially, charged with the responsibility to establish and commission LHWs as social enterprises, to take over the functions of LINks. Healthwatch England (HWE) was established as a sub-committee of the Care Quality Commission (CQC), to provide information and advice to the Secretary of State, the NHS Commissioning Board, Monitor and LAs on the views of people who use health and social care and the public, and the views of LHWs on the standard and improvements to health and social care provision. LHWs were also given a statutory seat on Health and Wellbeing Boards, potentially positioning them as a player in developing the focus on prevention and addressing of health inequalities, strengthening this facet of the PPI role.

These reforms built on those made under the previous administration with a further shift towards greater autonomy and local discretion, particularly in relation to FT membership and arrangements for OSCs. LAs responsibility for PPI was further enhanced by the requirement that they commission Independent Complaints Advocacy Service (ICAS), and independent mental health advocacy previously commissioned by PCTs. Furthermore, the relocation of public health from PCTs to LAs and their role in chairing Health and Wellbeing Boards was also seen as facilitating PPI (Peckham et al, 2014). Three key elements of the Coalition's reforms are discussed in more detail below.

'No decision about me, without me'

Co-opting the strapline from the disabled people's movement 'No decision about me, without me', the discourse of reshaping the relationship with service users, communities and health and social care was much in evidence in the Coalition's reforms. A patient-centred NHS was promoted, framed as increasing choices, in relation to treatment location and provider, and promoting shared decision-making with health professionals (Department of Health, 2010). The NHS Constitution was revised, setting out a series of rights and responsibilities, with service users positioned as 'joint providers of their own care' and expected to take responsibility for adhering to treatment and observing the implications for their lifestyles (Department of Health, 2012a). Service users as responsible consumers was further strengthened by the White Paper, Caring for our Future (HM Government, 2012a). Concerned with adult social care, this made it clear that 'people should be in control of their own care and support' and 'empowered to make the choices that are right for them'. The Care Act 2013 placed a market-shaping duty on LAs providing a context whereby service users could exercise greater choice. These themes were replayed in the Five Year Forward View (NHS England, 2014), which emphasised access to information, self-management, and increasing choices, with individuals managing their own budgets.

Despite this clear policy commitment for people to be more in control of their own health and evidence on how to do this, a recent review of such initiatives identified a general lack of systematic progress (Foot et al, 2014). This review identified that the extent of the choices and scope for control was limited by local factors, including CCG commissioning, a restricted range of providers, organisational commitment and professional attitudes to people exercising greater choice and control (Foot et al, 2014).

Healthwatch

The centrepiece of the coalition's PPI reforms, Healthwatch was described as 'a powerful new consumer champion' for health and for adult social care, as illustrated in Figure 15.1, with its branding and identity intended to enhance accountability, profile and transparency (Gilburt et al, 2015). Despite the consumerist language, the HW branding and model of involvement evoked comparisons with CHCs.

Drawing on volunteers, the key activities of LHWs were as follows (adapted from HWE, 2013):

- enabling local people to monitor and influence commissioning and service provision
- gathering intelligence and reporting on people's needs for and experiences of local care services

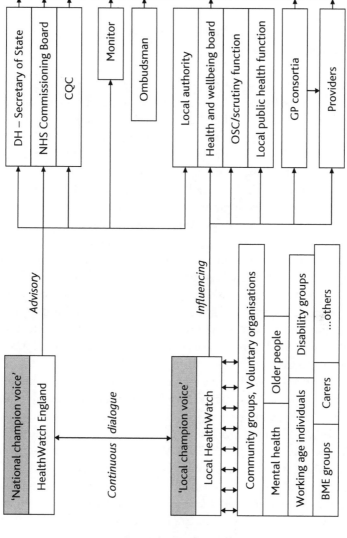

Figure 15.1: Summary of the PPI architecture as a consequence of the PPI reforms

Arrangements will ensure sharing of information to involve, consult and protect the public

DH – Secretary of State

NHS Commissioning Board

CQC

Monitor

Ombudsman

Local authority

Health and wellbeing board

OSC/scrutiny function

Local public health function

GP consortia

Providers

Advisory

Influencing

'National champion voice'

HealthWatch England

Continuous dialogue

'Local champion voice'

Local HealthWatch

Community groups, Voluntary organisations

Older people

Disability groups

...others

Mental health

Carers

Working age individuals

BME groups

The public and patient voice – their views and experiences – influencing better health and social care outcomes

Source: Department of Health, 2012b

- making reports and recommendations on how care services should be improved
- providing advice and information about local care services to support people in exercising choice
- formulating views on the standard of provision and improvements to care provision
- providing intelligence to HWE and making recommendations to HWE to advise the CQC to conduct special reviews or investigations

Predictably, in the absence of a defined model, a variety of approaches were taken to establishing LHWs. Underpinning these were differences in interpretation of the HWE role: 'an independent voice, rooted in the community ("the critic") or a strategic local partner working within the system ("the friend")' (Gilburt et al, 2015, 36). Carter and Martin (2016) argue that the ambiguity of the role of LHWs is a structural feature of this new architecture with a model of involvement suggestive of citizenship rather than consumerism.

The context within which LHW organisations were, and are still operating, are clearly challenging. They are aligned with LA boundaries but have to deal with a range of commissioners and providers whose administrative and geographical boundaries differ (Carter and Martin, 2016). As with LINks, their contractual arrangements with LAs potentially compromises their independence, compounded by the positioning of HWE within the CQC. Austerity and dramatic reductions in LA budgets have meant that LHWs were, and remain, vulnerable to threat of 'cream skimming' of PPI budgets (Watts, 2011). The impact of LHWs being subject to the vagaries of LA finance was identified as prejudicing its independence by Francis (2013: 585) and 'gagging the consumer voice just as it's starting to make a difference' by the HWE Chair, Anna Bradley, in 2013.[3] The central funding for HWE was top-sliced in 2013 (HWE, 2013) and further reductions were planned by LAs with proposed cuts ranging from 17.9% to 53.4% in the financial settlements for 2015/16.[4] This included areas where health inequities were well documented such as Blackpool where male life expectancy is the lowest in England (Office for National Statistics, 2015). There was also an expectation that LHWs would income generate, potentially increasing inequities between the most and least deprived areas of England, negatively impacting on participatory parity. In practice income generation may further compromise the independence of LHWs and constitutes a diversion of energy of LHWs away from its core functions.

There is little empirical evidence of the impact of LHWs under the Coalition. A Department of Health funded evaluation of the first 18–21 months of LHWs reported over three quarters considered they were particularly effective at directly influencing providers and were making good progress with influencing commissioners (Gilburt et al, 2015), although HWE subsequently observed that the engagement of LHWs with CCGs was poor. Furthermore, other commentators have pointed to the multiplicity of the arrangements for PPI; the diversity of providers, including in the voluntary and independent sector; the increasing complexity of local governance arrangements and inadequate resourcing serving to limit the impact of LHWs (Baggott and Jones, 2015; Carter and Martin, 2016).

PPI and commissioning

PPI in commissioning was strengthened by the 2012 Act but there was scepticism about whether this would be translated into practice, not least because GPs, now in the driving seat of the new commissioning arrangements, did not have history of engagement with their patients and communities (Petsoulas, 2015). The authorisation and assurance processes for CCGs included meaningful engagement with service users, carers and their communities as one of six domains on which they had to provide evidence (NHS England, 2013). A lack of clear guidance about the PPI arrangements in commissioning (Patients Association, 2011) and preoccupation with establishing new structures, processes and governance (Coleman et al, 2011) were identified as jeopardising the priority that CCGs would afford PPI. Furthermore, the increasing complexity of the commissioning context meant it was unclear how CCGs would develop appropriate methods and a conducive context for effective PPI (Petsoulas, 2015) and a concern that they would struggle to effectively engage with seldom heard groups (Patients Association, 2011). Early evidence suggests that PPI activity is peripheral to the main commissioning activities of the CCG, with a focus on getting structures and processes rights as opposed to the quality of involvement (Peckham et al, 2014).

Implications and future directions

The Coalition government built on the foundations for PPI laid by the previous government, and both administrations could be characterised by their reluctance to understand and address weaknesses in previous PPI arrangements. There was continuity in the direction of travel with Labour's reforms and reflected in the current Conservative government's approach to PPI: a shift to conceiving PPI in individualist terms, emphasising choice in tandem with marketisation and promoting greater local determination through pursuing devolution and localism. Drawing on the discussion on the purpose and conceptualisation of PPI discussed at the beginning of this chapter, it is possible to distill five interrelated challenges arising from the Coalition's reforms.

Individualising and responsibilising service users and the public

The focus of much active PPI activity is on individuals' experiences of services and treatment, with service users positioned as consumers (HWE, 2015). The language of consumerism pervades the PPI discourse, and coupling rights with responsibilities, positions service users and the public as a particular sort of consumer – the responsible consumer – responsible not only for making good choices about care services but also for complying with treatment and safeguarding personal health, with self-management gaining ascendancy as a concept (Mold, 2010; Foot et al, 2014), in tandem with health framed as a personal achievement. A focus on individual voce can undermine engaging with collective voices, which has always been a more challenging endeavour, dogged with concerns about representation and representativeness (Martin, 2008; Baggott and Jones, 2015). This focus, however, can create tensions with the role of strengthening the collective voice of local people, which LHWs are resolving differently (Carter and Martin, 2016).

The paradox of localism

The enhanced role of LAs and CCG duties in relation to PPI, and an associated focus on place, provides fertile ground for strengthening the role of local people in strategic and operational developments but is contingent on the political, social and organisational context. The impact of PPI can be muted as a consequence and, unsurprisingly, the status of PPI in the governance of FTs and commissioning activity is highly variable and typically weak (Maybin et al, 2011; Allen et al, 2012; Peckham et al, 2014). Furthermore, a lack of evidence of impact can leave PPI open to the charge that it is a costly investment and localities can exercise the discretion to reduce capacity, as is happening with LHWs. This has implications for sustaining and developing relationships with local communities and for addressing inequities in health and social care (Mold, 2010). The emphasis on localism is complicated by the lack of coterminosity of the boundaries of LAs with CCGs and provider organisations, and also PPI activity and rights activism that spans administrative boundaries and is reliant on solidarity and networks (Barnes et al, 2007). The question remains open as to whether there should be a basic national model for LHWs, as recommended by Francis (2013) and independent national oversight as previously provided by CPPIH.

Depowering the PPI engine

The power of the engine for PPI has been incrementally reduced since the abolition of CHCs through to LHWs, as illustrated in Table 15.2. Successive reorganisations have impacted on organisational memory and capacity for PPI, which with reductions in funding, under the Coalition, have increased its fragility (Peckham et al, 2014). These reorganisations have led to fragmentation of various functions – voice, choice, representation, scrutiny and redress – which has increased the complexity and potential duplication of effort, resulting in confusion and a loss of confidence for service users, the public and services (Carter and Martin, 2016).

Also of note is the removal of the power to refer issues of concern regarding service reconfigurations to the Secretary of State, with LHWs required to refer matters to LA OSCs. The likelihood of OSCs challenging NHS service reconfigurations is debatable, underscored by the reducing capacity of LAs for scrutiny and a disinclination of some to be involved in major projects because of opposition from senior officers (Centre for Public Scrutiny, 2015). Unease at wider public involvement in decision-making can also be discerned from the regulations which placed limits on the political activity of LHWs. The regulations do permit campaigning if the prime purpose is as a consumer champion (HM Government 2012b) but this is a far cry from the active campaigning role of CHCs, particularly in relation to service closures and PFI deals.

In and against the state[5]

Independence is repeatedly asserted as an important principle that underpins service users and the public having an effective voice: having the freedom to raise issues, speak out, campaign, resist changes and ensure their issues are on the agenda for decision-makers. PPI structures have increasingly been located within the state apparatus with their independence further compromised by the Coalition reforms, despite

Table 15.2: Comparison of the functions and powers of different PPI structures

Functions and statutory powers	CHCs	PPI forums	LINks	Healthwatch
Representation: statutory duty to represent public views	Yes	Yes	Yes in commissioning and provision	Yes in commissioning and provision
Scrutiny Monitor and review services	Yes	Yes	Yes. Observation and review of commissioning and FTs	Yes, including reports making recommendations about how local services could or should be improved.
Right of access and inspection	Access to NHS premises and power to inspect but could be refused	As previously	Power to inspect replaced by 'enter and view' but could be refused. Extended to social care.	Enter and view for health and social care provision[1] but could be refused. Can escalate concerns to CQC.
Right to be formally consulted on major service reconfiguration	Yes	No	No	No
Power to refer matters to the Secretary of State	Yes	No. Power to refer matters given to the Overview and Scrutiny Committee (OSC), which can refer matters to the Secretary of State	No. Power to refer to the OSC, which can refer matters to the Secretary of State	No. Power to refer matters to the OSC, which can refer matters to the Secretary of State. LAs afforded discretion in arrangements for OSCs.
Individual redress by supporting complainants and providing advocacy	Majority did but for NHS only	No	No	LHW the biggest provider of ICAS (HWE 2015) and securing contracts to provide other forms of advocacy for health and social care.

Note: [1] Excludes LA premises for young people under the age of 18.

concerns highlighted by the All Parliamentary Group on PPI (2011)[6] and Francis (2013). The contractual arrangements of LHWs with LAs is of particular significance, compromising their independence and potentially reducing their monitoring role, reflecting a shift from accountability and scrutiny, as with LINKs, to a source of intelligence about local needs and expectations (Tritter and Koivusalo, 2013). Thus, the organisational location of PPI, weak governance arrangements for PPI bodies such as LHWs (Foot et al, 2015) combined with the decentralisation of the accountability of PPI mechanisms to NHS Trusts and LAs makes them vulnerable to organisational commitment to PPI, austerity measures and political ideology.

This taming of PPI is potentially a problem for PPI if conceptualised as a mechanism for addressing the democratic deficit. As Fraser (1990) asserted, alternatives arenas, 'counterpublics', are an important element in democracy by expanding the discursive space and, thus, providing alternative accounts and norms to those officially sanctioned by the state. Social movements, voluntary and community sector organisations and organic coalitions of service users and the public, as in the campaign for a public inquiry into the Mid-Staffordshire NHS Foundation Trust and the campaigning by organisations such as 38 Degrees, are an important strand of PPI. User groups, voluntary sector and community sector organisations are increasingly being commissioned to provide services by local government, however, with implications for their capacity to challenge and campaign. Furthermore, their capacity and the wider context of welfare benefit changes will impact on involvement increasing the risk that the sector aligns more closely with government agendas (Baggott and Jones, 2015).

Pluralism and opening up discursive spaces

In discussion of PPI initiatives, the state is typically portrayed as powerful and service users, carers and the public as powerless (Conklin et al, 2010). Such an analysis risks ignoring the relational nature of PPI, adopting a top-down, linear approach to the policy process in which PPI adopts a monolithic character in order to enhance rational decision-making processes. An analysis of PPI that includes the expressive and relational aspects and recognises the agency of service users, carers and the public, however, will identify the potential of PPI to open up new discursive spaces and networks (Gibson et al 2012). This approach is likely to deliver the kinds of transformation to enable health and social care services to become more person centred.

The conditions for this will include investment in capacity of the PPI sector, not solely formal PPI structures; tolerance of ambiguity; and an acknowledgement that a plurality of approaches to PPI is an opportunity for democratising the power dynamic further. This represents a significant challenge for any government and experience to date indicates the focus required is on key functions, organisational culture of commissioners and providers, relationships, quality and depth of involvement and the environmental enabling influences rather than structures and processes per se (Meads et al, 2007).

Conclusion

PPI is an easy target for reform by government, but failure to learn from previous initiatives diverts attention and weakens effective arrangements. The Coalition's reforms promoted PPI at different levels but the sparse empirical data compromises evaluation of their impact. The reforms have built on previous initiatives and further shifted towards individual voice, responsibilising service users in a context of increased marketisation of health and care services. The introduction of HWE has restored a national profile for PPI, albeit with more limited powers than its predecessors, and an extended role to social care. The increasing emphasis on localism is both an opportunity and a threat, placing LHWs at risk of budget cuts, weakening their capacity and compromising their effectiveness. The complexity and fragmentation of the different aspects of PPI needs careful thought, and the question of whether there should be a national model with reintegration of these functions should be addressed.

Weakening the power of PPI arrangements will reduce their impact and this will place them at risk of a change of government, eager to demonstrate a new approach to PPI. Experience under the Labour administration, however, indicates that large scale reorganisation of PPI means that the focus on improving services, their quality and outcomes, and the networks and enthusiasm of local patients, service users and their communities can be seriously damaged. Evaluations of recent PPI initiatives re-emphasises its situated nature and the importance of adopting an approach that recognises and values the agency of service users, carers and the public and acts on their issues. This is also actively promoted by these groups and their communities and there is some evidence of new discursive spaces opening up. The Coalition government has, therefore, provided a policy direction that continues to support the role of PPI but has further weakened the foundations in its operalisation. The challenge for the Conservative government, from 2015 on, is to strengthen and sustain PPI, ensuring its independence, investing adequately in capacity building and shifting the focus to include the quality and depth of involvement, ensuring that service users, carers and the public are actively involved in both setting the agenda and in decision-making. Perhaps uncomfortably for the state, it also requires recognition of the value and commitment to the various forms of PPI, including activism and campaigning, in transforming health and social care to ensure the responsiveness and quality of the health and care system to the diversity of local people and their communities.

Notes

[1] Described by a former ACHEW Director as 'shabby' (Gerrard, 2006: 270).

[2] Rebadged as NHS England from March 2013.

[3] Healthwatch England's position on funding for local Healthwatch. Blog posted on 19/11/13, available http://www.healthwatch.co.uk/resource/funding-local-healthwatch (accessed 15th December 2015).

[4] See http://healthwatchtrafford.co.uk/news/health-and-care-watchdog-warns-10-councils-over-funding-cuts-that-could-mute-voice-of-patients/ (accessed 15th December 2015).

[5] Carter and Martin (2015).

[6] Debate at the APPG meeting in January 2011. Available at: http://www.patients-association.org.uk/policy-campaigns/all-party-parliamentary-group-patient-and-public-involvement/ [accessed 151215].

References

Alford, R, 1975, *Health care politics*, Chicago: University of Chicago

Allen, P, Townsend, J, Dempster, P, Wright, J, Hutchings, A, Keen, J, 2012, Organizational form as a mechanism to involve staff, public and users in public services: A study of the governance of NHS Foundation Trusts, *Social Policy and Administration* 46, 3, 239–57

Arnstein, SR, 1969, A ladder of citizen participation, *Journal of the American Institute of Planners* 35, 4, 216–24

Baggott, R, 2005, A funny thing happened on the way to the forum? Reforming patient and public involvement in the NHS in England, *Public Administration* 83, 3, 533-551

Baggott, R, Jones, K, 2015, The Big Society in an age of austerity: Threats and opportunities for Health Consumer and Patients' Organizations in England, *Health Expectations* 18, 6, 2164–73

Barnes, M, Newman, J, Sullivan, HC, 2007, *Power, participation and political renewal: Case studies in public participation*, Bristol: Policy Press

Beresford, P, 2002, User involvement in research and evaluation: Liberation or regulation? *Social Policy and Society* 1, 2, 95–105

Beresford, P, 2005, Developing the theoretical basis for service user/survivor-led research and equal involvement in research, *Epidemiologia e Psichiatrica Sociale* 14, 1, 4–8

Booker, S, Daykin, N, Powell, J, Taylor, P, Weil, S, 2008, *National evaluation of Patient Advice and Liaison Services (PALS): Final report*, Bristol: University of the West of England

Carel, H, Kidd, IJ, 2014, Epistemic injustice in healthcare: A philosophical analysis, *Medicine, Health Care and Philosophy* 17, 4, 529–40

Carter, P, Martin, G, 2015, Researching reforms of patient and public involvement in real time and at close range, Presentation at Health Services Management Centre seminar, *Evaluating Health Policy Reforms*, University of Birmingham, 24 April

Carter, P, Martin, G, 2016, Challenges facing Healthwatch: A new consumer champion in England, *International Journal of Health Policy Management* 5, 4, 259-263

Centre for Public Scrutiny, 2015, *Annual survey of overview and scrutiny in local government 2014–2015*, London: The Centre for Public Scrutiny

Clarke, J, 2005, New Labour's citizens: Activated, empowered, responsibilized, abandoned? *Critical Social Policy* 25, 4, 447–63

Coleman, A, Checkland, K, McDermott, I, Harrison, S, 2011, Patient and public involvement in the restructured NHS, *Journal of Integrated Care* 19, 4, 30–36.

Conklin, A, Morris, ZS, Nolte, E, 2010, *Involving the public in healthcare policy: An update of the research evidence and proposed evaluation framework*, Cambridge: Rand Europe

Council of Europe, 2000, Committee of Ministers: Recommendation No. R (2000) 5 of the Committee of Ministers to member states on the development of structures for citizen and patient participation in the decision-making process affecting health care, www.formazione.eu.com/_documents/governance/documenti/doc001.pdf

Department of Health, 2000, *The NHS Plan: A plan for investment, a plan for reform*, London: Department of Health (Cm 4818-I)

Department of Health, 2003, *Strengthening accountability: Involving patients and the public, Policy guidance, Section 11 of the Health and Social Care Act 2001*, London: Department of Health

Department of Health, 2009, Our health, our care, our say: A new direction for community services, London: Department of Health (Cm 6737)

Department of Health, 2009, *The NHS Constitution for England*, London: Department of Health

Department of Health, 2010, *Equity and excellence: Liberating the NHS*, Cm 7881), www.gov.uk/government/uploads/system/uploads/attachment_data/file/213823/dh_117794.pdf

Department of Health, 2012a, *NHS Constitution*, London: Department of Health

Department of Health, 2012b, *Healthwatch Transition Plan*, London: Department of Health

Elston, MA, 2009, Remaking a trustworthy medical profession in twenty-first century Britain, in J Gabe, M Calnan, M (eds), *The new sociology of the health service*, London: Routledge

Florin, D, Dixon, J, 2004, Public involvement in health care, *BMJ: British Medical Journal* 328, no. 7432, 2004, 159.

Foot, C, Gilburt, H, Dunn, P, Jabbal, J, Seale, B, Goodrich, J, Buck, D, Taylor, J, 2014, People in control of their own health and care: The state of involvement, *London: The Kings Fund.*

Francis, R, 2013, *Report of the Mid Staffordshire NHS foundation trust public inquiry*, London: The Stationery Office

Fraser, N, 1990, Rethinking the public sphere: A contribution to the critique of actually existing democracy, *Social Text* 25/26, 56–80

Fraser, N, Honneth, A, 2003, *Redistribution or recognition? A political–philosophical exchange*, New York: Verso

Gerrard, M, 2006, *A stifled voice: Community Health Councils in England, 1974–2003*, Brighton: Penn Press.

Gibson, A, Britten, N, Lynch, J, 2012, Theoretical directions for an emancipatory concept of patient and public involvement, *Health* 16, 5, 531–47

Gilburt, H, Dunn, P, Foot, C, 2015, *Local Health watch: Progress and promise*, www.gov.uk/government/uploads/system/uploads/attachment_data/file/417395/KF_Healthwatch_with_cover.pdf,

Gorsky, M, 2008, Community involvement in hospital governance in Britain: evidence from before the National Health Service, *International Journal of Health Services* 38, 4, 751–71

Health and Social Care (Community Health and Standards) Act 2003, c. 43, www.legislation.gov.uk/ukpga/2003/43/contents

Health and Social Care Act 2008, c. 14, www.legislation.gov.uk/ukpga/2008/14/contents

Health and Social Care Act, 2012, c. 7, www.legislation.gov.uk/ukpga/2012/7/contents/enacted

HWE (Healthwatch England), 2013, Understanding the legislation: The legal requirements for Healthwatch, www.healthwatch.co.uk/sites/healthwatch.co.uk/files/20130822_a_guide_to_the_legislation_affecting_local_healthwatch_final.pdf

HWE, 2015, 12 ways local Healthwatch have made a difference in 2015, http://www.healthwatch.co.uk/news/healthwatch-network-2015-year-review

HM Government, 2012a, *Caring for our future: Reforming care and support*, London: The Stationery Office

HM Government, 2012b, *The NHS Bodies and Local Authorities (Partnership Arrangements, Care Trusts, Public Health and Local Healthwatch) Regulations 2012: No. 2094*, London: The Stationery Office

Hogg, CN, 2007, Patient and public involvement: What next for the NHS? *Health Expectations*, 10(2), 129–138

Hogg, C, 2009, *Citizens, Consumers and the NHS: Capturing voices*, Basingstoke: Palgrave Macmillan

Local Government and Public Involvement in Health Act 2007, www.legislation.gov.uk/ukpga/2007/28/contents

Martin, GP, 2008, 'Ordinary people only': Knowledge, representativeness, and the publics of public participation in healthcare, *Sociology of health and illness* 30, 1, 35–54

Maybin, J, Addicott, R, Dixon, A, Storey, J, 2011, *Accountability in the NHS: Implications of the government's reform programme*, London: The King's Fund

Meads, GD, Griffiths, FE, Goode, SD, Iwami, M, 2007, Lessons from local engagement in Latin American health systems, *Health Expectations* 10, 4, 407–418

Mockford, C, Staniszewska, S, Griffiths, F, and Herron-Marx, S, 2012, The impact of patient and public involvement on UK NHS health care: A systematic review, *International Journal for Quality in Health Care* 24, 1, 28–38

Mold, A, 2010, Patient groups and the construction of the patient-consumer in Britain: An historical overview, *Journal of Social Policy* 39, 4, 505–21

National Health Service Reform and Health Care Professions Act 2002, www.legislation.gov.uk/ukpga/2002/17/section/25

NHS England, 2013, CCG Assurance Framework 2013/14, NHS England, www.england.nhs.uk/wp-content/uploads/2013/05/ccg-af.pdf

NHS England, 2014, *Five year forward view*, London: Department of Health

Office for National Statistics (2015). Life Expectancy at Birth and at Age 65 by Local Areas in England and Wales: 2012 to 2014, www.ons.gov.uk/peoplepopulationandcommunity/births deathsandmarriages/lifeexpectancies/bulletins/lifeexpectancy atbirthandatage65bylocalareasinenglandandwales/2015-11-04

O'Hara, G, 2013, The complexities of 'consumerism': Choice, collectivism and participation within Britain's National Health Service, c. 1961–c. 1979. *Social History of Medicine* 26, 2, 288–304

Parkinson, J, 2004, Hearing voices: Negotiating representation claims in public deliberation, *The British Journal of Politics and International Relations* 6, 3, 370–88

Parliament, House of Commons Health Select Committee, 2007, *Patient and public involvement in the NHS: Third Report of Session 2006–2007*, HC-278-1, www.publications.parliament.uk/pa/cm200607/cmselect/cmhealth/278/278i.pdf

Patients Association, 2011, Involving patients in commissioning: No decision about me, without me, www.patients-association.org.uk/wp-content/uploads/2014/07/Involving-Patients-in-Commissioning.pdf

Peckham, S, Exworthy, M, Greener, I, Powell, M, 2005, Decentralizing health services: More local accountability or just more central control? *Public Money and Management* 25, 4, 221–8

Peckham, S, Wilson, P, Williams, L, Smiddy, J, Kendall, S, Brooks, F, Reay, J, Smallwood, D, Bloomfield, L, 2014, *Commissioning for long-term conditions: Hearing the voice of and engaging users – a qualitative multiple case study,* Health Services and Delivery Research 2, 44, 1-195

Petsoulas, C, Peckham, S, Smiddy, J, Wilson, P, 2015, Primary care-led commissioning and public involvement in the English National Health Service: Lessons from the past, *Primary health care research and development* 16, 3, 289–303

Popay, J, 2006, Community Engagement, community development and health improvement, *A Background Paper prepared for the UK National Institute for Health and Clinical Excellence*, www.nice.org.uk/guidance/ph9/documents/community-engagement-final-scope2

South, J, 2007, Bridging the gap? A critical analysis of the development of the Patient Advice and Liaison Service (PALS), *Journal of health organization and management* 21, 2, 149–65

Stewart, E, 2013, What is the point of citizen participation in health care? *Journal of Health Services Research and Policy* 18, 2, 124–6

Tritter, JQ, McCallum, A, 2006, The snakes and ladders of user involvement: Moving beyond Arnstein, *Health Policy* 76, 2, 156–68

Tritter, JQ, 2009, Revolution or evolution: The challenges of conceptualizing patient and public involvement in a consumerist world, *Health Expectations* 12, 3, 275–87

Tritter, JQ, Koivusalo, M, 2013, Undermining patient and public engagement and limiting its impact: The consequences of the Health and Social Care Act 2012 on collective patient and public involvement, *Health Expectations* 16, 2, 115–18

Vincent-Jones, P, Hughes, D, Mullen, C, 2009, New Labour's PPI reforms: Patient and public involvement in healthcare governance? *The Modern Law Review* 72, 2, 247–71

Warsh, J, 2014, PPI: Understanding the difference between patient and public involvement, *The American Journal of Bioethics* 14, 6, 25–6

Watts, R, 2011, Guest editorial: A closer eye on HealthWatch, *Health Policy Insight*, 23 January

Williamson, L, 2014, Patient and citizen participation in health: The need for improved ethical support, *The American Journal of Bioethics* 14, 6, 4–16

World Health Organization, 1978, *Declaration of Alma-Ata*, Geneva: World Health Organization

SIXTEEN

'Groundhog Day': the Coalition government's quality and safety reforms

Martin Powell and Russell Mannion

Introduction

Quality and safety are defined and measured in different ways by academics, commentators and agencies, while the relationship between them are viewed in different ways (Leatherman and Sutherland, 2003; 2008; Raleigh and Foot, 2010; Vincent et al, 2013). The US Institute of Medicine (IoM, 2001) provides a 'long list' that healthcare is high quality if it is safe, effective, timely, person-centred, equitable and efficient (Raleigh and Foot, 2010; Gardner, 2015), but this has often been reduced to a 'short list' of three dimensions. Raleigh and Foot (2010) write that while the definitions of quality vary in different settings, some themes – safety, effectiveness and patient experience – are common to most quality frameworks (for example, IoM, 2001; DH, 2008; NQB, 2013), and are regarded as the three pillars of quality in healthcare (Doyle et al, 2013; NQB, 2013; Swinglehurst et al, 2015).

As Donaldson and Darzi (2012) put it, however, in the first 50 years of the NHS, quality was implied but not made explicit (but see Thorlby and Maybin, 2010), perhaps assumed not to be an issue due to the 'best in the world' mantra (see Chapters 3 and 17). Issues of quality and safety in healthcare became more central about the turn of the twenty-first century, with important reports in the UK and the USA (Kohn et al, 1999; IoM, 2001; DH, 2000b).

This chapter examines the three pillars of safety, effectiveness and patient experience (compare DH, 2008). After a brief review of earlier periods, it focuses on reforms in England under the Coalition government. It then explores the impact of reforms on quality and safety, providing a wider comparative perspective.

Historical background: quality in the NHS 1948–97

Although rarely explicitly addressed, there were occasional concerns over quality in the early NHS. Vincent et al(2013) provide a chronology of events related to patient safety in England in the twentieth century including the Confidential Enquiry into Maternal Deaths (1952), the Safety in Drugs Committee (1963), and inquiries into failures at Alder Hey Hospital; Ashworth Secure Hospital, and enquiries into doctors – Rodney Ledward and Harold Shipman (1990s). In 1969 Labour Secretary of State Richard Crossman seized the opportunity provided by a report revealing 'scandalous conditions' at Ely hospital to set up the Hospital Advisory Service, an inspectorate in all but name (Klein, 2013, 59), Over time, concerns of quality shifted to a new agenda: from the individual clinician to a collective clinical responsibility towards the consumer (Powell, 1997).

Reforms under the New Labour Government, 1997–2010

In this period, quality and safety issues were driven by a broad policy agenda together with a more specific safety agenda that was shaped more by 'events', which are described below (see Powell and Mannion, 2015). 'The New NHS' (DH, 1997) introduced clinical governance, new wider performance measurement systems, National Service Frameworks (NSFs); the National Institute of Clinical Excellence (NICE); and the Commission for Health Improvement (CHI) as a new regulator for quality. 'A First Class Service' (DH, 1998) placed quality at the centre of the NHS, introducing the National Clinical Assessment Authority, and the National Patient Safety Agency. A statutory 'duty of quality' shared by all providers of NHS services was established in the Health Acts of 1999 and 2003, with provider Chief Executive Officers accountable for quality as well as financial matters. The influential policy paper, *An organisation with a memory* (DH, 2000b), stated that the NHS needed to develop: unified mechanisms for reporting and analysis when things go wrong; a more open culture; a much wider appreciation of the value of the system approach in preventing, analysing and learning from errors; and mechanisms for ensuring that the necessary changes are put into practice. The NHS Plan (DH, 2000a) introduced a new performance measurement system that initially consisted of 'traffic lights' (red, amber, green) that were later replaced with star ratings for hospitals. The CHI changed its name to the Health Care Commission (HCC) in 2004, and reported new annual health checks. A Quality and Outcomes Framework (QOF) was introduced in 2003 as part of the general medical services contract between the NHS and general practitioners (GPs). The Darzi Report (DH, 2008) signalled 'a revivalist burst of enthusiasm for change in the name of quality' (Klein, 2013, 253). It stated that the NHS must have 'quality of care at its heart', and raised to importance three dimensions of quality: clinical effectiveness; safety; patient experience. It set out the 'National Quality Board', regional 'Quality Observatory' and local 'Quality Accounts' and Patient Reported Outcome Measures (PROMs), and outlined 'best practice tariffs' and 'Never Events'. In a 'Groundhog Day' re-run of the claim of DH (1997), quality was to be the 'organising principle' of the NHS.

Perhaps 'events' were more important, however. These included the Bristol Royal Infirmary, which involved the deaths of 15 children while, or after, undergoing cardiac surgery that, in effect, placed the medical profession on trial (Klein, 2013, 197); patient deaths from healthcare-acquired infections (HCAIs) at Stoke Mandeville Hospital in 2005 and at Maidstone and Tunbridge Wells in 2007, but the most important spur involved events at the Mid Staffordshire Foundation Trust (see below) (Vincent et al, 2013).

Reforms under the Coalition government, 2010–15

The terms 'quality' and 'safety' appear a great deal in the White Paper *Equity and excellence: Liberating the NHS* (DH, 2010). At one level, policy on these matters seems to be incremental such as 'building on Lord Darzi's work, in putting a stronger emphasis on quality' (NQB, 2013), and through a continuation of existing policies on regulation, choice and competition, and patient information. However, the document states that compared to other countries, the NHS has achieved relatively poor outcomes in some areas, claiming that rates of mortality amenable to healthcare, rates of mortality from some respiratory diseases and some cancers and some measures of stroke have been among the worst in the developed world (DH, 2010, 8). These claims have been criticised for being 'cherry picked' and ignoring that rates had fallen faster than in other countries (for example, Appleby, 2011; Davis et al, 2015, 39–40, but see below).

The White Paper introduced the NHS Outcomes Framework which was designed to be the primary assurance mechanism to assess the progress of NHS England at a national level, and aimed to improve quality throughout the NHS by encouraging a change in culture and behaviour focused on health outcomes not process (Nagendran et al, 2012). It has five domains (premature death, quality of life for chronic disease, recovery from illness or injury, patient experience of care, safety), derived from the Darzi (DH, 2008) definition of quality of effectiveness, patient experience and safety, which was enshrined into the Health and Social Care Act of 2012. It was claimed that 'patient safety is placed above all else at the heart of the NHS', and the (first) Francis Report (2010) on Mid Staffordshire (see below) was already being seen as a major spur to change.

The Mid Staffordshire hospital scandal and its aftermath

Stafford hospital was at the centre the most notorious hospital scandal in the history of the NHS. Although the scandal dates back to the previous Labour government, Stafford was to cast a long shadow over health policy under the Coalition government, and was the catalyst for several inquiries and reviews culminating in a raft of reforms and supporting policies designed to improve quality and safety across the NHS.

The Healthcare Commission (2009), the hospital inspectorate that preceded the Care Quality Commission (CQC), published a scathing report about the standards of care at Mid Staffordshire NHS Hospital Trust (Taylor, 2013) which largely corroborated the concerns of some local people that had been dismissed by the hospital, and local and national agencies (Bailey, 2012). It severely criticised the Trust's chaotic system of management and documented appalling conditions and manifest failings in professional practice at the hospital.

In July 2009, the Secretary State for Health, Andy Burnham, announced an independent inquiry into care provided by the Trust which was to be led by Robert Francis QC, a barrister with extensive experience of managing clinical negligence claims. It heard harrowing testimony from patients and their families about the appalling standards of care experienced at the hospital. These included examples of patients being left in excrement in soiled bed clothes for long periods, assistance not being provided with feeding for patients who could not eat without help, wards and toilet facilities left in a filthy condition, and staff treating patients and their families with indifference and a lack of basic kindness, respect and compassion.

The report (Francis, 2010) contained damning criticism of the standard of basic care in various departments at the Trust and painted a picture of an inward-looking organisation that suffered from a lack of new ideas and of nurturing a negative culture that became entrenched and had a deleterious impact on professional standards. The consultant body largely dissociated itself from management and there was low morale among staff. It pointed to an historic understaffing of nurses; a bullying culture at the trust; senior managers in denial about the extent of the problems. Staff and patient concerns were repeatedly ignored by senior management in favour of balancing the books, and managers were more focused on the organisation attaining foundation trust status than on quality of care. However, the report also flagged up failings that went beyond the trust, among the regulatory bodies, commissioners and wider management system.

The Trust Board and the Department of Health accepted the recommendations of the first Francis inquiry in full. In response, and to support the NHS to learn from and respond to the findings of the report, the Department of Health published three reports designed to help embed effective governance and prevent similar problems from happening again. *Review of Early Warning Systems in the NHS*, which detailed the key systems, values and behaviours related to detecting and preventing similar scandals. *Assuring the Quality of Senior NHS Managers* set out recommendations to further raise the standards of senior NHS managers as well as *The Healthy NHS Board*, which developed guidelines for improving NHS board effectiveness (NHS Leadership Academy, 2013; Mannion et al, 2015).

Members of the local patient pressure group – *Cure the NHS* – established by Julie Bailey, the daughter of one of the patients who had died at Mid Staffordshire, were, however, highly vocal in their criticisms of the first Francis inquiry. They complained that the inquiry was insufficient in scope and transparency and called for a full public inquiry. In June 2010, the incoming coalition government ordered a full public inquiry with a wider remit on the 'system', also chaired by Francis. As Taylor (2013, 205) put it, 'this is the NHS on trial'. It considered more than a million pages of evidence, and the 1,782 page report, with the 'executive summary' of 125 pages (Francis, 2013), provided 290 recommendations with major implications for all levels of the health service across England. It called for a 'fundamental culture change' across the health and social care system to put patients first at all times, with action across six core themes: culture, compassionate care, leadership, standards, information, and openness, transparency and candour.

The government's initial response, *Patients first and foremost* (DH, 2013a) was followed by a more detailed response, *Hard truths* (DH, 2013b). The first document reported a number of new initiatives and programmes. The CQC would appoint a Chief Inspector of Hospitals to identify problems and ensure that action was taken more effectively than before, and rate all hospitals. There would be a statutory 'duty of candour' making it a criminal offence for providers to supply false and misleading information about performance. It was proposed that every student who sought NHS funding for nursing degrees should first serve up to a year as a healthcare assistant (HCA), to promote frontline caring experience and values, as well as academic strength. HCAs would not face statutory regulation, as Francis had recommended, but they would be subject to national minimum training and a code of conduct.

The second document undertook to implement fully 204 of the 290 recommendations including, requiring trusts to publish ward staffing levels on a monthly basis and complaints data quarterly, a proposal to legislate to create a duty of candour for providers and the development of a criminal charge of wilful neglect. There should be transparent, monthly reporting of ward-by-ward staffing levels and other safety measures, a new national patient safety programme across England to spread best practice and build safety skills across the country, and 5,000 patient safety fellows will be trained and appointed in five years. In addition, there will be a new fit and proper person test, to act as a barring scheme for senior managers, and for every hospital patient to have the names of a responsible consultant and nurse above their bed.

The government commissioned six independent reviews to consider some of the key issues identified by the Inquiry: *Quality of care and treatment provided by 14 Hospital Trusts in England* (Keogh, 2013); *Healthcare assistants and support workers in the NHS and social care settings* (Cavendish, 2013); *Improving the safety of patients in England* (Berwick, 2013); *NHS hospitals complaints system* (Clwyd and Hart, 2013); *Challenging bureaucracy* (NHS Confederation, 2013); and *Children and young people's health outcomes forum* (Lewis and Lenehan, 2014). In addition, quality and safety issues have been explored by the House of Commons Health Committee (2013; 2015) and Public Administration Committee (2015).

All these reports produced recommendations, but we focus on arguably the most important areas. The 2013 Berwick report, *A promise to learn – a commitment to act*, set out a 'zero harm' target for the NHS and reignited the discussion about adequate or safe staffing levels. It made ten recommendations, including that all leaders concerned with NHS healthcare should place quality of care in general and patient safety in particular, at the top of their priorities and that that all non-personal data on quality and safety, whether assembled by government organisations, or professional societies, should be shared in a timely fashion with all parties who want it, including the public. However, the most important recommendations stated that it made no sense to punish someone who made an error, but that the NHS must be a learning organisation.

The 2013 Keogh review examined 14 NHS Trusts that displayed a pattern of poor performance, based on their mortality rates. Following its publication, 11 trusts were placed into 'special measures'. A 'special measures' regime was introduced to help improve their services. The measures for poorly performing trusts involved closer scrutiny from Monitor (for foundation trusts) or the NHS Trust Development Authority (for NHS trusts), the appointment of an improvement director, and linking with a partner (or buddy) trust that is performing well in areas where improvement was required.

The Cavendish Review was tasked with finding a solution to what could be done to ensure that unregistered staff treat all patients and clients with care and compassion. Key recommendations made in the report included that the CQC should require HCAs and health and support workers in social care to have completed the 'Certificate of Fundamental Care' before they can work unsupervised. Trusts should empower Directors of Nursing to take greater Board level responsibility for the recruitment, training and management of HCAs.

The government later asked the ubiquitous Sir Robert Francis to lead the *Freedom to Speak Up* Review which aimed to provide advice and recommendations to ensure that NHS staff feel safe to raise concerns, confident that they will be listened to and that the concerns raised will be acted on. This was in light of various national surveys indicating that NHS staff often felt reluctant to raise concerns for fear of reprisals. For example, the 2014 NHS National Staff Survey (Picker Institute, 2015) shows that the while 93 per cent of NHS staff would know how to report any concerns they have about unsafe clinical practice, 68 per cent would feel secure raising these concerns about unsafe clinical practice and just over half (57 per cent) would feel confident that their organisation would address their concern. Sir Robert spoke to hundreds of NHS whistleblowers and managers as part of his review and considered nearly 20,000 submissions. The report (Francis, 2015) set out 20 principles with specific actions, including:

- a common policy and procedure for raising concerns, including better investigations and promoting a model of good practice in the handling of concerns
- training for managers and all staff in the raising and handling of concerns
- cultural change towards open, transparent and learning cultures which value communication and engagement

- Freedom to Speak Up Guardians to be appointed to each NHS organisation, supported by an Independent National Officer (INO)
- legal change to anti-discrimination law to protect whistleblowers from discrimination in recruitment
- additions to the list of prescribed persons to whom protected disclosures can be made.

A year after the second Francis Report, Francis considered that 'all but a very few of the Public Inquiry's recommendations were accepted in full by the Department of Health, and all were in principle' (in Thorlby et al, 2014).

Yet another report, *Culture change in the NHS: Applying the lessons of the Francis Inquiries* (DH, 2015a) set out progress, which included a new, rigorous CQC inspection regime for hospitals, GPs and adult social care, extra clinical staff working in the NHS and the special measures regime for failing trusts.

Taylor (2013, vii) writes that the name of Mid Staffordshire has been 'hung around the neck of the NHS as a badge of shame'. However, around this time other areas within the NHS have experienced quality and safety issues. For example, there were other specific concerns about the abuse of vulnerable patients in hospitals and other care settings, raised for example by reports on the Winterbourne View case (DH, 2012). Following concerns over serious incidents in Furness General Hospital's maternity department covering January 2004 to June 2013, the report of the investigation into University Hospitals of Morecambe Bay NHS Foundation Trust (*The Report of the Morecambe Bay Investigation*, 2015) concluded that the maternity unit was dysfunctional and that serious failures of clinical care led to avoidable and tragic deaths of mothers and babies.

All this has led to a crowded quality and safety agenda (see NQB, 2013). There is no shortage of ambition. For example, in January 2014, NHS England (2014) launched 'the biggest patient safety initiative in the history of the NHS' creating a countrywide network of 'collaboratives' to improve patient safety across England. Gregory et al (2012) review policies under headings of patient safety, clinical effectiveness and patient experience. For patient safety, they note changes to national structures such as the abolition of the NPSA, with its functions transferred to the NHS Commissioning Board (now NHS England); the NHS Outcomes Framework; the development of an 'NHS Safety Thermometer' , which measures four 'high-volume' patient safety issues such as pressure ulcers, falls while in care, urinary infections in patients with a catheter, and treatment for venous thromboembolism; the continuation of the 'Commissioning for Quality and Innovation' (CQUIN) payment programme and of the 'Never Events Framework'; tackling healthcare associated infections; regulating providers; and creating a safety culture inside organisations. Under clinical effectiveness, they note the Outcomes Framework (particularly domains 1 and 3): incentivising clinical effectiveness through payment mechanisms; increased transparency and publication of information; the continuation of patient-reported outcome measures (PROMs); clinical networks and senates; and centralising specialist acute services. Policies under Patient Experience include measuring progress through domain 4 of the NHS Outcomes Framework ('ensuring that people have a positive experience of care'); other frameworks, standards and measures (for example, NICE and NQB); shared decision-making; patient choice; and patient involvement.

Conservative government (2015–)

In July 2015, the Secretary of State set out the direction of reform for the future NHS (Hunt, 2015). He discussed a number of measures such as an 'international buddying scheme', seven-day working, and from 2016 becoming the first country in the world to publish avoidable deaths by hospital trust. He stated that around 6,000 people lose their lives every year due to the lack of a proper seven-day service in hospitals, and that you are 15 per cent more likely to die if you are admitted on a Sunday compared to being admitted on a Wednesday. A new organisation with safety and quality at the heart of its remit, NHS Improvement, will replace Monitor and TDA. It will have two early safety priorities: working with the Chief Nursing Officer to complete the work started by NICE on safe staffing levels, and setting up a new Independent Patient Safety Investigation Service modelled on the Air Accident Investigation Branch used by the airline industry, where a 'no blame' learning culture has led to dramatic reductions in both fatalities and cost. He argued that the NHS needs a profound transformation in its culture, and – yet again – stressed the importance of a 'learning organisation': 'The world's fifth largest organisation needs to become the world's largest learning organisation' (Hunt, 2015).

The government's response to three reports (FSU, PASC, and Morecombe Bay) (DH, 2015c) stated that there were common themes across the reports: openness, honesty and candour; listening to patients, families and staff; finding and facing the truth; learning from errors and failures in care; people and professionalism; and the right culture from top to bottom. The government claims that it was continuing to build a culture that listens, learns and speaks the truth, arguing that since the Francis Report (2013) the landscape of policy and legislation to ensure safe, effective, respectful and compassionate care had been transformed.

The impact of reforms on quality and safety

A number of studies have charted changes in quality, and explored the relationship between reforms and quality. First, there are 'official' accounts. In NHS England Annual Report (2015), NHS Chief Executive Simon Stevens writes that 2014–15 was a year in which the Health Service responded – largely successfully – to wide-ranging operational pressures, with most goals of the 25 objectives of the government's Mandate for 2014–15 'met or were close to being met'. The CQC (CQC, 2015) reported the results of its 'new tougher approach' of inspection. Of the 38 acute trusts inspected, nine were rated good, improvement was required at 24, and five were inadequate. It stated that safety was the biggest concern: four out of every five safety ratings were inadequate or required improvement. However, it stressed that these figures were not representative as it focused on higher risk acute trusts first. It inspected GP practices for the first time in 2013/14, and found variations in the quality of care. The majority of the services were safe, effective, caring, responsive and well-led. The quality of dental care was generally good, and continued to be lower risk than most other sectors. It found wide variation in care between trusts, between hospital sites, between hospital services and within each service, from outstanding to inadequate. It stated that this variation in the quality and safety of care in England is too wide and unacceptable.

According to Monitor (2015), the number of FTs breaching at least one of the three standards increased when compared to the same period of the previous year from 24 to 53. The total number of reported Clostridium difficile (C difficile) cases saw an increase in 2014/15 compared to 2013/14 (806 compared to 676). By the end of March 2015, 29 FT (or 19 per cent of the total) were in breach of their licence and subject to regulatory action by Monitor. In the previous 12 months, ten more FTs were in breach of their licence, while eight FTs demonstrated sufficient improvements to be removed from formal action. Twelve FTs are in special measures or have been during last year, while three have exited.

The Department of Health (DH, 2015b) provided an annual assessment of NHS England's performance during 2014–15. It agrees with the assessment of NHS England's annual report for 2014–15 that, in a challenging year, with the majority of the 68 indicators of the NHS outcomes framework showing improvements in outcomes over the past year, more progress in some areas was still required. This does not appear to be a particularly focused or rigorous assessment, similar to a rather vague school report card. Moreover, it is not clear who assesses the assessors, or what actions result if progress is unsatisfactory.

Second, there are a number of independent commentaries on quality and safety. The King's Fund interim assessment (Gregory et al, 2012) drew on the criteria of Thorlby and Maybin (2010) for a high-performing health system, including safety; clinical effectiveness; and patient experience to conduct a mid-term assessment of the Coalition government. In terms of patient safety, they note reductions in the rates of MRSA and C difficile; a rise in the number of reported safety incidents; higher hospital death rates for weekend admission; rises in claims of clinical negligence; and that 14 per cent of NHS hospitals inspected between April 2010 and July 2011 did not meet CQC standards relating to safe management of medicine. Some clinical effectiveness measures predate the Coalition government, although broadly continuing falls in cancer mortality still compares poorly with the OECD average. Finally, patient experience of NHS inpatient and outpatient services showed little change; one-fifth of NHS acute hospitals inspected by the CQC in 2011 did not meet essential standards in nutrition and dignity for older people; a number of major reports have highlighted serious failures in the quality of care received by vulnerable patients in hospitals and in long-stay residential settings; and the number of written complaints to hospitals and community services rose. The King's Fund final assessment (Appleby et al, 2015) is structured as a conventional 'production path', which makes it difficult to focus on quality and safety issues. However, they report that one of the traditional indicators of safety in hospitals, HCAI, has continued to fall in recent years and has now broadly stabilised at an historically low rate, which is a significant achievement given the high rates reported a decade ago. Patient satisfaction with the care received has remained generally high on a number of measures, and public satisfaction with the NHS has increased, after a fall in 2011.

QualityWatch (2015) presents three main conclusions. First, many indicators of quality are improving. However, second, there are clear signals that performance in many areas is declining, with some continuing trends of deteriorating access to hospital, mental health and social care services. Third, there is a substantial risk that the current staffing situation in both health and social care may be reducing the quality of care received by patients and service users.

Gardner (2015) examines nearly 300 indicators which can be used to monitor changes over time in the quality of services provided. He points out that there is no single answer as to whether quality is better or worse across every patient, in every service and in every care setting across the NHS in England. He writes that 'there are two sides to every story' (both positive and negative changes). There are wide variations in safety both between and within NHS organisations. Progress continues to be made in tackling some key harms in hospitals, but we still know very little about safety in other settings such as general practice. He concludes that the NHS has done extraordinarily well to maintain and improve quality across a range of areas in the face of growing pressure from increased demand and financial constraints. However, it is not possible to say definitively whether overall quality of care in the NHS got better or worse between 2010 and 2015, or to attribute any changes to policy and legislation.

Finally, the NHS can be compared to other health systems. First, the English NHS can be compared with other systems within the UK (see Chapter 17). Bevan et al (2014) state that there is little sign that one country is consistently moving ahead of the others. Much of the data does not extend much beyond 2010, but it appears that England, compared to the other nations, has lowest rates of HCAI, and amenable mortality, medium quality of stroke care and good (that is, lowest) waiting times for hospital admission and ambulance response.

Second, the English NHS can be compared to health systems outside the UK. There are many different studies (Kossarova et al, 2015), but international comparisons are problematic, as different studies at different times stress different measures and produce rather different results. The NHS does not appear to do particularly well in terms of outcomes. For example, it came twenty-third out of 166 countries in terms of population outcomes (EIU, 2014). In a later study of 30 countries with a wider range of measures based on data from around 2012, the UK was ranked third on equity and access; fourteenth on disease outcomes, sixteenth on expenditure; seventeenth on healthcare costs; nineteenth on population health outcomes; and twenty-eighth on healthcare resources (EIU, 2015). Kossarova et al (2015) use Organisation for Economic Co-operation and Development (OECD) data to explore care in four sectors (primary care, hospital care, cancer care and mental health) across 15 countries over the period 2000–13. The UK does not consistently over-perform or under-perform when compared with the pool of the other 14 countries. Absolute and relative trends (that is, whether the UK is improving or deteriorating and how it is performing in relation to other countries) are also mixed. The UK is stable or improving on 25 out of 27 indicators, but performs worse than most countries on 14 out of 27 indicators, and performance is deteriorating on two indicators.

Niemietz (2014) states that, since the early 2000s, the NHS has improved according to most measures of quality and performance. Survival rates for major diseases have increased, waiting lists have been shortened, and the prevalence of hospital infections has been reduced, but this improvement has come from a very low base so that the performance of the NHS is still poor in international terms. For example, the UK ranks twentieth out of 24 developed countries for cancer survival and nineteenth out of 23 for mortality amenable to healthcare.

The Commonwealth Fund study (Davis et al, 2014) ranks health systems according to five categories (quality, access, efficiency, equity, outcomes). It ranked the NHS best of 11 countries on overall rank and for 9 of 11 criteria as structurally designed to favour an NHS-style model of healthcare. However Niemietz (2014) claims that this study is different from most others in two respects. It is mostly based on inputs and procedures as opposed to outcomes, and it is mostly based on doctors' and patients' survey responses as opposed to clinical data. Only one category is concerned with outcomes, and in that category, the UK comes out second to last. He cites the Guardian's (presumably non-ironic) verdict that 'the only serious black mark against the NHS was its poor record on keeping people alive'.

According to the OECD (2015), indicators on the quality of care show that the UK has low levels of expenditure and staffing, and lags behind in key areas, including coming twenty-first out of 23 countries on cervical cancer survival, twentieth out of 23 countries on breast and bowel cancer survival, nineteenth out of 31 countries on stroke survival, and twentieth out of 32 countries on heart attack deaths. It is also a 'middling to low performer' on three out of four key health areas, including quality of care and life expectancy.

Conclusion

The quality and safety agenda has been shaped by many reports and recommendations, and has been largely reactive. It can be argued that quality is in the eye of many conflicting beholders. This results in conflicting divisions of responsibility and courses of action. Gregory et al (2012) write that there is much to be clarified under the new NHS structures with regard to patient safety. It could be argued that quality and safety is everybody's business but nobody's responsibility.

It is unclear if different emphasis is being placed on the three pillars of quality of safety, effectiveness and patient experience, although the stress on patient experience may be increasing (Donaldson and Darzi, 2012; Doyle et al, 2013). Similarly, it is unclear if there are virtues in simplicity such as the simple, single question about experience borrowed from a consumer notion of customer service of the 'Friends and Family Test' ('Would you recommend to family and friends the service you have received?') or the multidimensional (for example, the 300 measures of Gardner (2015)). Donaldson and Darzi (2012) warn that it is clear that the much more easily quantifiable measures – money and activity – were the true priority for managers of the system: 'No matter how often the language of quality and safety is spoken by those assessing performance, the true lingua franca of healthcare is financial.' They argue that metrics must be acceptable to clinicians, collectable from management systems and understandable by the public, but this simple triad is hard to reconcile.

While most commentators conclude that quality and safety has improved over time, it is probably too early to causally link specific Coalition reforms with any changes (Powell and Mannion, 2015). Gardner (2015) writes that it is not possible to say definitively whether overall quality of care in the NHS got better or worse between 2010 and 2015, or to attribute any changes to policy and legislation. Moreover, while it is not fully clear if particular mechanisms work to improve quality, it is even less clear *how* they improve quality (for example, 'selection', 'change' and 'reputation' pathways (Raleigh and Foot, 2010)).

The current situation reflects a possible paradox of largely positive studies pointing to improvements in quality with reports highlighting widespread problems. Given the 'seminal document' of An Organisation with a Memory (OWAM) (DH, 2000b), the 'Ten-year Quality Agenda' of 1997–98 (Leatherman and Sutherland, 2003), and that the NHS seems to be the only healthcare system in the world with a definition of quality enshrined in legislation (Keogh, 2013), scandals such as Mid Staffordshire are difficult to explain. It is possible that this is due to greater transparency and scrutiny. QualityWatch (2013) states that the quality of NHS care in England has been scrutinised more in the past year than in any other since 1948.

According to the Health Select Committee (2013), the failings at Stafford General Hospital have cast a shadow over the reputation of the NHS for safe, high-quality patient care. If Bristol put the medical profession on trial (Klein, 2013), then Mid Staffs put the NHS on trial (Taylor, 2013, 205). It may be unfair to judge the NHS on what it gets wrong rather than what it does right, as a series of scandals such as Ely, Bristol, Shipman, Alder Hey, Winterbourne View and so on show that every period of the NHS has experienced some serious deficiencies. However, there is an element of 'Groundhog Day' as 'quality' is periodically rediscovered as a major theme in the NHS and recommendations of previous inquiries being recycled, with resonances of 'deja vu all over again' as history repeats itself as tragedy rather than farce. Quality is periodically rediscovered such as by Darzi, and after Mid Staffordshire (see for example Klein, 2013, 259, 296), and solutions sometimes reinvent the wheel. For example, organisational learning has been advanced many times (for example, DH, 2000b; 2015a; 2015c; Kennedy, 2001; NAO, 2005; Berwick, 2013; Hunt, 2015).

Newdick and Danbury (2013) cite the *British Medical Journal* editorial response to Bristol that the NHS would be 'all changed, changed utterly', but the Francis Inquiries (2010; 2013) suggest nothing changed at all. As Professor Sir Ian Kennedy (2001, 159) warned: 'the history of the NHS is littered with the reports of Inquiries and Commissions: most have soon been consigned to gather dust on shelves…It will only be a matter of time therefore, before the same, or a similar set of problems arises again.' Similarly, Francis (2013, para 2.164) writes that for all the 'fine words' about candour, and willingness to remedy wrongs, 'there lurks within the system an institutional instinct which, under pressure, will prefer concealment, formulaic responses and avoidance of public criticism'.

Sir Brian Jarman notes that the word 'hindsight' was used 456 times in the testimony to the Francis public inquiry (Taylor, 2013, 184). However, some degree of foresight may be possible. For example, Spiegelhalter et al (2003) demonstrated that risk-adjusted monitoring of outcomes could have led to earlier detection of two notable failures of care in the NHS: paediatric cardiac surgery deaths at Bristol Royal Infirmary and the murders of elderly patients by GP Harold Shipman. It seems that the NHS has much to learn in becoming a learning organisation. At times the NHS appears to be an organisation *without* a memory. 'Sorry' may be the hardest word, but learning and implementation appear to be the hardest activities.

References

Appleby, J, 2011, Does poor health justify NHS reform?, *British Medical Journal*, 342:d566

Appleby, J, Baird, B, Thompson, J, Jabbal, J, 2015, *The NHS under the coalition government. Part two: NHS performance*, London: King's Fund

Bailey, J, 2012, *From ward to Whitehall: The disaster at Mid-Staffs*, Stafford: Cure the NHS

Berwick, D, 2013, *The National Advisory Group on the Safety of Patients in England. A promise to learn – a commitment to act: Improving the safety of patients in England*, London: Department of Health

Bevan, G, Karanikolos, M, Exley, J, Nolte, E, Connolly, S, Mays, N, 2014, *The four health systems of the United Kingdom: How do they compare?*, London: Health Foundation/Nuffield Trust

Cavendish, C, 2013, *The Cavendish review: An independent review into healthcare assistants and support workers in the NHS and social care settings*, London: Department of Health

Clwyd, A, Hart, T, 2013, *A review of the NHS hospitals complaints system: Putting patients back in the picture*, London: Department of Health

CQC (Care Quality Commission), 2015, *The state of health care and adult social care in England 2013/14*, London and Newcastle upon Tyne: CQC

Davies, HTO, Mannion, R, 2013, Will prescriptions for cultural change improve the NHS?, *British Medical Journal* 346:f1305

Davis, J, Lister, J, Wrigley, D (eds), 2015, *NHS for sale: Myths, lies and deception*, London: Merlin Press

Davis, K, Stremikis, K, Squires, D, Schoen, C, 2014, *Mirror, mirror on the wall: How the performance of the US health care system compares internationally*, New York: Commonwealth Fund, www.commonwealthfund.org/ publications/fund-reports/2014/jun/mirror-mirror

DH (Department of Health), 1997, *The new NHS – modern, dependable*, London: The Stationery Office

DH (Department of Health), 1998, *A first class service – quality in the new NHS*, London: The Stationery Office

DH (Department of Health), 2000a, *The NHS plan – a plan for investment, a plan for reform*, London: The Stationery Office

DH (Department of Health), 2000b, *An organisation with a memory*, London: The Stationery Office

DH (Department of Health), 2001, *Building a safer NHS for patients: Implementing an organisation with a memory*, London: The Stationery Office

DH (Department of Health), 2008, *High quality care for all* (Final Darzi Report), London: The Stationery Office

DH (Department of Health), 2010, *Equity and excellence: Liberating the NHS*, London: The Stationery Office

DH (Department of Health), 2012, *Transforming care: A national response to Winterbourne View hospital – Final report*, London: Department of Health

DH (Department of Health), 2013a, *Patients first and foremost: The initial government response to the report of the Mid Staffordshire NHS Foundation Trust public inquiry*, London: The Stationery Office

DH (Department of Health), 2013b, *Hard truths: The journey to putting patients first*, London: The Stationery Office

DH (Department of Health), 2015a, *Culture change in the NHS: Applying the lessons of the Francis Inquiries*, Cm 9009, London: Department of Health

DH (Department of Health), 2015b, *Annual assessment of the NHS Commissioning Board (known as NHS England, 2014–15)*, London: Department of Health

DH (Department of Health), 2015c, *Learning not blaming: The government response to the Freedom to Speak Up consultation, the Public Administration Select Committee report 'Investigating Clinical Incidents in the NHS', and the Morecambe Bay investigation*, Cm 9113, London: Department of Health

Donaldson, L, Darzi, A, 2012, Quality measures: Bridging the cultural divide, *British Medical Journal Quality Safety*, 1–4, doi:10.1136/bmjqs-2012-001477

Doyle, C, Lennox, L, Bell, D, 2013, A systematic review of evidence on the links between patient experience and clinical safety and effectiveness, *British Medical Journal Open* 3:e001570

EIU (Economist Intelligence Unit), 2014, *Health outcomes and cost: A 166-country comparison*, London: EIU, www.eiu.com/healthcare

EIU (Economist Intelligence Unit), 2015, *The NHS: How does it compare?*, London: EIU, www.eiu.com/healthcare

Francis, R, 2010, *Independent Inquiry into care provided by Mid Staffordshire NHS Foundation Trust January 2005–March 2009, Volume I*, HC 375-I, London: The Stationery Office

Francis, R, 2013, *Report of the Mid Staffordshire NHS Foundation Trust Public Inquiry*, London: The Stationery Office

Francis, R, 2015, *Freedom to speak up review*, London: The Stationery Office

Gardner, T, 2015, *Swimming against the tide? The quality of NHS services during the current parliament*, London: The Health Foundation

Gregory, S, Dixon, A, Ham, C (eds), 2012, *Health policy under the coalition government: A mid-term assessment*, London: King's Fund

Ham, C, Baird, B, Gregory, S, Jabbal, J, Alderwick, H, 2015, *The NHS under the coalition government Part one: NHS reform*, London: King's Fund

House of Commons Health Committee, 2013, *After Francis: Making a difference*, Third Report of Session 2013–14, HC 657, London: The Stationery Office

House of Commons Health Committee, 2015, *Complaints and raising concerns*, Fourth Report of Session 2014–15, HC 350, London: The Stationery Office

House of Commons Public Administration Select Committee, 2015, *Investigating clinical incidents in the NHS*, Sixth Report of Session 2014–15, HC 886 London: The Stationery Office

Hunt, J, 2015, Speech, 16 July, *Making healthcare more human-centred and not system-centred*, London: Department of Health, www.gov.uk/government/speeches/making-healthcare-more-human-centred-and-not-system-centred

IoM (Institute of Medicine), 2001, *Crossing the quality chasm: A new health system for the 21st century*, Washington, DC: National Academy Press

Kennedy, Sir I, 2001, *Learning from Bristol*, Cm 5207, London: The Stationery Office

Keogh, Sir B, 2013, *Review into the quality of care and treatment provided by 14 Hospital Trusts in England: Overview report*, London: NHS

Klein, R, 2013, *The new politics of the NHS*, 7th edn, London: Radcliffe Publishing

Kohn, L, Corrigan, J, Donaldson, M (eds), 1999, *To err is human: Building a safer health systems for better care*, Washington, DC: National Academy Press

Kossarova, L, Blunt, I, Bardsley, M, 2015, *Focus on: International comparisons of healthcare quality. What can the UK learn?*, London: Health Foundation/Nuffield Trust

Leatherman, S, Sutherland, K, 2003, *The quest for quality in the NHS: A mid-term evaluation of the ten-year quality agenda*, London: Nuffield Trust

Leatherman, S, Sutherland, K, 2008, *The quest for quality: Refining the NHS reforms*, London: Nuffield Trust

Lewis, I, Lenehan, C, 2014, Report of the children and young people's health outcomes forum 2013/14, https://www.gov.uk/government/uploads/system/uploads/attachment_data/file/307011/CYPHOF_Annual_Report_201314_FORMAT_V1.5.pdf

Mannion, R, Davies, H, Millar, R, Freeman, T, Jacobs, R, Kasteridis, P, 2015, Overseeing oversight: Governance of quality and safety by hospital boards in the English NHS, Journal of Health Services Research and Policy 20, 15, 9–16

Monitor, 2015, *Annual report and accounts 1 April 2014 to 31 March 2015*, HC 237, London: The Stationery Office

The Report of the Morecambe Bay Investigation (the Kirkup Report), 2015, London: The Stationery Office

Nagendran, M, Maruthappu, M, Raleigh, V, 2012, Is the new NHS outcomes framework fit for purpose?, *British Medical Journal Quality Safety*, 21:524e527

NAO (National Audit Office), 2005, *A safer place for patients: Learning to improve patient safety*, London: The Stationery Office

Newdick, C, Danbury, C, 2013, Culture, compassion and clinical neglect: Probity in the NHS after Mid Staffordshire, *Journal of Medical Ethics* 1–7

NHS (National Health Service) Confederation, 2013, *Challenging bureaucracy*, London: NHS Confederation, http://www.nhsconfed. org/~/media/Confederation/Files/Publications/Documents/ challenging-bureaucracy.pdf

NHS (National Health Service) England, 2014, The biggest patient safety initiative in the history of the NHS – Mike Durkin, www. england.nhs.uk/2014/01/21/mike-durkin-3/

NHS (National Health Service) England, 2015, *Annual Report and Accounts 2014–15*, HC 109, London: NHS England

NHS (National Health Service) Leadership Academy, 2013, *The healthy NHS board 2013: Principles for good governance*, Leeds: NHS Leadership Academy

Niemietz, K, 2014, Health check, *Institute of Economic Affairs (IEA) Discussion Paper* 54, London: IEA

NQB (National Quality Board), 2013, *Quality in the new health system*, London: Department of Health

OECD (Organisation for Economic Co-operation and Development), 2015, *Health at a glance 2015: OECD indicators*, Paris: OECD Publishing, doi: http://dx.doi.org/10.1787/health_glance-2015-en

Picker Institute, 2015, Briefing Note: Issues highlighted by the 2014 NHS Staff Survey in England, ST14 NHS staff survey_ nationalbriefing_2014 Final MW/CK 24/02/2015 Unclassified

Powell, M, 1997, *Evaluating the National Health Service*, Buckingham: Open University Press

Powell, M, Mannion, R, 2015, England in J Braithwaite, Y Matsuyama, R Mannion, J Johnson (eds) *Healthcare reform, quality and safety*, pp 227–36, Farnham: Ashgate

QualityWatch, 2013, *Is the quality of care in England getting better?*, QualityWatch Annual Statement 2013, London: Health Foundation/ Nuffield Trust

QualityWatch, 2015, *Closer to critical?*, London: Health Foundation/ Nuffield Trust

Raleigh, V, Foot, C, 2010, *Getting the measure of quality*, London: King's Fund

Spiegelhalter, D, Grigg, O, Kinsman, R, et al, 2003, Risk-adjusted sequential probability ratio tests: Applications to Bristol, Shipman and adult cardiac surgery, *International Journal Quality in Health Care* 5:7e13

Swinglehurst, D, Emmerich, N, Maybin, J, Park, S, Qulligan, S, 2015, Confronting the quality paradox, *BMC Health Services Research* 15, 240

Taylor, R, 2013, *God bless the NHS*, London: Faber and Faber

Thorlby, R, Maybin, J (eds), 2010, *A high-performing NHS? A review of progress 1997–2010*, London: King's Fund

Thorlby, R, Smith, J, Williams, S, Dayan, M, 2014, *The Francis Report: One year on*, London: Nuffield Trust

Vincent, C, Burnett, S, Carthey J, 2013, *The measurement and monitoring of safety*, London: Health Foundation

SEVENTEEN

A view from abroad: a New Zealand perspective on the English NHS health reforms

Robin Gauld

Introduction

The English NHS is of significance among health policy observers around the globe for various reasons. The NHS is particularly noteworthy for the fact that, for many, it represents the high-income world's best attempt to have built and maintained a 'national' health system with a focus on universal access to care that is free at point of service. Compared with, say, the United States, with its multiple competing health insurers and funding mechanisms paying multiple competing providers, the NHS is a very straightforward system: national government funds, generated through taxes, are paid over to a predominantly public system of providers (albeit with various caveats such as GPs who are mostly private business owners, but funded largely by the NHS) (Wendt et al, 2009). Despite the 'Obamacare' reforms in the US, implementation of which commenced around the turn of the decade, thousands of North Americans continue to die every year through inability to pay for the costs of required healthcare. Many thousands more go bankrupt. Indeed, studies have shown that inability to pay healthcare costs as the number one reason for bankruptcy in the US (Himmelstein et al, 2005; 2009). By comparison, the NHS has historically represented values of civility and compassion for the fact that it is designed on, and underpinned by, principles that no-one should miss out from needed care simply because they do not have the personal funds or insurance required to pay a provider's invoice. This said, these values have come into question in recent times, notably via the Frances inquiry into lapses in patient care at the Mid-Staffordshire NHS trust (Francis, 2013; Spence, 2013) (Chapter 16).

The NHS and US health systems are, in many ways, polar opposites. The NHS is often categorised as a 'national' health system (Blank and

Burau, 2010) in which healthcare is viewed as a state responsibility. The NHS is effectively a large government department which traditionally has delivered services in a one-size-fits-all model in that government has provided the directions for everything from policy around structure and goals of hospitals through to pay scales and payroll services for its very large workforce. There has also, historically, been a focus on delivering the same standard services in the same way across the entire country. For its part, the US is the most prominent example in the high-income world of a 'market' system with few rules or certainties (Blank and Burau, 2010). US healthcare providers mostly work on a fee for service basis with inbuilt incentives to raise fees, see more patients and overprovide services. Its administrative costs are high (Exworthy and Freeman, 2009; Morra et al, 2011).

The NHS has been in transition for several years. Many commentators have highlighted the role and influence of US market ideals in this transition, with various UK governments clearly pushing this agenda. But the agenda has also been laced with other ideas, such as the need to improve quality and patient safety, to better coordinate and integrate care, to move services closer to patients in the community, and to involve patients and the public in planning and decision making (Chapters 9, 15, 16). Some of these ideas sit behind policy shifts in parts of the US. In other countries more closely comparable to England, such as New Zealand (NZ), they are at the core of present policy directions. While some observers look at how ideas from the market can help improve the NHS, it is often useful to look to countries with similar health systems and policies for comparison with a view to improvement. This chapter takes such an approach in looking at the NHS from abroad. It draws upon the case of NZ which, in many ways, is very similar to England when it comes to health policy and the healthcare system. In doing so, it aims to provide a critique of the NHS reforms and demonstrate that there are alternatives to the policies and structures being pursued for the English NHS by the coalition government (2010–15).

First, the chapter discusses why we might look to NZ rather than, say, the US to bring a view from abroad on the NHS reforms. Second, it describes how, despite a historical bond and similarities, the two countries are diverging in present health policy directions. Third, it draws on research into the large number of NHS trained doctors resident in NZ to provide a window into how the NHS reforms are affecting front line services. Finally, the chapter looks at the trajectories of the health policies and systems of the two countries into the future and asks what one might learn from the other.

Why compare the NHS and New Zealand?

There has been rapid growth in the field of comparative health policy and system studies in the past generation (Aspalter et al, 2012; Gauld, 2005; Marmor et al, 2009; Marmor and Wendt, 2012). A question often asked of such studies is why the comparator countries or systems were selected. Sometimes it is due to convenience; sometimes as comparable data are available; sometimes because there is something, such as a specific policy initiative, of interest which is present in each; and sometimes in the search for lessons from abroad that may inform domestic policy. The NHS is routinely the subject of comparative studies. Mostly, the comparators are EU, North American, or a range of OECD countries. Despite stark differences between the two countries, the US has been particularly prominent in many recent comparative studies (Exworthy and Freeman, 2009). Studies have also looked to compare the four separate NHS systems of Ireland, Scotland, Wales and England, highlighting considerable differences across various dimensions (Bevan et al, 2014) (Chapter 7).

Other than as part of a larger group of comparison countries, rarely are the NHS and NZ compared despite a long history of close relationships between the two and a number of similarities (see Table 17.1) (Mein Smith et al, 2009). NZ remains an active Commonwealth

Table 17.1: England and NZ background data

	England	NZ
Land area	130,395 km²	268,021 km²
Population	63.489 million (July 2014)	4.617 million (September 2015)
Capital city	London*	Wellington
Government	Westminster (bi-cameral)	Westminster (uni-cameral)
Infant mortality rate per 1,000 live births	3.8*	5.2
Life expectancy at birth (male/female)	79.2/82.9*	79.5/83.2
Total health expenditure as % of GDP	8.5*	9.5
Government expenditure as % of total health expenditure	86.6*	79.8
Total health expenditure per capita (US$ PPP)	3,235*	3,328
Practising physicians per 1000 population	2.8*	2.8

Notes: * United Kingdom; GDP: gross domestic product; PPP: purchasing power parity

Sources: latest available data (Government statistics in both countries; OECD Health Data, 2015)

member and its system of government is derived from the Westminster parliamentary model. Despite its distance, NZ's primary source of inward migration remains the UK, especially England, and a vast majority of NZers have at least some UK ancestry. This means that the societal values and many traditions in England and NZ are very similar.

When it comes to healthcare, the NHS and NZ have more in common than most countries. Both are considered to have 'national' health systems but the extent of this varies between the two. In 1938, some ten years ahead of the UK, NZ made the world's first attempt to create a 'national' health service. The government wished to remove barriers to care, especially financial, and create universal access. Other goals included creating integrated services, with no discernable gaps between primary and hospital care, and focusing on preventive rather than curative services. These goals were, in many ways, visionary and continue to be health policy aims today in many countries. For NZ, they were derailed owing to medical resistance. Doctors, largely in private practice at the time, were opposed to state control. NZ's current health system has roots in a historic compromise made shortly after 1938 between the government and the NZ branch of the British Medical Association. This was that hospital doctors would be employed on salary but also be allowed to maintain a private practice. General practitioners (GPs) would retain their private status and businesses and right to charge patients at the point of service, but receive a government subsidy to reduce direct patient fees. The resulting institutional arrangements remain to this day. GPs (and associated primary care) and hospitals remain siloed with a lack of system integration, and many hospital specialists are in dual practice, while the national health service vision was never achieved (Gauld, 2013). NZ diverges from the NHS in that there is no 'system', conceptually, for the public to grasp hold of, as there is in England: debates around 'our NHS' are not tenable in NZ as the health services have never been promoted by policy makers or enshrined in legislation in this way.

NZ and the NHS have much in common, however. First, there is a strong focus on primary care and GP services as first point of patient contact. GPs are the gatekeepers of the system and coordinate referrals and other aspects of patient care. Like the NHS, GPs are in private practice and have a formal list of patients on their books. GPs tend to refer most patients to public hospitals for specialist treatments although waiting lists for non-urgent services along with government funding shortfalls mean many patients may not be seen. This means GPs will often refer patients to private hospitals, where waiting times are minimal, so long as they are able to pay the full costs of service.

Public hospitals dominate the health system as private hospitals provide only non-urgent services. Second, healthcare in NZ is tax-funded with a strong tradition of public services provision. In 2015, almost 80 per cent of total health expenditure was public, not quite as much as in the UK. Like the NHS, the NZ government uses a population based formula to allocate funding to 20 districts (Penno et al, 2013). These districts plan and fund services for their respective populations. The emphasis is on prevention, as a district's only source of income is via the government. Third, health professional training programmes and regulation of professionals are similar in both countries. Doctors trained in the UK have a very straightforward path to registration in NZ, owing to reciprocal recognition of qualifications and training standards and very close historical relationships between medical schools and registration authorities. NZ has always relied on the UK for doctor supply, and this reliance has increased in recent years. Presently, around a quarter of NZ's doctors are UK born or trained in a medical workforce that, at 44 per cent, has the highest proportion of international medical graduates among OECD countries (Gauld and Horsburgh, 2015; Health Workforce New Zealand, 2014). Fourth, central government is heavily involved in driving health policy and its implementation. As in the UK, NZ governments from both sides of the political spectrum have presided over successive large-scale reforms since the 1980s. Such reforms have often been ideologically driven, with limited evidence suggesting that reform was needed or that proposed changes would deliver on proposed goals (Gauld, 2009b). These reforms have come at a huge cost, leaving the health workforce doubtful about the motivations and knowledge of politicians and their advisers (Gauld, 2003; Gower et al, 2003).

NZ experienced four rounds of major reforms through the 1990s (Gauld, 2009b). These included a move to devolve planning and decision making to local areas (late-1980s); an endeavour to create an internal market of government funded purchasers and competition between public hospitals and other providers for service contracts (1991–96); a national purchasing model focused on national planning, goals and consistency across local services (1996–99); and a move back to devolution of planning and funding to the local district level (the present system in place since 2000). While some benefits of the various reforms emerged, many unforeseen, these have been outweighed by negatives. An important lesson for NZ has been that health reforms imposed from the top-down need to be approached with extreme caution due to the costs involved, particularly on health professionals who have become disengaged over the years.

Various changes have taken place in NZ driven by health professionals themselves, especially GPs. Most important has been the creation of Independent Practitioner Associations (IPAs) which are networks of GPs across a region (Malcolm and Mays, 1999; Malcolm and Powell, 1996). These formed to facilitate contracting with government purchasers in the 1990s and quickly became a vehicle for clinical governance and leadership. GPs showed that, with organisation, they could improve patient services across networked practices and focus more closely on preventive care. While some IPA advances were sidelined as a result, in the early 2000s, the government sought to further such organisation by funding Primary Health Organisations (PHOs). These feature a range of primary care professionals, with a focus on an enrolled population via GPs (Gauld and Mays, 2006). Like the NHS, NZ has emphasised clinical governance and leadership for several years now. However, the IPA movement has provided particular reason for policy makers in NZ to fertilise the ground for bottom–up policy. This is a current focus of NZ health policy.

The NZ current system of 20 District Health Boards, as noted, has been in place since 2000. These are not dissimilar to the recently-abandoned English Primary Care Trusts, with some subtle differences. Perhaps most important is that DHBs are predominantly elected bodies which plan and fund services for their populations. Thus, they must undertake needs assessments for their populations and then fund and coordinate a full spectrum of services. DHBs own the public hospitals in their region and favour these in funding decisions. DHBs also fund the Primary Health Organisations and GPs in their catchment area. Despite the planning and coordination role, and ongoing efforts, DHBs have mostly failed to traverse the historic divide between primary and hospital services meaning integration remains largely aspirational (Cumming, 2011; Ministerial Review Group, 2009). This is, arguably, due to firmly embedded institutional arrangements founded in the post-1938 compromise

Beyond structural similarities, NZ has long borrowed policy ideas from the NHS. Prime examples include the competitive internal market policy of the 1990s. NZ was, of course, at that time heavily influenced by neoliberal economic ideas and new public management of the type espoused under Margaret Thatcher and her successors (Boston et al, 1999; 1996). Other policies include quality and patient safety policies, with NZ now having an independent Health Quality and Safety Commission (similar to the CQC), and clinical governance and leadership with key policy advice coming almost straight from the NHS (Scally and Donaldson, 1998). NZ's medical council has always looked closely at its UK counterpart, the GMC, for new methods of regulating and upholding professional standards. Finally, a significant number of senior government officials and DHB managers are 'NHS refugees'. While the exact number has never been tallied up, it is very unusual for there not to be at least one UK (especially English) accent in a policy meeting at the national or local level. This means there is a natural flow of ideas into the NZ health system at various levels.

How the English NHS and NZ are diverging and why

Of interest to this chapter is the question of how the NHS and NZ health systems and policies have developed over time. This section describes developments since the Conservative-led coalition government came to power in the UK in 2010 and, in New Zealand, from the election of the present National Party-led coalition government (politically, broadly similar to the Conservatives) in 2008. As the NHS is covered extensively elsewhere in this book, NZ receives more emphasis.

The NHS

The watershed development in the NHS was the 2012 Health and Social Care Act. Viewed from abroad, this act (and the incentives it represents) seemed to counter the capacity to deliver on the goals for a national health system, and smacked of policy amnesia. Widely debated both before and since its highly controversial passage (Chapters 6 and 18), the 2012 act spelled radical changes for the NHS. Written into the act are ideals of competition and the increasing involvement of private providers in the delivery of NHS services (Paton, 2014). Such ideas have been shown to fail. NZ tried this in the 1990s, with poor results, as had the UK government previously. In NZ's case, politicians drew advice primarily from prominent business people and consultancies (Gauld, 2009b; Goldfinch, 1998). They, in turn, derived their thinking from early experience with restructuring of public utilities such as postal services and electricity supply (corporatisation produced some gains initially; over the longer-term performances were at best mediocre). There are many other examples from around the world which demonstrate the limits of competition (Devereaux et al, 2004; Tuohy et al, 2004).

The nub of the 2012 act was that the NHS would remain an 'insurer' of public access to healthcare, but that providers would be subject to increasing competitive pressure. This would come in the bid for patients, following the policy that they be given a 'choice' of hospital and health service providers, and for service delivery contracts in much the same way as in the US. In England, a commissioning role was created with establishment of a new body, NHS England (Chapter 5). In theory, this meant key allocation decisions would be de-politicised through a shift from central government. Heavily opposed by many and politically difficult for the coalition government, the competition policy, as written into the 2012 act, was subsequently juxtaposed with a policy focus on service integration and quality improvement (Chapters 9 and 16). By 2015, these areas formed much of the policy core. Indeed, ideas of integration and collaboration among multiple providers, particularly around patients with chronic conditions, were at the centre of the *Five Year Forward View* released in late 2014 (Chapter 5).

In structural terms, the 2012 act spelled massive and disruptive change. With reference to NZ having endured successive reforms (see below), widescale change rarely delivers expected results; mostly, it leads to considerable system damage and undermining of morale, especially among front-line health professionals who often cannot see the rationale for change nor any potential for benefits (Chapter 13). The commissioning responsibility was shifted from the 'meso' level with PCTs having relative independence from hospitals, GPs and other services, and a responsibility for the spectrum of care, to GP control with CCGs responsible for funding services from a range of providers (Chapter 8). In principle, this shift in the commissioning landscape is not a bad one. However, from NZ's experience, GPs themselves needed to be in the driving seat of such a shift, with a commitment to clinical leadership and robust, population focused, primary care development. Compelling GPs through legislation to form CCGs is an example of 'top-down' policy, known to carry considerable costs in order to meet a series of conditions for 'perfect implementation' (Hill and Hupe, 2002; Hogwood and Gunn, 1984). Better would have been a 'bottom-up' approach, with GPs engaged in and even leading policy development from the outset, shown to have worked in NZ in the 1990s (Malcolm and Mays, 1999).

New Zealand

Through a NZ lens and health reform experience, a range of observations around the coalition government's reforms can be made. First, NZ's current policy agenda has parallels with that of England's NHS, at least in terms of basic goals. The post-2008 agenda has been one of efficiency, with the National government seeing considerable administrative overlaps and transactions costs across the 20 DHBs, each working in parallel, albeit with different regional populations to serve. There has also been a focus on quality and integration, on bolstering primary care, on revitalising clinical governance and leadership, and on centralisation of some administrative activities (Gauld, 2012). However, the means for pursuing these goals has differed somewhat from the coalition's approach.

Like the UK coalition government, NZ's National government came to power in 2008 with a reform agenda. However, politically, the 20 DHBs are difficult to reform, given their locally elected and embedded nature. There is also an unwritten recognition among the political parties, often stated by politicians, that the health sector is tired of radical reform and that this does more damage than good, especially when forced upon the sector without strong supporting evidence. This is probably, in itself, an important lesson for the NHS. There is, however, a widespread view in NZ, backed by evidence and reviews commissioned by the government, that the DHBs are reactive, lacking capacity to drive service improvements and mired in bureaucratic process (Ministerial Review Group, 2009). The electoral system does not necessarily deliver boards with the right skill mix or understanding of health services and their improvement (Laugesen and Gauld, 2012). The financial situation for most DHBs is no different from that facing the NHS, with 'deficit' a frequently mentioned word and driver of many local decisions as failure to come in on budget results in government-imposed financial sanctions. Because of this, the Ministry of Health is very closely involved in DHB operational activities, planning and decision making processes, which further constrains local innovation and flexibility. As such, most DHBs have failed over time to deliver on their overarching objective laid down in 2000, which is to integrate care and work with other social and local services, and involve the public in planning and decision making (the rationale for the elected boards). Instead, they have focused mostly on hospital and associated services only, and particularly on budget control, and have been relatively passive funders of PHOs and other services.

Despite the pressures on government spending resulting from the global financial crisis and its aftermath, which saw the National government cut expenditure across the public sector, it gave health separate treatment by continuing to invest at around or just above general inflation. The post-2008 government also eschewed competition, choosing instead to promote cross-sectoral collaboration and to listen closely to health professionals in the policy development process, in keeping with its clinical governance focus. This approach came from considerable contemplation on the impact of the period of wholesale reforms in the 1990s and the potential for negative and unintended consequences, especially for the workforce and public confidence. While in opposition, senior National party politicians had also consulted closely with front-line health professionals and their unions, and therefore sought to involve them in policy development once in government.

What followed has been a series of 'quiet' reforms, compared with the 'big bang' approach in England (Klein, 1995). A National Health Board was created through a carving out of the Ministry of Health. With broad parallels to NHS England, but a closeness to the Ministry of Health, its focus has been on improving operational performance of the DHBs, freeing the Ministry to focus on policy advice and sector monitoring. Other agencies noted above were also created to bring attention to quality and safety, to provide national coordination of health IT which had been allowed to develop from the bottom up via the 20 DHBs and multiple PHOs, and to improve health workforce planning. The primary care sector endured some change, with DHBs instructed to reduce the number of PHOs through mergers from around 80 pre-2008 to a present 30. At the regional level, 2010 amendments to the Public Health and Disability Services Act (originally passed in 2000), required DHBs to coordinate their plans and where possible share services. Thus, there are now four regional alliances each of which features around five DHBs. These are working to better coordinate services for specific populations, such as those with certain cancers, to plan services using pooled resources of multiple DHBs, and join up various back office functions such as development of IT systems and health pathways (clinically-led patient referral guidelines).

At the local DHB level, there was very little change in service organisation with DHBs and PHOs continuing to work in a relatively siloed manner, despite planning and delivering services for common populations. Perhaps most significant was the government's 'clinical governance and leadership' policy (2009) which required every DHB to implement internal structural changes to develop and promote this (Gauld et al, 2011; Ministerial Task Group on Clinical Leadership, 2009). Since 2013, when the government amended the national contract that DHBs sign with PHOs to require an 'alliance' between the two, change has been in motion. Again, this reform has been almost by stealth and consequent changes incremental. However, alliancing spells perhaps the most fundamental shift in the institutional arrangements in NZ's health sector for many decades. This means the key funders and service providers in the local health system must, for the first time since the abovementioned 1938 Social Security Act was passed, work together with a focus on the whole system, rather than the specific part of the system they may represent. In theoretical terms, alliances might be considered a model of 'experimental' governance as sketched out by Klein:

> Instead of a top-down, hierarchical rule-based system where failures to adhere are sanctioned, or unregulated market-based approaches, the new governance school posits a more participatory and collaborative model of regulation in which multiple stakeholders, including, depending on the context, government, civil society, business and nonprofit organizations, collaborate to achieve a common purpose. In order to encourage flexibility and innovation, 'new governance' approaches favor more process-oriented political strategies like disclosure requirements, benchmarking, and standard-setting, audited self-regulation, and the threat of imposition of default 'regulatory regimes' to be applied where there is a lack of good-faith effort at achieving desired goals. (Klein, 2007)

The aim of the alliance model is to break down the traditional silos and institutional arrangements that exist within the health system through a mix of service delivery redesign, joined-up planning and trust-building between the different partners.

The alliance policy was derived from National's pre-election health strategy entitled *Better, Sooner, More Convenient Healthcare* (commonly referred to as 'BSMC') which has guided policy since 2008 (Ryall, 2008). This made the case for services to be increasingly delivered in community settings, including various specialist services traditionally requiring a visit to a hospital outpatient clinic, and for closer integration between different providers and sites of care. In 2010, the government agreed to fund nine BSMC pilots, which effectively promised new integrated care models and systems with a particular focus on older populations, chronic disease management and primary care enhancement. These were selected from over 70 business case submissions received by the government. Each of the nine served quite different populations and geographic areas. But each had in common an alliance governance structure which, in the NZ context, has origins in alliance contracting which is common to large construction projects. The basic premise is that different companies enter into an alliance as each has a common goal: to complete the project on time and within budget. In turn, alliance partners agree to collaborate and assist one another, including sharing resources, to ensure the end-goal is achieved. NZ's health alliances have similar aims of connecting providers in a region to build a common focus and mechanism for working together (Lovelock et al, 2014).

As noted, the principal partners of an alliance are the DHB and PHO who had never previously had a formal arrangement for collaborating despite the former providing substantial funding to the latter. There are various structural and compositional expectations for alliances. For example, membership of the 'alliance leadership team', the overarching governance body, should be a mix of health professionals and managers, ideally including the CEO of both the DHB and PHO and other senior administrative staff. Health professionals should include senior leaders such as the chief medical officer, chief nurse and chief of allied health for the DHB and GP and nursing members from the PHO. Many alliances also involve contracted services such as ambulance services, as well as appointees from within the Maori and Pacific communities who bear a disproportionate burden of disease and have shorter life expectancy. The idea is to build an alliance of both those holding resources and those providing care. Members are appointees who work on behalf of the local health system and patients and must put aside any notion that they are representatives and, therefore, protectors of their particular profession or organisation. What is important is that they must have respect among professional and other colleagues and be able to engage them in discussions around new models of care and modes of working. In this regard, getting the right people, who see the value in alliancing, at the alliance leadership team table is critical (Gauld, 2014).

The way an alliance conducts it work differs from that of the partner organisations. An Alliance Charter spells out the 'rules of engagement' and binds members to these as each signs the charter in the presence of the others. The Charter states that members will work collaboratively with a genuine focus on how patients would like to see services delivered; that members will respect one another's roles in the local system; that they will work actively to redesign care using the whole of system approach and draw on the respective contributions to the care delivery process of alliance member organisations and professionals; and that they will also (re)allocate resources to ensure alliance decisions are implemented. Alliances are, therefore, potentially game changing.

They offer considerable practical potential in terms of system design by allowing GPs and hospital specialists, for instance, to talk about their roles in a care spectrum and which components of patient care might be better delivered by a GP in a primary care setting with appropriate support and resourcing from the hospital.

How much influence NZ's alliances have is an important question. The answer is that all the local power sits around the table, with a mandate to redesign care. The local DHB has reserve powers but it is unlikely that these would be invoked as DHB leaders are involved in alliance discussions and decisions. The test of alliance influence is in the extent to which the focus and activities of the provider member organisations changes over time. This might be seen, for example, in the extent to which hospitals focus on primary care in the context of the broader local health system, and shifting services and funding support for these from hospital to primary care settings. Impact, of course, might also be quantifiable via indicators such as ambulatory sensitive hospitalisations for people with known chronic conditions, or the percentage of patients discharged from hospital with a care plan in place.

In terms of service planning and design, the alliance leadership team effectively delegates authority to a series of 'service level alliance teams' (SLATs), or 'clinical networks', as these are variously called in different parts of NZ. These are where clinical governance is fully operationalised as membership is almost entirely health professionals. Again, a spectrum of professionals and organisations are represented in accordance with the focus of the SLATs, along with patient representatives and with support staff in attendance. Common SLATs are in areas such as older persons health, long-term conditions, child and youth health, rural health, pharmaceuticals, clinical pathways and urgent care. A typical SLAT will focus on identifying major problems or challenges in the area of focus, such as patients with multiple long-term conditions, then work on a plan for care that involves all providers working in collaboration with a goal of improved patient management and service integration. Once such plans have been agreed, the recommendations to the alliance leadership team are effectively binding as they have been clinically-led and designed by SLAT members with interaction along the way with the broader health provider community and the alliance leadership team. Because of this consultative and iterative process, surprises or unacceptable recommendations and lack of support for redesigned models of care are unlikely.

In terms of resourcing alliance decisions, beyond the commitment of the partners to implementation, the government has permitted so-called 'flexible funding'. This allows the PHO to redirect funding that is historically allocated on a national and standard basis specifically for health promotion, for reducing patient access barriers, and for managing patients with chronic diseases into new locally-agreed alliance initiatives. The DHB and other partners are also expected to direct funds into the flexible funding pool. As flexible funding evolves over time, increasing portions of the budgets of alliance members will be combined and used for common purposes.

Perhaps most compelling, and highly-relevant to the English NHS, is that alliancing has an inherent public service and equity orientation. This is due to the collaborative and localised nature of the endeavour, and the focus on patients and communities ahead of the interests of individual providers. Alliancing thus offers considerable scope for delivering on traditional 'national' health service goals.

In sum, the English NHS and NZ appear to be on quite different trajectories although there are many similar developments and long-term goals across the two systems. There have been moves in some NHS regions toward developing alliance arrangements, and these are likely to be propelled by the NHS Five Year Forward View (Addicott, 2014). Probably, much of the similarity in terms of structures, agencies and some areas of policy has come from a one-way flow of ideas from the NHS to NZ, with NZ drawing on what have been seen to be useful initiatives. The key divergence between the two systems would appear to have been in the broader policy tools, philosophical underpinnings of these and resulting structures.

One way of explaining the divergence might be offered via the lens of 'socialised neoliberalism' (Gauld, 2009a). This posits that there has been a public policy struggle in high-income democratic countries over the decades from around the 1980s. In some cases, there has been an overlap between different policies, some of which are layered on top of existing arrangements. The policy struggle has been between emphasis on social democracy, with aims of participation, equity and community development, and a tendency to favour public sector services and government intervention; and neoliberalism with its counter-attack on social democratic ideals and preference for bolstering private markets and competition in delivery of public services. Socialised neoliberalism suggests that governments, in England, NZ and elsewhere, have sought both social democratic and neoliberal goals in tandem, sometimes due to path dependency, and in other cases as one philosophical approach and associated policies – for example, neoliberalism – is seen as a means for achieving social democratic objectives. The coalition government was clearly applying such logic in the 2012 Health and Social Care

Act. For its part, NZ's National government has pursued policy means and institutional arrangements that could be considered more closely in line with social democratic principles, despite being a government that is 'conservative' in nature. In both countries, it could be argued that various governments from different sides of the political spectrum have pursued different aspects of the socialised neoliberalism agenda, meaning a blurring of 'left' and 'right' in politics.

Why NZ's conservatives have taken a path more toward the social democratic end of the spectrum, rather than the neoliberal-influenced approach of the UK Conservative-led government, is an important question. The answer is probably two-fold. First, NZ's electoral system, once described as an 'elective dictatorship' in that it delivered single-party government, has produced coalition governments since 1996 when a mixed-member proportional voting system was introduced. This has made it considerably more difficult for governments to introduce unpopular and radical policy and, arguably, anchored much of policy in the political centre owing to the considerable amount of bargaining required between different parties in forming a post-election coalition. Thus, the main political parties and governments in recent years have tended to differ largely around the margins on health policy, with relative agreement on basic structures and directions. Second, the National party listened closely to and involved health professionals, especially those in public employment, in its policy deliberations. As such, NZ's trajectory is strongly anchored in professionally-led ideas. Health policy tensions today have tended to arise when local managers or national policy makers have failed to properly engage professionals in planning and decision making, or when there have been restrictions around access to services in the perpetual context of austerity.

The perspective of 'NHS refugees' in NZ

As with any significant changes, the impact of the NHS reforms on the workforce cannot be overlooked. Indeed, one reason why governments in NZ have, more recently, approached reform with trepidation is 'reform fatigue' from the decade of the 1990s, which remains a strong memory for many, and the sheer costs of this politically and on workforce engagement. There have been increasing reports of the NHS being under 'stress', with the coalition's reforms having a negative impact on workforce stress levels.

A 2014 study of UK-trained doctors registered and practicing in NZ provides some insights into this impact. The study's findings have been reported elsewhere (Gauld and Horsburgh, 2015). All UK-trained doctors registered with the Medical Council of NZ who had arrived within the previous ten years were invited to complete a survey (n=1354); 47 per cent (n=632) responded. Sixteen of these doctors were also interviewed.

Asked about motivations for the move to NZ, 65 per cent of survey respondents indicated a 'desire to leave the UK NHS', with one-third of all respondents indicating that this was 'highly important'. Only 38 per cent agreed that 'more attractive salary and incentives' motivated their move, with less than 10 per cent saying this was highly important. Regression analyses indicated that younger doctors (20–30 years of age) were around four times as likely as older doctors (aged 51 and over) to agree that 'desire to leave the NHS' was behind their move to NZ. Some 80 per cent of respondents agreed that 'The New Zealand health system is better to work in compared to the UK system', with over 40 per cent strongly agreeing with this statement. Regression results showed males and older respondents (41 years and over) were less likely to agree.

Asked about motivations to leave the NHS, both GP and specialist interviewees pointed to various factors. Commonplace was a stressful working environment with a high volume of patients and very limited time for each and a desire to leave behind stress and frustration. Said one: 'the constant re-organisation and a lot of constant directives coming from above. It didn't seem to really relate to patient needs, just kind of political objectives.' Another said: 'I think work conditions [in NZ] are vastly superior to the UK – at the moment. I enjoy working here and I suspect I would be quite burnt out if I had remained in the UK.'

Conclusion: two futures and potential lessons

Cross-country comparisons have the capacity to provide all-important lessons for how policy issues might be approached. Where the US has often been viewed as a source of lessons for the NHS, this chapter has argued that NZ perhaps provides a more useful and appropriate reference point. The health policy and system goals in the NHS and NZ appear similar, as is the country and cultural context. Arguably, the US is not useful for comparison and lesson-drawing. A range of conclusions might be drawn from the discussions in this chapter.

First, is that the post-2008 NZ health reform experience illustrates that the UK coalition government had other options available rather than the blunt tool of competition. The health policy goals in both countries are similar, but the means for pursuing these at the outset were very different. While considerable damage may well have been wrought via the coalition's Health and Social Care Act, their agenda now appears to be closer to that of NZ. If so, an aim for the Conservative-led government and NHS leaders now might be to analyse closely the NZ alliance experience which is both clinically-driven but also leverages off the incentives and values that are germane to the NHS and NZ health systems. Earlier studies comparing elements of the US health system with the NHS had a high impact, despite questions around the comparators and different context. Arguably, such studies contributed to the case that competition would be good for the NHS. Lesson drawing from a more closely comparable country ought to be given a high media profile and have similar influence. Second, in terms of framing the NHS and NZ experiences, 'socialised neoliberalism' provides a potential heuristic tool. The Conservative-led government has, since 2012, retracted from the harder end of neoliberalism, while the NZ National government has been largely social democratic in aim and approaches. The NZ experience tends to suggest that this is more appropriate if integrated care, quality improvement and equity are overarching goals. Third, the impact on professionals cannot be dismissed. Finally, this view from abroad sees the challenge for the research and policy community as one of continuing to look for models that counter the prominent US-guided critique of the NHS.

References

Addicott, R, 2014, *Commissioning and contracting for integrated care*, London: The King's Fund

Aspalter, C, Yasuo, U, Gauld, R (eds), 2012, *Health care systems in Europe and Asia*, Abingdon: Routledge

Bevan, G, Karanikolos, M, Exley, J, Nolte, E, Connolly, S, Mays, N, 2014, *The four health systems of the United Kingdom: how do they compare?*, London: Nuffield Trust

Blank, RH, Burau, V, 2010, *Comparative Health Policy, 3rd edition*, Houndmills: Palgrave Macmillan.

Boston, J, Dalziel, P, St John, S (eds), 1999, *Redesigning the welfare state in New Zealand: Problems, policies, prospects*, Auckland: Oxford University Press

Boston, J, Martin, J, Pallot, J, Walsh, P, 1996, *Public management: The New Zealand model*, Auckland: Oxford University Press

Cumming, J, 2011, Integrated care in New Zealand, *International Journal of Integrated Care*, 11(November), http://doi.org/10.5334/ijic.678

Devereaux, PJ, Heels-Ansdell, D, Lacchetti, C, Haines, T et al, 2004, Payments for care at private for-profit and private not-for-profit hospitals: A systematic review and meta-analysis, *Canadian Medical Association Journal* 170, 12, 1817–24

Exworthy, M, Freeman, R, 2009, The United Kingdom: Health policy learning in the National Health Service, in T Marmor, R Freeman, K Okma (eds) *Comparative Studies and the politics of modern medical care*, p 153–79, New Haven, CT: Yale University Press

Francis, R, 2013, *Robert Francis Inquiry Report into Mid-Staffordshire NHS Foundation Trust*, London: The Stationery Office

Gauld, R, 2003, The impact on officials of public sector restructuring: The case of the New Zealand Health Funding Authority, *International Journal of Public Sector Management* 16, 4, 303–19

Gauld, R (ed), 2005, *Comparative health policy in the Asia-Pacific*, Maidenhead: Open University Press

Gauld, R, 2009a, *The New Health Policy*, Maidenhead: Open University Press.

Gauld, R, 2009b, *Revolving doors: New Zealand's health reforms – the saga continues*, Wellington: Institute of Policy Studies and Health Services Research Centre

Gauld, R, 2012, New Zealand's post-2008 health system reforms: Toward re-centralization of organizational arrangements, *Health Policy* 106, 110–13

Gauld, R, 2013, Questions about New Zealand's health system in 2013, its 75th anniversary year, *New Zealand Medical Journal* 126, 1380, 1–7

Gauld, R, 2014, What should governance for integrated care look like? New Zealand's alliances provide some pointers, *Medical Journal of Australia* 201, 3, s267–s268

Gauld, R, Horsburgh, S, 2015, What motivates doctors to leave the UK NHS for a 'life in the sun' in New Zealand; and, once there, why don't they stay?, *Human resources for health* 13, 1, 75

Gauld, R, Mays, N, 2006, Reforming primary care: Are New Zealand's new primary health organisations fit for purpose?, *British Medical Journal* 333, 1216–18

Gauld, R, Horsburgh, S, Brown, J, 2011, The Clinical Governance Development Index: results from a New Zealand study, *BMJ Quality and Safety* 20, 11, 947–53

Goldfinch, S, 1998, Remaking New Zealand's economic policy: Institutional elites as radical innovators 1984–1993, *Governance* 11, 2, 177–207

Gower, S, Finlayson, M, Turnbull, J, 2003, Hospital restructuring: The impact on nursing, in R Gauld (ed), *Continuity amid chaos: Health care management and delivery in New Zealand*, Dunedin: University of Otago Press

Health Workforce New Zealand, 2014, *The health of the Health Workforce*, Wellington: Health Workforce New Zealand

Hill, M, Hupe, P, 2002, *Implementing public policy*, London: Sage

Himmelstein, D, Warren, E, Thorne, D, Woolhandler, S, 2005, Illness and injury as contributors to bankruptcy, *Health Affairs*, Web exclusive, w5-63–w65-73

Himmelstein, DU, Thorne, D, Warren, E, Woolhandler, S, 2009, Medical bankruptcy in the United States, 2007: Results of a national study, *The American Journal of Medicine* 122, 8, 741–6

Hogwood, B, Gunn, L, 1984, *Policy analysis for the real world*, Oxford: Oxford University Press

Klein, A, 2007, Judging as nudging: New governance approaches for the enforcement of constitutional social and economic rights, *Columbia Human Rights Law Review* 39, 351

Klein, R, 1995, Big Bang health care reform: Does it work? The case of Britain's 1991 National Health Service reforms, *Milbank Quarterly* 73, 3, 299–337

Laugesen, M, Gauld, R, 2012, *Democratic governance and health: Hospitals, politics and health policy in New Zealand*, Dunedin: Otago University Press

Lovelock, K, Martin, G, Cumming, J, Gauld, R, Derrett, S, 2014, *The evaluation of the better, sooner, more convenient business cases in MidCentral and the West Coast District Health Boards, Report to the Health Research Council*, January 2014, Otago and Victoria: University of Otago and Victoria University of Wellington

Malcolm, L, Mays, N, 1999, New Zealand's independent practitioner associations: A working model of clinical governance in primary care?, *British Medical Journal* 319, 1340–2

Malcolm, L, Powell, M, 1996, The development of independent practice associations and related groups in New Zealand, *New Zealand Medical Journal* 109, 184–7

Marmor, T, Wendt, C, 2012, Conceptual frameworks for comparing healthcare politics and policy, *Health policy* 107, 1, 11–20

Marmor, T, Freeman, R, Okma, K (eds), 2009, *Comparative studies and the politics of modern medical care*, New Haven, CT: Yale University Press

Mein Smith, P, Hempenstall, P, Goldfinch, S, 2009, *Remaking the Tasman world*, Christchurch: Canterbury University Press

Ministerial Review Group, 2009, *Meeting the challenge: Enhancing sustainability and the patient and consumer experience within the current legislative framework for health and disability services in New Zealand*, Wellington: Minister of Health

Ministerial Task Group on Clinical Leadership, 2009, *In good hands: Transforming clinical governance in New Zealand*, Wellington: Ministerial Task Group on Clinical Leadership

Morra, D, Nicholson, S, Levinson, W, Gans, DN, Hammons, T, Casalino, LP, 2011, US physician practices versus Canadians: Spending nearly four times as much money interacting with payers, *Health Affairs* 30, 8, 1443–50

OECD, 2015, OECD Health Data. Paris: OECD

Paton, C, 2014, *At what cost? Paying the price for the market in the English NHS*, London: Centre for Health and the Public Interest

Penno, E, Gauld, R, Audas, R, 2013, How are population-based funding formulae for healthcare composed? A comparative analysis of seven models, *BMC Health Services Research* 13, 470

Ryall, T, 2008, Better, sooner, more convenient healthcare, *Health discussion paper*, Wellington: National Party

Scally, G, Donaldson, L, 1998, Clinical governance and the drive for quality improvement in the new NHS in England, *British Medical Journal* 317, 7150, 61–5

Spence, D, 2013, Mid-Staffs shames us all, *British Medical Journal* 346, 1927

Tuohy, CH, Flood, CM, Stabile, M, 2004, How does private finance affect public health care systems? Marshaling the evidence from OECD nations, *Journal of Health Politics, Policy and Law* 29, 3, 359–96

Wendt, C, Frisina, L, Rothgang, H, 2009, Healthcare system types: A conceptual framework for comparison, *Social Policy and Administration* 43, 1, 70–90

Section E:
Conclusions

EIGHTEEN

Never again?
A retrospective and prospective view
of English health reforms

Martin Powell and Mark Exworthy

This Chapter takes retrospective and prospective perspectives on health reforms in English NHS. Retrospectively, we offer a precis of the preceding chapters, taking stock of the cumulative lessons from the significant body of evidence that has been presented in this book. Moreover, we seek to explain the 'how and why' of these reforms, using a specific conceptual model (multiple streams approach (MSA)). Prospectively, we consider the direction of health policy in the English NHS, and the research agenda which might inform this process.

What have we learnt so far?

We have presented 16 chapters of evidence across a diverse range of policy or thematic topics. Some of these (such as commissioning) have been standard topics in previous collections of evidence (Robinson and Le Grand, 1994; Le Grand et al, 1998; Mays et al, 2011) although the more recent emphasis has been upon 'clinical' commissioning (Chapter 8). Other topics are either novel to such collections of evidence (for example, equity, staffing and PPI: Chapters 12, 13 and 15) or are specific to the temporal context of the first and second decade of the twenty-first century (for example, fiscal austerity: Chapter 3). To organise the evidence (and to aid the reader), we grouped these chapters into three thematic sections: national health policy, commissioning and service provision, and governance.

National health policy

Over the past 25 years, the NHS has been the subject of a massive 'natural experiment' in reorganising, seeking to install the tenets of new public management (NPM). Specifically, this has entailed markets, competition, decentralisation and managerialisation. While the effects of these multiple reforms continue to play out, they have been overlain by the recent reforms since 2010. Archetypes such as the 'bureaucratic' NHS have been sedimented by newer ones (such as marketisation) which may distort and reinforce the effects of any single reform (Addicott et al, 2007).

The financial crisis of 2008 precipitated the conditions for fiscal austerity during the Coalition government (2010–15). Charlesworth and colleagues (Chapter 3) discuss the recent period of NHS austerity with reference to different sectors within the NHS, specific elements (such as agency pay), comparisons between the four nations of the UK, and wider international comparisons. Bojke and colleagues (Chapter 4) explore how the productivity impact of the declining inputs to the NHS have affected its outputs. With the impact of austerity policies, the output growth had fallen to 2.8 per cent during the Coalition government. These two chapters set the context for the ways in which recent national health policy was formulated.

A key facet of the Health and Social Care Act (HSCA) of 2012 was to reformulate the relationship between the Secretary of State for Health and the NHS by removing the latter's responsibility for providing a comprehensive health service (Chapter 5). This seemed to be in line with efforts to dismantle the existing NHS structures, in favour of a more autonomous network of local agencies. However, Greener (Chapter 6) notes that the rhetoric and reality of any policy is likely to be different, which is why the discursive approach of Parliamentary (and other) debates are vital to understanding the way in which these reforms were constituted. The Coalition reforms have exacerbated even further the differences between the nations of the UK. While most attention has been paid to the English health reforms, Hughes (Chapter 7) offers a counterbalance by noting the differences between nations *before* 2010 and the continued policy divergence since.

In regard to national health policy, the overall effect of the reforms seems to have been to decentre the NHS, by hollowing out the centre's ability to steer the health system (Bevir and Rhodes, 2001). Yet, it also points to the greater reliance of a network of national bodies (such as Monitor, CQC, NHS England et al) to ensure overall strategic direction to the NHS.

Commissioning and service provision

The ways in which the Coalition reforms have been played out across the (English) NHS is explored in the second section, through analysis of commissioning, health and social care integration, public health, plurality of service provision, and the impact of these upon equity.

Commissioning has been a constant feature of reforms since 1991 but its recent reincarnation incorporated GPs into decision-making of CCGs (Chapter 8). That said, the role of commissioning (within the purchaser–provider split) seems less relevant in 2016 than any time in the last 25 years. This shift in emphasis is manifest in the discussion of integration (Chapter 9). However, they reiterate the challenge of matching the rhetoric of integration with its reality as implemented in practice. Specifically, the recent emphasis on integration appears incompatible with the notion of diversity in service provision. This is especially significant in the ways in which the salience of markets and competition (notably with the private sector) has waxed and waned over time (Chapter 11). We balance the focus on commissioning and provision by including public health (Chapter 10). The historic transition of public health functions from the NHS to local government place it in a precarious position. It could either create the opportunity to tackle more effectively the social determinants of health or public health could become marginalised within a sector which has multiple competing demands upon its resources. Yet, equity seems to have been an afterthought in the Coalition reforms, drawing the conclusion that CCGs will struggle to tackle health inequality better than PCTs did (Chapter 12).

Governance

The governance of the NHS has come under strain as a result of greater emphasis on transparency and patient safety, together with the implementation of reforms. For example, the managerialisation in the NHS, pointing towards new forms of entrepreneurialism (Chapter 13). Likewise, Health and Wellbeing Boards are articulating the interests of different institutions and in doing so, creating a new form of planning (Chapter 14). Set against this is a familiar refrain of patient and public involvement, which remains an easy target for reform but evidence of improvement still remains sparse (Chapter 15). Arguably, quality and patient safety has become the primary discourse for health service improvement in the UK (and internationally) (Chapter 16). In England, this agenda has largely been shaped by a series of 'scandals' and subsequent reports, most the egregious of which was Mid-Staffordshire. However, such scrutiny and transparency might generate further challenge to improve quality. Finally, it is useful to place these reforms in an international context (Chapter 17 in relation to New

Zealand). Both countries drew on each other, especially in relation to marketisation. However, these comparators now illustrate divergent tendencies.

Overall, the Coalition reforms marked a pivotal moment in the NHS. Arguably, it is either the reinvention of the NHS or it denotes the logical extension of NPM (see Powell, 2015). The evidence is not always clear-cut. Often, the historical template of previous reforms have created a path dependency which has set the NHS on a particular course, from which it has hardly deviated. Whether this amounts to a dismantling of the NHS is contested. While the efforts have been made to stem the fragmentation of the NHS (around integration of health and social care, for example), the combination of Coalition policies and the legacy of previous reforms indicates that the NHS is becoming (and indeed may already have become) a much looser network of organisations, albeit still working under the title of the NHS. The impact of devolution and integration policies (in England) has yet to play out, but both might further exacerbate efforts to retain the cohesion of the NHS as an institution.

How can the Coalition government health reforms be explained?

Given the accumulation of evidence in this book, we are still left with two compelling questions: how and why did these reforms happen? As we have seen, the Coalition reforms have been viewed by some commentators as the biggest reform in the history of the NHS. They have also largely been viewed critically. For example, Timmins (2012, 7) states that it is widely seen as a 'car crash' in terms of both policy and politics, while the website 'Conservative Home' called for the bill to be dropped (D'Ancona 2014, 115; Timmins, 2012, 111). It was admitted in 2014 that NHS reforms were the government's 'worst mistake' (Davis et al, 2015, 271) and, according to D'Ancona (2014), a 'Downing street source' suggested that Lansley should be 'taken out and shot'. The 'NHS debacle' has been viewed by some as the biggest cock-up of Cameron's premiership (Seldon and Snowdon, 2015, 181).

There is a puzzle, therefore, about how and why did the Health and Social Care Act (HSCA) come about at all. First, Andrew Lansley developed a broad reform plan in his long period as Shadow Secretary of State for Health, while David Cameron attempted to reassure the public and 'de-toxify' the Conservative brand on health (Chapter 2; Timmins, 2012). As the 2010 general election approached, talk of reassurance trumped change. After the election, Coalition partners attempted to blend their health plans, resulting in a pledge in the Programme for Government to rule out any 'top-down reorganisation'. Lansley regarded this as an unworkable policy fudge, and essentially ignored it to produce a top-down reorganisation. Growing criticism of his health reforms necessitated some concessions, an unprecedented 'pause', many amendments, and extensive debate in the House of Commons and the Lords to produce the HSCA of 2012. There appears to be less agreement over the second issue. Jarman and Greer (2015) write that one remarkable thing about Coalition health policy has been its sheer improbability: of all the problems facing the UK (let alone the NHS) in 2010, the reorganisation of the NHS could not have been a big one. This section of the chapter explores how the HSCA got on the agenda through the lens of the 'multiple streams' model (Kingdon, 2011; Zahariadis, 2014; see for example, Jones et al, 2016).

The multi streams approach

Kingdon (2011) argues that an issue reaches the agenda when the policy window opens (sometimes through a policy entrepreneur) to allow the coupling of three independent streams – policy, problem and politics. This means that the approach has five major categorical concepts: three distinct streams, policy entrepreneurs and policy windows (see Zahariadis, 2014; Jones et al, 2016).

Problem stream

Kingdon (2011) argues that the problem stream involves indicators, focusing events and policy feedback. Indicators concern how actors identify and monitor potential problems, including metrics and anecdotes. Focusing events are jarring and sudden, and become attached to particular problems. Feedback provides information on current performance which may not square with intended goals or suggest unanticipated consequences.

Indicators

The indicators were the subject of significantly different interpretations. On the one hand, Lansley claimed that the NHS needed to change on the basis of finance and comparative mortality. On the other hand, his critics argued that the NHS was performing well (for example, Leys and Player, 2011, 148–9; Davis et al, 2015, 39–41; Toynbee and Walker, 2015, 213). As a result, there was no clear message or narrative for reform (Timmins, 2012; D'Ancona, 2014; Seldon and Snowdon, 2015). According to former Conservative Health Secretary, Ken Clarke, 'the reason Andrew failed was because he couldn't explain it' (in Timmins and Davies, 2015, 63). Timmins (2012, 139–40) compares the Lansley reforms unfavourably with the NHS Plan (DH, 2000), which clearly argued the need for change, and attempted to obtain ownership as far as possible from the public, the staff and key interest groups before the white paper. The same might also be said the 'Five year forward view' (NHS England, 2014).

Focusing Events

There does not appear to be a clear seminal event (or events) which focused attention within the policy network. While Mid-Staffordshire was briefly mentioned in 'Liberating the NHS' (DH, 2010), it perhaps became a focusing event only after the second Francis Report of 2013 (see Powell and Mannion, 2015, also Chapter 16 in this book). The lack of such events constricts the problem stream in explaining the 'how and why' of the reforms.

Feedback

This factor depends on whether, at the macro level, Labour's reforms are seen as 'analogous programmes' (see Chapter 2). In this case, Lansley's reforms can be seen as evolution of market-based reforms rather than revolution, and completing Labour's agenda (see Timmins, 2012), with CCGs as following the trail of earlier initiatives such as GPFH (see Goldacre, 2015).

Political stream

Kingdon (2011, 162) states that the political stream is composed of factors such as swings of national mood, election results, changes of administration, changes of ideological or partisan distributions in legislatures and interest group pressure campaigns.

National mood

Many critics claim that the national mood supported neither the Coalition reforms nor broader market-based reforms (for example, Leys and Player, 2011; Davis et al, 2015). It is apparent that the

Conservatives went into the 2010 election offering absolute reassurance on the NHS while plotting one of the most dramatic reforms in its 62-year history (D'Ancona, 2014, 104; Timmins, 2012). However, some opinion polls show significant opposition to markets, competition and 'privatisation', while others suggest that voters are more relaxed about who provides services so long as they are free at the point of use.

Party ideology

Ever since 1945, when the Conservatives voted against the establishment of the NHS, the health service had essentially been a Labour issue (Timmins, 2012). It has been claimed that there is a similarity and growing convergence between the health policy of Labour and Conservative since about 2000 (Leys and Player, 2011; Timmins, 2012; Davis and Tallis, 2013; Davis et al, 2015). Timmins (2012) notes that, by 2010, the message of reassurance about health had worked so well that while Labour was still rated to have the best policies on healthcare, the gap was narrow and the smallest it had been at almost any point since 1997. Timmins (2012, 40–1) points to the similarly between the 2010 election manifestos, writing that given the bitter controversy to come, all three parties endorsed at least a degree of choice, competition and use of the private sector in the provision of NHS care. However, the Liberal Democrat part of the Coalition did not have a clear and settled health policy. As the HCSA progressed, this was fought over both inside parliament and at grass roots level, and also seems to have opened up unhealed wounds within the Labour party (Timmins, 2012). There is, however, a significant difference of view between commentators who argue that the Liberal Democrats had a significant impact on the Bill (for example, Timmins, 2012; Glennerster, 2015; Walker and Yong, 2012; D'Ancona, 2014; Carrier and Kendall, 2015) and those who consider their influence to be minimal (for example, Jarman and Greer, 2015; Davis et al, 2015; Davis and Tallis, 2013). Finally, Timmins (2012, 142) states that the Act is a prime illustration of just how important the Lords has become as the amending chamber – and arguably even more important given that there is a coalition: 'all the changes of substance were made in the Lords'.

Interest group campaigns

According to Walker and Yong (2012, 177), a notable feature was the role of interest groups outside Parliament and of 'NHS professionals' in causing a rethink. Timmins (2012, 89) points to the importance of 38 Degrees, the web-based membership campaign that has used Twitter and Facebook to assemble petitions and campaigns. He claims that this was the first piece of government legislation to be seriously battered by the internet (p 142). However, others suggest a limited role for interest groups. For example, Tallis (2013, 2–3) argues that the NHS was betrayed by politicians, journalists, the unions and, perhaps most culpably, the leaders of the medical profession. The Act would not have been possible without the active collusion, passive acquiescence or incompetence of all these players.

Others suggest that, far from opposing the bill, interest groups associated with the 'private health lobbying industry' were the main shapers of the Bill. In particular, they stress the 'revolving door' between the public and private sector leading to the infiltration of NHS by 'private sector cheerleaders' (Davis et al, 2015, 213) and the 'privatisation of policy making' by management firms such as McKinsey – 'the firm that hijacked the NHS' (p 216). Huitson (2013, 152) points to the role of the private healthcare industry in drafting and 'cheerleading' the bill, concluding that the bill was 'a near perfect vision of Westminster's appropriation by high commerce' (p 152). They point to conflict of interests at both central and local level, asking who stood to profit, and concluding that MPs, peers, Tory party donors and CCG members, such as GPs, who had a financial stake in a private company which provides services to their own CCG (for example, Leys and Player, 2011; Davis and Tallis, 2013; Davis et al, 2015). Leys and Player (2011) argue that within the health policy 'community' (a cluster of linked organisations inside and outside the NHS: for example, Kings Fund, Nuffield Trust), the market agenda became the only agenda. According to Toynbee and Walker (2015, 222), now the private interests that had backed Lansley's Act wanted their pounds of flesh. While critics argue that the policy community were broadly supportive of markets, competition and choice, Timmins (2012, 66, 84) argues that there were few voices in favour of the reforms. The government did not even find friends in places where it might have expected them, with criticism from places where it might more normally have expected support such as think tanks (Shaw et al, 2014).

Policy stream

Kingdon (2011) argues that ideas float around in the 'policy primeval soup', with the generation of alternatives and proposals resembling a process of biological natural selection. The criteria for survival consist of technical feasibility, value acceptability within the policy community, tolerable cost, anticipated public acquiescence, and a reasonable chance for receptivity among elected decision-makers (p 131).

Value acceptability

Many critics argue that the broad values of markets, competition and choice were accepted by the 'policy community', and the reforms can be seen as evolution from earlier reforms (Chapter 2).

Technical feasibility

It could be argued that the reforms were technically feasible, but likely to be disruptive and costly as suggested by the group termed 'the incredulous' by Klein (2013). The past record suggests reorganisations do not solve problems (Walshe, 2010)

Tolerable cost

Paton (2014) considers that the official figure of the non-recurring cost of the current reforms of £1.4 billion is likely to be at least £3 billion, and estimates that at least £5 billion of the NHS's recurrent running costs relate to the market. According to Walshe (2014), Lansley's successor, Jeremy Hunt, claimed that they had cost £1.5 billion to implement but had saved £1 billion a year in NHS administrative costs. However, the claim that reorganisations save money appears problematic on the evidence of past reorganisations (Walshe, 2010).

Anticipated public acquiescence

The public did not expect such a significant reform (Timmins, 2012; D'Ancona, 2014). While there was significant criticism from interest groups (above), the polls were less clear and consistent, perhaps reflecting D'Ancona's (2014) 'white noise'. Certainly, the NHS was not a major issue at the 2015 election.

Receptivity among elected decision-makers

The reforms broadly fitted with the market-based policies of the last two decades, although some sections of the Liberal Democrats and Labour MPs voiced major criticism (but not perhaps as vociferously as their grass roots). However, D'Ancona (2014, 117) states that there were only a handful of true believers in the upper echelons of government: Lansley, Oliver Letwin and (possibly) Steve Hilton.

Policy windows

Kingdon (2011, 165) writes that the policy windows open when the separate streams come together at critical times: 'a problem is recognized, a solution is developed…a political change makes it the right time for policy change'. Policy windows are thus opened either by the appearance of compelling problems ('problem windows') or by happenings in the political stream ('political windows'). There appeared to be no 'compelling problem', so the HSCA seems to more reflect the opening of a political window. Lansley was convinced that he had a solution and, in the absence of significant expertise or challenge, he forged ahead.

Policy entrepreneurs

According to Kingdon (2011, 180–1), three qualities contribute to the success of policy entrepreneurs: some claim to a hearing (expertise, an ability to speak for others, and an authoritative position); political connections or negotiating skill; and 'probably most important', persistency. Oborn et al (2011) point out that the literature lacks a clear definition of 'policy entrepreneur' who may be singular or plural; and insider or outsider. This section is problematic as it is unclear if there was a policy entrepreneur. Regarding the 'outsider' perspective, there was no obvious policy entrepreneur, unlike Lord Darzi for Labour reforms (Oborn et al, 2011). This may be seen as a vital missing ingredient. The 'insider' perspective sees Lansley as the policy entrepreneur.

Claim to a hearing

Cameron largely left Ministers to make policy. Lansley clearly had expertise, reflecting his long tenure as Shadow Health Secretary, and was trusted on health matters. Both Cameron and Osborne had worked for him in the Conservative Research Department, and both considered him a reassuring figure on the NHS who knows his subject backwards (Seldon and Snowdon, 2015, 181–2; Glennerster, 2015, 292), giving him an 'authoritative decision-making position'.

Political connections or negotiating skill

Lansley had good political connections. However, commentators point to his lack of presentational or negotiating skills. Timmins (2012, 130) states that as Lansley was not a natural communicator, huge swathes of his parliamentary colleagues had no real idea what he planned. This can be contrasted with the communication style of Earl Howe in the House of Lords. He was also, in the words of one civil servant, an 'emollient genius'. Lord Warner, the Labour former health minister, says 'his silky skills got the bill through' (Timmins, 2012, 114).

There was a general lack of expertise on health issues, meaning that there was little challenge (D'Ancona, 2014; Glennerster, 2015; Timmins, 2012; Walker and Yong, 2012). Timmins (2012, 139) points to the problem of building a consensus; or at least some support, with Lansley largely declining to engage with his critics, and being 'all transmission, no reception'.

Persistence

A significant degree of persistence was present. Lansley's plans had been formed during his unprecedented six-and-a-half years' tenure as Shadow Secretary of State. Timmins (2012) points out that pretty much all of his ideas had been presented in dozens of speeches and documents.

In short, it would appear that the MSA points to the conclusion that HCSA should not have happened (see Table 18.1)! The fact that it did is open to interpretation. It may perhaps be testament to the ways in which the streams both combine (in different ways and with varying intensity over time) but also the synergistic confluence, creating an outcome is that is not simply a sum of the parts. It does not necessarily invalidate the model itself. For example, it might signify the lack of a coherent alternative to proposals, rather than an endorsement of the proposals themselves.

Future directions in health policy and research

It is invidious to point to future directions in health policy from the evidence presented here. We have discussed the contingencies of policy formulation and implementation across the NHS and so, to draw simple conclusions is misleading. However, the intention of this book has been to place the Coalition health reforms in a wider context and not simply consider them shortly after the end of the

Table 18.1: Summary of the components of the MSA model applied to the HSCA

Problem stream	
Indicators	Disputed
Focusing events	Mid Staffordshire scandal later
Feedback	Debate over impact of previous market-based reform in general, and over primary care commissioning in particular
Political stream	
National mood	No clear (public) mandate for market-based reform
Party ideology	All major parties pro-market, but debates within Labour and Liberal Democrats
Interest group campaigns	Private health lobby; and limited effectiveness by medical profession
Policy stream	
Value acceptability	Markets, competition and choice broadly accepted within policy community
Technical feasibility	Limited but disputed evidence
Tolerable cost	Claimed long-term savings unlikely
Anticipated public acquiescence	Lack of clear mandate for market-based reform trumped by 'free at point of use' and 'white noise'?
Receptivity among elected decision-makers	Broadly in line with direction of market-based reform, but few 'true believers'
Policy windows	
Problem window	No clear 'compelling problem' to be solved
Political window	Lansley was convinced that he had a solution, but unclear if 'the right time for policy change'
Policy entrepreneurs	
Key individual(s)	Lansley as policy entrepreneur
Claim to a hearing	Expertise; trusted among politicians and policy-makers
Political connections or negotiating skill	Good connections, but limited negotiating skills
Persistence	Plans developed during long tenure as Shadow Health Secretary

Coalition government. Not only would it be difficult to discern any attributable impact to any of these policies at this stage but is also misses the point that these reforms form part of a longer-term trend towards reforming the UK public sector and specifically the NHS. For some, this consists of a decentring of the state being played out in terms of devolution and to some extent, in internationalisation (through direct comparison and importing specific organisations and their practices). For others, it is a more severe dismantling of the NHS, through its 'privatisation' (in whatever form). For others still, it consists of a reconfiguration of the relationship between the service (its professionals and institutions) and the public (whether as patients or citizens). In any event, it is likely to be a combination of all these (and possibly, others).

In its seventh decade, the NHS is being transformed as fast and as extensively now as at any other point in its history. The motives and implications of such reorganisation have been explored in this book. While we have been able to present the parameters of this debate, its emergent impacts and its potential (often, dysfunctional) consequences, the ways in which these will be played out in the coming years will reflect the interaction between individuals (state and non-state actors (including the public) at all levels), the institutions within which they work, and the ideas with which they engage.

To make sense of these reforms, now and in the future, there is a pressing need for on-going research programmes which track specific policies. Inevitably, this agenda reflects our own specific social science perspective but it is, we believe, one which can shape a robust future for an equitable, accessible and sustainable NHS. The agenda is based upon the following four principles:

- *Long-term*: short-term evaluations serve a purpose but they shed relatively little light on the wider processes shaping the emergent outcomes of policy reform. Evaluation of pilot projects may not foster better use of evidence into policy-making or local decision-making (Ettelt et al, 2015).
- *Multi-method*: it is fair to say that qualitative methods have tended to dominate health policy research in research. While this may reflect the UK experience (and not necessarily other countries), we need to be mindful of the ways in which mixed methods can offer more compelling accounts of policy reform.
- *Inter-disciplinary*: this book has drawn on several disciplines; for example, economics, health services research, organisation studies, political science, social policy and sociology. In this way, we hope to have shown how an inter-disciplinary approach can provide insights in a way that single disciplines alone cannot.
- *Multi-level*: much of the health (policy) research taking place in recent years has focused at the micro level (of individual service, patient interactions and organisational change). While these are laudable, we also call for a multi-level approach which considers political aspects of policy-making, intermediary actors and the interpretation of and meaning given to such policy by local actors. This contextually-based approach has not been such a dominant

paradigm though signs of change are promising (Exworthy et al, 2011).

The outcome of the policies we have examined (and the research agenda we have proposed) may not be fully apparent for some time but we hope that this book has contributed to a more evidence-based debate to the future of the NHS. While the Coalition market-based reforms have significant similarities with those of previous Conservative and Labour governments, there are also clear differences, including the consolidation and extension of earlier reforms during a period of austerity, and Lansley's intention to make his changes irreversible. However, unless politicians, policy-makers and practitioners learn from such evidence as presented here or elsewhere, it is not clear if the outcome of the content and/or process of the Coalition reforms can be characterised, in the terms of Timmins (2012), as 'Never Again'.

References

Addicott, R, McGivern, G, Ferlie, E, 2007, The distortion of a managerial technique?: The case of NHS Cancer Networks, *British Journal of Management* 18, 93–105

Bevir, M, Rhodes, RAW, 2001, Decentring tradition: Interpreting British government, *Administration and Society* 33, 2, 107–32

Carrier, J, Kendall, I, 2015, *Health and the National Health Service*, 2nd edn, London: Routledge

D'Ancona, M, 2014, *In it together: The inside story of the Coalition government*, London: Penguin

Davis, J, Tallis, R (eds), 2013, *NHS SOS*, London: OneWorld

Davis, J, Lister, J, Weigley, D, 2015, *NHS for Sale*, London: Merlin.

DH (Department of Health), 2000, *The NHS Plan*, London: The Stationery Office

DH (Department of Health), 2010, *Liberating the NHS*, London: The Stationery Office

Ettelt, S, Mays, N, Allen, P, 2015, The multiple purposes of policy piloting and their consequences: Three examples from national health and social care policy in England, *Journal of Social Policy* 44, 2, 319–37

Exworthy, M, Peckham, S, Powell, M, Hann, A (eds), 2011, *Shaping health policy: Case study methods and analysis*, Bristol: Policy Press

Glennerster, H, 2015, Health and social care, in A Seldon, M Finn (eds) *The coalition effect 2010–2015*, Cambridge: Cambridge University Press

Goldacre, B, 2015, *I think you'll find it's a bit more complicated than that*, London: Fourth Estate

Huitson, O, 2013, Hidden in plain sight, in J Davis, R Tallis (eds) *NHS SOS*, pp 150–73, London: OneWorld

Jarman, H, Greer, S, 2015, The big bang: Health and social care reform under the coalition, in M Beech, S Lee (eds) *The Conservative–Liberal coalition*, pp 50–67, Basingstoke: Palgrave

Jones, M, Peterson, H, Pierce, J, Herweg, N, Bernal, A, Raney, H, Zahariadis, N, 2016, A river runs through it: A multiple streams meta-review, *The Policy Studies Journal*, 44, 1, 13-36

Kingdon, JW, 2011, *Agendas, alternatives and public policy*, 2nd edn (first published 1984), Boston, MA: Longman

Klein, Rudolf, 2013, The twenty-year war over England's National Health Service: A report from the battlefield, *Journal of Health Politics, Policy and Law* 38, 4, 849–69

Le Grand, J, Mays, N, Mulligan, J-A (eds) (1998) *Learning from the NHS internal market: A review of the evidence*. London; King's Fund

Leys, C, Player, S, 2011, *The plot against the NHS*, Pontypool: Merlin Press

Mays, N, Dixon, A, Jones, L (eds) (2011) *Understanding New Labour's market reforms of the NHS*. London: King's Fund

NHS England (2014) *Five year forward view*, London: NHS England, www.england.nhs.uk/wp-content/uploads/2014/10/5yfv-web.pdf

Oborn, E, Barrett, M, Exworthy, M, 2011, Policy entrepreneurship in the development of public sector strategy: The case of London health reform, *Public Administration* 89, 2, 325–44

Paton, C, 2014, *At what cost? Paying the price for the market in the English NHS*, London: Centre for Health and the Public Interest

Powell, M, 2015, Who killed the English National Health Service?, *International Journal of Health Policy and Management* 4, 267–9

Powell, M, Mannion, R, 2015, England, in J Braithwaite, Y Matsuyama, R Mannion, J Johnson(eds) *Healthcare reform, quality and safety*, pp 227–36, Farnham: Ashgate

Robinson, R, Le Grand, J (eds)(1994) *Evaluating the NHS reforms*. London: King's Fund Institute

Seldon, A, Snowdon, P, 2015, *Cameron at 10*, London: William Collins

Shaw, SE, Russell, J Greenhalgh, T, Korica, M, 2014, Thinking about think tanks in health care: A call for a new research agenda, *Sociology of Health and Illness* 36, 3, 447–61

Tallis, R, 2013, Introduction, in J Davis, R Tallis (eds), *NHS SOS*, pp 1–16, London: OneWorld

Timmins, N, 2012, *Never again? The story of the Health and Social Care Act 2012*, London: The King's Fund and the Institute for Government

Timmins, N, Davies, E (eds), 2015, *Glaziers and window breakers: The role of the Secretary of State for Health in their own words*, London: Health Foundation

Toynbee, P, Walker, D, 2015, *Cameron's coup*, London: Guardian Faber

Walker, P, Yong, B, 2012, Case Studies II: Tuition fees, NHS reform and nuclear policy, in R Hazell, B Yong (eds) *The politics of coalition: How the Conservative-Liberal Democrat government works*, pp 172–89, Oxford: Hart

Walshe, K, 2010, Reorganisation of the NHS in England, *British Medical Journal 341, c384*

Walshe, K, 2014, Counting the cost of England's NHS reorganisation, *British Medical Journal 349, g6340*

Zahariadis, N, 2014, Ambiguity and Multiple Streams, in P Sabatier, CM Weible (eds) *Theories of the policy process*, pp 25–58, first published in 1999, Boulder, CO: Westview Press

Index